P9-DYY-736

PN Nursing Care of Children
REVIEW MODULE EDITION 11.0

Contributors

Debborah Williams MSN, RN

LaKeisha Wheless MSN, RN

Sheryl Sommer PhD, RN, CNE

Janean Johnson MSN, RN, CNE

Marsha Barlow MSN, RN

Kellie Wilford MSN, RN

Consultants

Christi Blair DNP, RN

Dr. Teresa M. Conte PhD, CPNP

Judith Drumm DNS, RN, CPN

REPRINTED NOVEMBER 2021

Director of content review: Kristen Lawler

Director of development: Derek Prater

Project management: Tiffany Pavlik

Coordination of content review: Debborah Williams, LaKeisha Wheless

Copy editing: Kelly Von Lunen, Kya Rodgers

Layout: Maureen Bradshaw, Bethany Phillips

Illustrations: Randi Hardy

Online media: Brant Stacy, Ron Hanson, Britney Fuller, Trevor Lund

Cover design: Jason Buck

Interior book design: Spring Lenox

IMPORTANT NOTICE TO THE READER

User's Guide

Welcome to the Assessment Technologies Institute® PN Nursing Care of Children Review Module Edition 11.0. The mission of ATI's Content Mastery Series® Review Modules is to provide user-friendly compendiums of nursing knowledge that will:
- Help you locate important information quickly.
- Assist in your learning efforts.
- Provide exercises for applying your nursing knowledge.
- Facilitate your entry into the nursing profession as a newly licensed nurse.

This newest edition of the Review Modules has been redesigned to optimize your learning experience. We've fit more content into less space and have done so in a way that will make it even easier for you to find and understand the information you need.

ORGANIZATION

This Review Module is organized into units covering the foundations of nursing care of children, nursing care of children who have systems disorders, and nursing care of children who have other specific needs. Chapters within these units conform to one of four organizing principles for presenting the content.
- Nursing concepts
- Growth and development
- Procedures
- System disorders

Nursing concepts chapters begin with an overview describing the central concept and its relevance to nursing. Subordinate themes are covered in outline form to demonstrate relationships and present the information in a clear, succinct manner.

Growth and development chapters cover expected growth and development, including physical and psychosocial development, age-appropriate activities, and health promotion, including immunizations, health screenings, nutrition, and injury prevention.

Procedures chapters include an overview describing the procedure(s) covered in the chapter. These chapters provide nursing knowledge relevant to each procedure, including indications, nursing considerations, interpretation of findings, and complications.

System disorders chapters include an overview describing the disorder(s) and/or disease process. These chapters address assessments, including risk factors, expected findings, laboratory tests, and diagnostic procedures. Next, you will focus on patient-centered care, including nursing care, medications, therapeutic procedures, interprofessional care, and client education. Finally, you will find complications related to the disorder, along with nursing actions in response to those complications.

ACTIVE LEARNING SCENARIOS AND APPLICATION EXERCISES

Each chapter includes opportunities for you to test your knowledge and to practice applying that knowledge. Active Learning Scenario exercises pose a nursing scenario and then direct you to use an ATI Active Learning Template (included at the back of this book) to record the important knowledge a nurse should apply to the scenario. An example is then provided to which you can compare your completed Active Learning Template. The Application Exercises include NCLEX-style questions, such as multiple-choice and multiple-select items, providing you with opportunities to practice answering the kinds of questions you might expect to see on ATI assessments or the NCLEX. After the Application Exercises, an answer key is provided, along with rationales.

NCLEX® CONNECTIONS

To prepare for the NCLEX-PN, it is important to understand how the content in this Review Module is connected to the NCLEX-PN test plan. You can find information on the detailed test plan at the National Council of State Boards of Nursing's website, www.ncsbn.org. When reviewing content in this Review Module, regularly ask yourself, "How does this content fit into the test plan, and what types of questions related to this content should I expect?"

To help you in this process, we've included NCLEX Connections at the beginning of each unit and with each question in the Application Exercises Answer Keys. The NCLEX Connections at the beginning of each unit point out areas of the detailed test plan that relate to the content within that unit. The NCLEX Connections attached to the Application Exercises Answer Keys demonstrate how each exercise fits within the detailed content outline. These NCLEX Connections will help you understand how the detailed content outline is organized, starting with major client needs categories and subcategories and followed by related content areas and tasks. The major client needs categories are:
- Safe and Effective Care Environment
  - Management of Care
  - Safety and Infection Control
- Health Promotion and Maintenance
- Psychosocial Integrity
- Physiological Integrity
  - Basic Care and Comfort
  - Pharmacological and Parenteral Therapies
  - Reduction of Risk Potential
  - Physiological Adaptation

An NCLEX Connection might, for example, alert you that content within a unit is related to:
- Physiological Adaptation
  - Alterations in Body Systems
    - Identify clinical manifestations and incubation periods of infectious diseases.

QSEN COMPETENCIES

As you use the Review Modules, you will note the integration of the Quality and Safety Education for Nurses (QSEN) competencies throughout the chapters. These competencies are integral components of the curriculum of many nursing programs in the United States and prepare you to provide safe, high-quality care as a newly licensed nurse. Icons appear to draw your attention to the six QSEN competencies.

Safety: The minimization of risk factors that could cause injury or harm while promoting quality care and maintaining a secure environment for clients, self, and others.

Patient-Centered Care: The provision of caring and compassionate, culturally sensitive care that addresses clients' physiological, psychological, sociological, spiritual, and cultural needs, preferences, and values.

Evidence-Based Practice: The use of current knowledge from research and other credible sources, on which to base clinical judgment and client care.

Informatics: The use of information technology as a communication and information-gathering tool that supports clinical decision-making and scientifically based nursing practice.

Quality Improvement: Care related and organizational processes that involve the development and implementation of a plan to improve health care services and better meet clients' needs.

Teamwork and Collaboration: The delivery of client care in partnership with multidisciplinary members of the health care team to achieve continuity of care and positive client outcomes.

ICONS

Icons are used throughout the Review Module to draw your attention to particular areas. Keep an eye out for these icons.

(N) This icon is used for NCLEX Connections.

(G) This icon indicates gerontological considerations, or knowledge specific to the care of older adult clients.

Qs This icon is used for content related to safety and is a QSEN competency. When you see this icon, take note of safety concerns or steps that nurses can take to ensure client safety and a safe environment.

QPCC This icon is a QSEN competency that indicates the importance of a holistic approach to providing care.

QEBP This icon, a QSEN competency, points out the integration of research into clinical practice.

QI This icon is a QSEN competency and highlights the use of information technology to support nursing practice.

QQI This icon is used to focus on the QSEN competency of integrating planning processes to meet clients' needs.

QTC This icon highlights the QSEN competency of care delivery using an interprofessional approach.

M◇ This icon appears at the top-right of pages and indicates availability of an online media supplement, such as a graphic, animation, or video. If you have an electronic copy of the Review Module, this icon will appear alongside clickable links to media supplements. If you have a hard copy version of the Review Module, visit www.atitesting.com for details on how to access these features.

FEEDBACK

ATI welcomes feedback regarding this Review Module. Please provide comments to comments@atitesting.com.

As needed updates to the Review Modules are identified, changes to the text are made for subsequent printings of the book and for subsequent releases of the electronic version. For the printed books, print runs are based on when existing stock is depleted. For the electronic versions, a number of factors influence the update schedule. As such, ATI encourages faculty and students to refer to the Review Module addendums for information on what updates have been made. These addendums, which are available in the Help/FAQs on the student site and the Resources/eBooks & Active Learning on the faculty site, are updated regularly and always include the most current information on updates to the Review Modules.

Table of Contents

When reviewing the following chapters, keep in mind the relevant topics and tasks of the NCLEX outline, in particular:

Safety and Infection Control

ACCIDENT/ERROR/INJURY PREVENTION
Assist in and/or reinforce education to the client about safety precautions.

Identify client factors that influence accident/error/injury prevention.

Identify and facilitate correct use of infant and child car seats by client.

HOME SAFETY: Reinforce client education on home safety precautions.

Health Promotion and Maintenance

AGING PROCESS
Provide care that meets the needs of the newborn less than 1 month old through the infant or toddler client through 2 years.

Provide care that meets the needs of the preschool, school–age, and adolescent client ages 3 through 17 years.

DATA COLLECTION TECHNIQUES
Collect data for health history.

Collect baseline physical data.

Report client physical examination results to the health care provider.

DEVELOPMENTAL STAGES AND TRANSITIONS
Identify barriers to communication.

Identify occurrence of expected body image changes.

Compare client to developmental milestones.

Modify approaches to care in accordance with the client's development stage.

HEALTH PROMOTION/DISEASE PREVENTION
Identify clients in need of immunizations.

Identify precautions and contraindications to immunizations.

Provide assistance for screening examinations.

Monitor incorporation of healthy behaviors into lifestyle by the client.

Basic Care and Comfort

NUTRITION AND ORAL HYDRATION: Monitor and provide for nutritional needs of client.

REST AND SLEEP
Provide measures to promote sleep/rest.

Identify client usual rest and sleep patterns

CHAPTER 1
Family-Centered Nursing Care

Families are groups that should remain constant in children's lives. Family is defined as what an individual considers it to be.

Families often include individuals with a biological, marital, or adoptive relationship, but in the absence of these characteristics, families also consist of individuals who have a strong emotional bond and commitment to one another.

Due to the expanding concepts of family, the term household is sometimes used.

Positive family relationships are characterized by parent-child interactions that show mutual warmth and respect.

COMPONENTS OF CARE

Family-centered nursing care includes the following. Qpcc
- Agreed-upon partnerships between families of children, nurses, and providers, in which the families and children benefit.
- Respecting cultural diversity and incorporating cultural views in the plan of care.
- Understanding growth and developmental needs of children and their families.
- Treating children and their families as clients.
- Working with all types of families.
- Collaborating with families regarding hospitalization, home, and community resources.
- Allowing families to serve as experts regarding their children's health conditions, usual behaviors in different situations, and routine needs.

PROMOTING FAMILY-CENTERED CARE

Nurses should perform comprehensive family data collection to identify strengths and weaknesses.

Characteristics of healthy families
- Members communicate well and listen to each other.
- There is affirmation and support for all members.
- There is a clear set of family rules, beliefs, and values.
- Members teach respect for others.
- There is a sense of trust.
- Members play and share humor together.

- Members interact with one another.
- There is a shared sense of responsibility.
- There are traditions and rituals.
- There is adaptability and flexibility in roles.
- Members seek help for their problems.

NURSING ACTIONS
- Nurses should pay close attention when family members state that a child "isn't acting right" or has other concerns.
- Children's opinions should be considered when providing care.

FAMILY THEORIES

FAMILY SYSTEMS

The family is viewed as a whole system, instead of the individual members.
- A change to one member affects the entire system.
- The system can both initiate and react to change.
- Too much and too little change can lead to dysfunction.

FAMILY STRESS

Describes stress as inevitable.
- Stressors can be expected or unexpected.
- Explains the reaction of a family to stressful events.
- Offers guidance for adapting to stress.

DEVELOPMENTAL

Views families as small groups that interact with the larger social system.
- Emphasizes similarities and consistencies in how families develop and change.
- Uses Duvall's family life cycle stages to describe the changes a family goes through over time.
- How the family functions in one stage has a direct effect on how the family will function in the next stage.

FAMILY COMPOSITION

Traditional nuclear family: Married couple and their biologic children (only full brothers and sisters)

Nuclear family: Two parents and their children (biologic, adoptive, step, foster)

Single-parent family: One parent and one or more children

Blended family (also called reconstituted): At least one stepparent, stepsibling, or half-sibling

Extended family: At least one parent, one or more children, and other individuals (might not be related)

Gay/lesbian family (LGBT): Two members of the same sex who have children and a legal or common-law tie

Foster family: A child or children who have been placed in an approved living environment away from the family of origin, usually with one or two parents

Binuclear family: Parents who have terminated spousal roles but continue their parenting roles

Communal family: Individuals who share common ownership of property and goods, and exchange services without monetary consideration

Changes that occur with the birth (or adoption) of the first child

- Parents' sense of self as they transition to the new parental role
- Division of labor and roles within the relationships of couples
- Relationships with grandparents
- Work relationships
- Increased financial responsibilities and possible loss of income
- Necessary sleep habit changes

PARENTING STYLES

TYPES OF PARENTING

Authoritarian

Parents try to control the child's behaviors and attitudes through unquestioned rules and expectations.

> The child is never allowed to watch television on school nights.

Permissive

Parents exert little or no control over the child's behaviors, and consult the child when making decisions.

> The child assists with deciding whether they will watch television.

Authoritative

Parents direct the child's behavior by setting rules and explaining the reason for each rule setting.

> The child can watch television for 1 hr on school nights after completing all homework and chores.

Parents negatively reinforce deviations from the rules.

> The privilege is taken away but later reinstated based on new guidelines.

GUIDELINES FOR PROMOTING ACCEPTABLE BEHAVIOR IN CHILDREN

- Set clear and realistic limits and expectations based on the developmental level of the child.
- Validate the child's feelings, and offer sympathetic explanations.
- Provide role modeling and reinforcement for appropriate behavior.
- Focus on the child's behavior when disciplining the child.

FAMILY DATA COLLECTION

History: Medical history for parents, siblings, and grandparents

Structure: Family members (mother, father, son)

Developmental tasks: Tasks a family works on as the child grows (parents with a school-age child helping her to develop peer relations)

Family characteristics: Cultural, religious, and economic influences on behavior, attitudes, and actions

Family stressors: Expected (birth of a child) and unexpected (illness, divorce, disability, or death of a family member) events that cause stress

Environment: Availability of and family interactions with community resources

Family support system: Availability of extended family, work and peer relationships, as well as social systems and community resources to assist the family in meeting needs or adapting to a stressor

Application Exercises

1. A nurse on a pediatric unit is assisting the manager with preparing an education program on working with families for a group of newly hired nurses. Which of the following should the nurse include when discussing the developmental theory?

   A. Describes that stress is inevitable

   B. Emphasizes that change with one member affects the entire family

   C. Provides guidance to assist families adapting to stress

   D. Defines consistencies in how families change

2. A nurse is assisting a group of guardians of adolescents to develop skills that will improve communication within the family. The nurse hears one guardian state, "My son knows he better do what I say." Which of the following parenting styles is the parent exhibiting?

   A. Authoritarian

   B. Permissive

   C. Authoritative

   D. Passive

3. A nurse is assisting with performing family data collection. Which of the following should the nurse include? (Select all that apply.)

   A. Medical history

   B. Parents' education level

   C. Child's physical growth

   D. Support systems

   E. Stressors

Active Learning Scenario

A nurse is assisting providing anticipatory guidance to the mother of a toddler. The nurse learns that the household includes the mother, toddler, an older brother, and a grandmother. Use the ATI Active Learning Template: Basic Concept to complete this item.

RELATED CONTENT: Describe the composition of this family.

UNDERLYING PRINCIPLES: Describe two ways the parent can promote acceptable behavior in the child.

NURSING INTERVENTIONS: Include two additional family data collection the nurse should perform.

Application Exercises Key

1. A. The family stress theory describes that stress is inevitable.
   B. The family systems theory emphasizes that change with one member affects the entire family.
   C. The family stress theory provides guidance to assist families adapting to stress.
   D. **CORRECT:** Include that the developmental theory defines consistencies in how families change.

   Ⓝ NCLEX® Connection: Health Promotion and Maintenance, Developmental Stages and Transitions

2. A. **CORRECT:** This parent is exhibiting an authoritarian parenting style. The parent controls the adolescent's behaviors and attitudes through unquestioned rules and expectations.
   B. This parent is not exhibiting a permissive parenting style. Using this style, the parent exerts little or no control over the adolescent's behaviors, and consults the adolescent when making decisions.
   C. This parent is not exhibiting an authoritative parenting style. Using this style, the parent directs the adolescent's behavior by setting rules and explaining the reason for each rule setting.
   D. This parent is not exhibiting a passive parenting style. Using this style, the parent is uninvolved, indifferent, and emotionally removed.

   Ⓝ NCLEX® Connection: Health Promotion and Maintenance, Developmental Stages and Transitions

3. A. **CORRECT:** Include a medical history on the parents, siblings, and grandparents when performing family data collection.
   B. **CORRECT:** Include the family structure, which includes family members, family size, roles/position within the family, and occupation and education of family members when performing a family assessment.
   C. Include the child's physical growth when performing an individual assessment on the child.
   D. **CORRECT:** Include support systems to determine the availability of extended family, work and peer relationships, and social systems and community resources to assist the family in meeting needs when performing a family assessment.
   E. **CORRECT:** Include stressors, both expected and unexpected, when performing a family assessment.

   Ⓝ NCLEX® Connection: Health Promotion and Maintenance, Data Collection Techniques

Active Learning Scenario Key

Using the ATI Active Learning Template: Basic Concept

RELATED CONTENT: This is an extended family, which includes at least one parent, one or more children, and other individuals who are either related or not related.

UNDERLYING PRINCIPLES: Promoting acceptable behavior
- Validate the child's feelings, and offer sympathetic explanations.
- Provide role modeling and reinforcement for acceptable behavior.
- Set clear and realistic limits and expectations based on the child's developmental level.
- Focus on the behavior when implementing discipline.

NURSING INTERVENTIONS: Family data collection
- Medical history on parents, siblings, and grandparents
- Family structure for roles/position within the family, as well as occupation and education of family members
- Developmental tasks a family works on as the child grows
- Family characteristics (cultural, religious, and economic influences on behavior, attitudes, and actions)
- Family stressors, (expected [birth of a child] and unexpected [illness of a child, divorce, disability or death of a family member] events that cause stress)
- Availability of and family interactions with community resources
- Family support systems (availability of extended family; work and peer relationships; and social systems and community resources to assist the family in meeting needs or adapting to a stressor)

Ⓝ NCLEX® Connection: Health Promotion and Maintenance, Aging Process

CHAPTER 2   *Physical Data Collection Findings*

Alter exams to accommodate chronological age and developmental needs. Involve children and family members in examinations. Praise children for cooperation during exams. ⦾PCC

Observe for behaviors (interacting with nurse, making eye contact, permitting physical touch, and willingly sitting on the examination table) to determine the child's readiness to cooperate.

Language, cognition, physical, social, and emotional development can be screened using a variety of standardized tools. A combination of data collected from psychosocial and medical histories and a physical examination is used to determine the need to initiate a referral for further evaluation.

NURSING ACTIONS

- Keep the room warm and well lit.
- Perform examinations in nonthreatening environments. Keep medical equipment out of sight.
- Provide privacy. Determine whether older school-age children and adolescents prefer a caregiver to remain during examination.
- Take time to play and develop rapport prior to beginning an examination.
- Observe for behaviors that demonstrate child's readiness to cooperate (interacting with nurse, making eye contact, permitting physical touch, and willingly sitting on the examination table).
- Explain each step of the examination to the child.
  - Use age-appropriate language.
  - Demonstrate what will happen using dolls, puppets, or paper drawings.
  - Allow the child manipulate and handle equipment.
  - Encourage the child to use equipment on others.
- Examine the child in a secure, comfortable position. For example, a toddler can sit on a parent's lap if desired.
- Proceed to examine the child in an organized sequence when possible.
- If the child is uncooperative, determine reasons, be firm and direct about expected behavior, complete the examination quickly, and use a calm voice.
- Encourage the child and family to ask questions during physical exams. Discuss findings with family after the examination.

PHYSIOLOGIC AND GROWTH MEASUREMENTS

TEMPERATURE

2.1 Temperature by age

	EXPECTED LEVEL	RECOMMENDED ROUTES
3 months	37.5° C (99.5° F)	• Axillary • Rectal (if exact measurement necessary)
6 months		
1 year	37.7° C (99.9° F)	
3 years	37.2° C (99.0° F)	• Axillary • Tympanic • Oral (if child cooperative) • Rectal (if exact measurement necessary)
5 years	37.0° C (98.6° F)	
7 years	36.8° C (98.2° F)	• Oral • Axillary • Tympanic
9 years	36.7° C (98.1° F)	
11 years		
13 years	36.6° C (97.9° F)	

PULSE RATE

Newborn (birth to 4 weeks): 110 to 160/min

Infant (1 to 12 months): 90 to 160/ min

Toddler (1 to 2 years): 80 to 140/min

Preschooler (3 to 5 years): 70 to 120/min

School aged (6 to 12 years): 60 to 110/min

Adolescent (13 to 18 years): 50 to 100/min

Values listed are general guidelines and may vary according to reference, as well as the child's specific age and activity level.

RESPIRATIONS

Newborn (birth to 4 weeks): 30 to 60/min

Infant (1 to 12 months): 25 to 30/min

Toddler (1 to 2 years): 25 to 30/min

Preschooler (3 to 5 years): 20 to 25/min

School aged (6 to 12 years): 20 to 25/min

Adolescent (13 to 18 years): 16 to 20/min

Values listed are general guidelines and may vary according to reference, as well as the child's specific age and activity level.

BLOOD PRESSURE

- Readings should be compared with standard measurements (National High Blood Pressure Education Program Working Group on High Blood Pressure in Children and Adolescents). ⦾EBP
- Age, height, and sex all influence blood pressure readings. **(2.3)**

GROWTH

Growth can be evaluated using weight, length/height, body mass index (BMI), and head circumference. Growth charts are tools that can be used to determine the overall health of a child.

- It is recommended to use the World Health Organizations (WHO) growth standards for infants and children ages 0 to 2 in the United States and CDC growth charts for children 2 years and older.
- To see growth charts by age and sex, visit the website for the Centers for Disease Control and Prevention. ⦾EBP

EXPECTED PHYSICAL FINDINGS

GENERAL APPEARANCE

- Appears undistressed, clean, well-kept, and without body odors.
- Muscle tone: Erect head posture is expected in infants after 4 months of age.
- Makes eye contact when addressed (except infants).
- Follows simple commands as age-appropriate.
- Uses speech, language, and motor skills spontaneously.

SKIN, HAIR, AND NAILS

Skin

- Variations in skin color are expected.
- Temperature should be warm or slightly cool to the touch.
- Skin texture should be smooth and slightly dry, not oily.
- Skin turgor exhibits brisk elasticity with adequate hydration.
- Lesions are unexpected findings.
- Skin folds should be symmetric.

Hair and scalp

- Hair should be evenly distributed, smooth, and strong.
  - Manifestations of nutritional deficiencies include hair that is stringy, dull, brittle, and dry.
  - Hair loss or balding spots on infants can indicate the child is spending too much time in the same position.
- Scalp should be clean and absent from any scaliness, infestations, and trauma.
- Examine children approaching adolescence for the presence of secondary hair growth.

Nails

- Pink over the nail bed and white at the tips
- Smooth and firm (but slightly flexible in infants)

LYMPH NODES

Lymph nodes should be nonpalpable. Lymph nodes that are small, palpable, nontender, and mobile can be an expected finding in children.

HEAD AND NECK

Head

- The shape of the head should be symmetric.
- Fontanels should be flat. The posterior fontanel usually closes by 8 weeks of age, and the anterior fontanel usually closes between 12 and 18 months of age.

Face

- Symmetric appearance and movement
- Proportional features

Neck

- Short in infants
- No palpable masses
- Midline trachea
- Full range of motion present whether elicited actively or passively

EYES

Eyebrows should be symmetric and evenly distributed from the inner to the outer canthus.

Eyelids should close completely and open to allow the lower border and most of the upper portion of the iris to be seen.

Eyelashes should curve outward and be evenly distributed with no inflammation around any of the hair follicles.

Conjunctiva
- Palpebral fissures and conjunctiva are pink.
- Bulbar conjunctiva are transparent.

Lacrimal apparatus is without excessive tearing, redness, or discharge.

Sclera should be white.

Corneas should be clear.

Pupils should be:
- Round
- Equal in size
- Reactive to light
- Accommodating

Irises should be round with the permanent color manifesting around 6 to 12 months of age.

2.3 Expected blood pressure ranges by age and sex

		Average (50th Percentile)		Hypertension (95th Percentile)	
		SYSTOLIC (mm Hg)	DIASTOLIC (mm Hg)	SYSTOLIC GREATER THAN (mm Hg)	DIASTOLIC GREATER THAN (mm Hg)
NEWBORN (FULL TERM: BIRTH TO 4 WEEKS)		64	41	n/a	
INFANT (1 MONTH TO 12 MONTHS)		85	50	n/a	
TODDLER (1 YEAR TO 2 YEARS)	MALE	85 to 91	37 to 46	103 to 109	56 to 65
	FEMALE	86 to 89	40 to 49	104 to 107	58 to 67
PRESCHOOLER (3 TO 5 YEARS)	MALE	91 to 98	46 to 53	109 to 112	65 to 72
	FEMALE	89 to 93	49 to 52	107 to 110	67 to 72
SCHOOL AGED (6 TO 12 YEARS)	MALE	96 to 106	55 to 62	114 to 123	74 to 81
	FEMALE	94 to 105	56 to 62	111 to 123	74 to 80
ADOLESCENT (13 TO 18 YEARS)		less than 120	less than 80	n/a	

Visual acuity

- Can be difficult to determine in children younger than 3 years of age.
- Visual acuity in infants can be checked by holding an object in front of the eyes and checking to see whether the infant is able to fix on the object and follow it.
- Use the tumbling E or HOTV test to check visual acuity of children who are unable to read letters and numbers.
- Older children should be tested using a Snellen chart or symbol chart.

Peripheral visual fields should be:
- Upward 50°
- Downward 70°
- Nasally 60°
- Temporally 90°

Extraocular movements

- Might not be symmetric in newborns.
- Corneal light reflex should be symmetric.
- Cover/uncover test should demonstrate equal movement of the eyes.
- Six cardinal fields of gaze should demonstrate no nystagmus.

Color vision

- Should be determined using the Ishihara color test or the Hardy-Rand-Rittler test.
- The child should be able to correctly identify shapes, symbols, or numbers.

Internal exam

- Red reflex should be present in infants.
- Arteries, veins, optic discs, and maculae can be visualized in older children and adolescents.

EARS

Alignment: The top of the auricles should meet in an imaginary horizontal line that extends from the outer canthus of the eye.

External ear

- The external ear should be free of lesions and nontender.
- The ear canal should be free of foreign bodies or discharge.
- Cerumen is an expected finding.

Internal ear

- In infants and toddlers, pull the pinna down and back to visualize the tympanic membrane.
- In children older than 3 years of age, pull the pinna up and back to visualize.
- The ear canal should be pink with fine hairs.
- The tympanic membrane should be pearly pink, or gray.
- The light reflex should be visible.

Hearing

- Newborns should have intact acoustic blink reflexes to sudden sounds.
- Infants should turn toward sounds.
- Older children can be screened by whispering a word from behind to see whether they can identify the word.

NOSE

- The position should be midline.
- Patency should be present for each nostril without excessive flaring.
- Sense of smell can be determined in older children.

Internal structures

- The septum is midline and intact.
- The mucosa is deep pink in light-skinned clients and various shades of brown or gray in dark-skinned clients. The mucosa should be moist without evidence of discharge.

MOUTH AND THROAT

Lips

- Darker pigmented than facial skin
- Smooth, soft, moist, and symmetric

Gums

- Coral pink in light-skinned clients, and various shades of brown or gray in dark-skinned clients
- Tight against the teeth

Mucous membranes

- Without lesions
- Moist, smooth, and glistening. Pink in light-skinned clients and various shades of brown or gray in dark-skinned clients

Tongue

- Infants can have white coatings on their tongues from milk that can be easily removed. Oral candidiasis coating is not easily removed.
- Children and adolescents should have pink, symmetric tongues that they are able to move beyond their lips.

Teeth

- Infants should have six to eight teeth by 1 year of age.
- Children and adolescents should have teeth that are white and smooth, and begin replacing the 20 deciduous teeth with 32 permanent teeth.

Hard and soft palates: Intact, firm, and concave

Uvula: Intact and moves with vocalization

Tonsils

- Infants: Might not be able to visualize
- Children: Barely visible to prominent, same color as surrounding mucosa

Voice

- Infants: Strong cry
- Children and adolescents: Clear and articulate

THORAX AND LUNGS

Chest shape

- Infants: Shape is almost circular with anteroposterior diameter equaling the transverse or lateral diameter.
- Children and adolescents: The transverse diameter to anteroposterior diameter changes to 2:1.

Ribs and sternum: More soft and flexible in infants; symmetric and smooth, with no protrusions or bulges

Movement

- Symmetric, no retractions.
- Infants: Irregular rhythms are common.
- Children younger than 7 years: More abdominal movement is seen during respirations.

Breath sounds

- Inspiration is longer and louder than expiration.
- Vesicular, or soft, swishing sounds, are heard over most of the lungs.

Breasts

- Newborns: Breasts can be enlarged during the first few days.
- Children and adolescents: Nipples and areolas are darker pigmented and symmetric.
  - Females: Breasts typically develop between 10 to 14 years of age. The breasts should appear asymmetric, have no masses, and be palpable.
  - Males can develop gynecomastia, which is unilateral or bilateral breast enlargement that occurs during puberty.

CIRCULATORY SYSTEM

A comprehensive examination of the circulatory system includes checking the pulses, capillary refill time, neck veins, clubbing of fingers, peripheral cyanosis, edema, blood pressure, and respiratory status.

Heart sounds

- Auscultation should be done in both a sitting and reclining position.
- S_1 and S_2 heart sounds should be clear and crisp. S_1 is louder at the apex of the heart. S_2 is louder near the base of the heart. Physiologic splitting of S_2 and S_3 heart sounds are expected findings in some children. Sinus arrhythmias that are associated with respirations are common.

Pulses

- Infants: Brachial, temporal, and femoral pulses should be palpable, full, and localized.
- Children and adolescents: Pulse locations and expected findings are the same as those in adults.

Abdomen

- Without tenderness, no guarding. Peristaltic waves can be visible in thinner children.
- Shape: Symmetric and without protrusions around the umbilicus.
  - Infants and toddlers have rounded abdomens.
  - Children and adolescents should have flat abdomens.
- Bowel sounds should be heard every 5 to 30 seconds.

GENITALIA

Anus: Surrounding skin should be intact with sphincter tightening noted if the anus is touched. Routine rectal exams are not done with the pediatric population.

MALE: Hair distribution is diamond shaped after puberty in adolescent males. No pubic hair is noted in infants and small children.

- **Penis**
  - Penis should appear straight.
  - Urethral meatus should be at the tip of the penis.
  - Foreskin might not be retractable in infants and small children.
  - Enlargement of the penis occurs during adolescence.
  - The penis can look disproportionately small in males who are obese because of skin folds partially covering the base.

- **Scrotum**
  - The scrotum hangs separately from the penis.
  - The skin on the scrotum has a rugose appearance and is loose.
  - The left testicle hangs slightly lower than the right.
  - The inguinal canal should be absent of swelling.
  - During puberty, the testes and scrotum enlarge with darker scrotal skin.

2.4 Infant reflexes

	EXPECTED FINDING	EXPECTED AGE
Sucking and rooting reflexes	Elicited by stroking an infant's cheek or the edge of an infant's mouth The infant turns their head toward the side that is touched and starts to suck.	Birth to 4 months
Pincer grasp	Infant will pick up small objects with their thumb and finger.	8 to 10 months
Palmar grasp	Elicited by placing an object in an infant's palm The infant grasps the object.	Birth to 4 months
Plantar grasp	Elicited by touching the sole of an infant's foot The infant's toes curl downward.	Birth to 8 months
Moro reflex	Elicited by allowing the head and trunk of an infant in a semi-sitting position to fall backward to an angle of at least 30° The infant's arms and legs symmetrically extend, then abduct while fingers spread to form C shape.	Birth to 4 months
Tonic neck reflex (fencer position)	Elicited by turning an infant's head to one side The infant extends the arm and leg on that side and flexes the arm and leg on the opposite side.	Birth to 3 to 4 months
Babinski reflex	Elicited by stroking the outer edge of the sole of an infant's foot up toward the toes The infant's toes fan upward and out.	Birth to 1 year
Stepping	Elicited by holding an infant upright with his feet touching a flat surface The infant makes stepping movements.	Birth to 4 weeks

FEMALE: Hair distribution over the mons pubis should be documented in terms of amount and location during puberty. Hair should appear in an inverted triangle. No pubic hair should be noted in infants or small children.
- **Labia:** Symmetric, without lesions, moist on the inner aspects
- **Clitoris:** Small, without bruising or edema
- **Urethral meatus:** Slit-like in appearance with no discharge
- **Vaginal orifice:** Hymen can be absent or completely or partially cover the vaginal opening prior to sexual intercourse.

MUSCULOSKELETAL SYSTEM

Length, position, and size of extremities are symmetric.

Joints

Stable and symmetric with full range of motion and no crepitus or redness

Spine

Infants: Spines should be without dimples or tufts of hair. They should be midline with an overall C-shaped lateral curve.

Toddlers appear squat with short legs and protuberant abdomens.

Preschoolers appear more erect than toddlers.

Children should develop the cervical, thoracic, and lumbar curvatures like that of adults.

Adolescents should remain midline (no scoliosis noted).

Gait

Toddlers and young children: A bowlegged or knock-knee appearance is a common finding. Feet should face forward while walking.

Older children and adolescents: A steady gait should be noted with even wear on the soles of shoes.

NEUROLOGIC SYSTEM

Infant reflexes (2.4)

Cranial nerves (2.5)

Deep tendon reflexes

Deep tendon reflexes should demonstrate the following.
- Partial flexion of the lower arm at the biceps tendon
- Partial extension of the lower arm at the triceps tendon
- Partial extension of the lower leg at the patellar tendon
- Plantar flexion of the foot at the Achilles tendon

Cerebellar function (children and adolescents)

Finger to nose test: Rapid coordinated movements

Heel to shin test: Able to run the heel of one foot down the shin of the other leg while standing

Romberg test: Able to stand with slight swaying while eyes are closed

2.5 Cranial nerves: expected findings

	INFANTS	CHILDREN AND ADOLESCENTS
I Olfactory	Difficult to test	Identifies smells through each nostril individually
II Optic	Looks at face and tracks with eyes	Has intact visual acuity, peripheral vision, and color vision
III Oculomotor	Blinks in response to light Has pupils that are reactive to light	Has no nystagmus and PERRLA is intact
IV Trochlear	Looks at face and tracks with eyes	Has the ability to look down and in with eyes
V Trigeminal	Has rooting and sucking reflexes	Is able to clench teeth together Detects touch on face with eyes closed
VI Abducens	Looks at face and tracks with eyes	Is able to move eyes laterally toward temples
VII Facial	Has symmetric facial movements	Has the ability to differentiate between salty and sweet on tongue Has symmetric facial movements
VIII Acoustic	Tracks a sound Blinks in response to a loud noise	Does not experience vertigo Has intact hearing
IX Glossopharyngeal	Has an intact gag reflex	Has an intact gag reflex Is able to taste sour sensations on back of tongue
X Vagus	Has no difficulties swallowing	Speech clear, no difficulties swallowing Uvula is midline
XI Spinal Accessory	Moves shoulders symmetrically	Has equal strength of shoulder shrug against examiner's hands
XII Hypoglossal	Has no difficulties swallowing Opens mouth when nares are occluded	Has a tongue that is midline Is able to move tongue in all directions with equal strength against tongue blade resistance

Application Exercises

1. A nurse is preparing to examine a preschooler during a well-child visit. Which of the following actions should the nurse take to prepare the child?

   A. Allow the child to role-play using miniature equipment.

   B. Use medical terminology to describe what will happen.

   C. Separate the child from the caregiver during the examination.

   D. Keep medical equipment visible to the child.

2. A nurse is checking the vital signs of a 3-year-old child during a well-child visit. Which of the following findings should the nurse report to the provider?

   A. Temperature 37.2° C (99.0° F)

   B. Heart rate 106/min

   C. Respirations 35/min

   D. Blood pressure 88/54 mm Hg

3. A nurse is using an otoscope to examine a child's ears. Which of the following findings should the nurse expect?

   A. Light reflex is located at the 2 o'clock position.

   B. Tympanic membrane is red in color.

   C. Bony landmarks are not visible.

   D. Cerumen is present bilaterally.

4. A nurse is collecting data from a 6-month-old infant. Which of the following reflexes should the nurse expect the infant to exhibit?

   A. Moro

   B. Plantar grasp

   C. Stepping

   D. Tonic neck

5. A nurse is checking the trigeminal nerve of an adolescent client. Which of the following responses should the nurse expect? (Select all that apply.)

   A. Clenching teeth together tightly

   B. Recognizing sour tastes on the back of the tongue

   C. Identifying smells through each nostril

   D. Detecting facial touches with eyes closed

   E. Looking down and in with the eyes

Active Learning Scenario

A nurse is preparing to examine a preschooler during a well-child visit. Use the ATI Active Learning Template: Basic Concept to complete this item.

UNDERLYING PRINCIPLES: Describe two behaviors that indicate the child is ready to cooperate.

NURSING INTERVENTIONS

- Describe two actions to take if child is uncooperative.

- Include three actions to promote the child's comfort during the examination.

Application Exercises Key

1. A. **CORRECT:** Allow the child to role-play or manipulate actual or miniature equipment to reduce anxiety and fear related to the examination.
   B. Use neutral words and avoid overestimating the child's understanding of words when describing what will happen.
   C. Encourage parental presence during the examination.
   D. Keep medical equipment out of sight unless showing or using it on the child.

   Ⓝ *NCLEX® Connection: Health Promotion and Maintenance, Developmental Stages and Transitions*

2. A. A temperature of 37.2° C (99.0° F) is within the expected reference range for a 3-year-old child and should not be reported to the provider.
   B. A heart rate of 106/min is within the expected reference range for a 3-year-old child and should not be reported to the provider.
   C. **CORRECT:** Respirations of 35/min is above the expected reference range for a 3-year-old child and should be reported to the provider.
   D. A blood pressure of 90/52 mm Hg is within the expected reference range for a 3-year-old child and should not be reported to the provider.

   Ⓝ *NCLEX® Connection: Health Promotion and Maintenance, Data Collection Techniques*

3. A. The light reflex should be located around the 5 or 7 o'clock position.
   B. The tympanic membrane should be a pearly pink, or gray color.
   C. Bony landmarks should be visible.
   D. **CORRECT:** The presence of cerumen bilaterally is an expected finding.

   Ⓝ *NCLEX® Connection: Reduction of Risk Potential, Potential for Alterations in Body Systems*

4. A. The Moro reflex is exhibited by infants from birth to the age of 4 months.
   B. **CORRECT:** The plantar grasp is exhibited by infants from birth to the age of 8 months.
   C. The stepping reflex is exhibited by infants from birth to the age of 4 weeks.
   D. The tonic neck reflex is exhibited by infants from birth to the age of 3 to 4 months.

   Ⓝ *NCLEX® Connection: Health Promotion and Maintenance, Developmental Stages and Transitions*

5. A. **CORRECT:** Clenching teeth together tightly is an expected response by the adolescent when checking the trigeminal cranial nerve.
   B. Recognizing sour tastes on the back of the tongue is an expected response by the adolescent when checking the glossopharyngeal cranial nerve.
   C. Identifying smells through each nostril is an expected response by the adolescent when checking the olfactory cranial nerve.
   D. **CORRECT:** Detecting facial touches with eyes closed is an expected response by the adolescent when checking the trigeminal cranial nerve.
   E. Looking down and in with the eyes is an expected response by the adolescent when checking the trochlear cranial nerve.

   Ⓝ *NCLEX® Connection: Health Promotion and Maintenance, Data Collection Techniques*

Active Learning Scenario Key

Using the ATI Active Learning Template: Basic Concept

UNDERLYING PRINCIPLES
- Child is ready to cooperate.
- Interacting with nurse.
- Making eye contact.
- Permitting physical touch.
- Willingly sitting on examination table.
- Accepting and handling equipment.

NURSING INTERVENTIONS
- Actions to take if child is uncooperative
  - Determine reasons for being uncooperative.
  - Engage both the child and parent.
  - Be firm and direct about expected behavior.
  - Complete the examination as quickly as possible.
  - Use a calm voice.
- Actions to enhance child's comfort
  - Perform examination in nonthreatening environment.
  - Take time to play and develop rapport prior to beginning the examination.
  - Keep the room warm and well lit.
  - Keep medical equipment out of sight until needed.
  - Provide privacy.
  - Explain each step of the examination to the child.
  - Examine the child in a secure, comfortable position.
  - Examine the child in an organized sequence when possible.
  - Encourage the child and family to ask questions during the examination.

Ⓝ *NCLEX® Connection: Health Promotion and Maintenance, Developmental Stages and Transitions*

CHAPTER 3 *Health Promotion of Infants (2 Days to 1 Year)*

EXPECTED GROWTH AND DEVELOPMENT

GENERAL MEASUREMENTS OF FULL-TERM NEWBORN

Head circumference: The head circumference averages between 33 and 35 cm (13 and 14 in).

Crown to rump length: The crown to rump length is 31 to 35 cm (12.5 to 14 in), approximately equal to head circumference.

Length: Head to heel length averages 48 to 53 cm (19 to 21 in).

Weight: Newborn weight averages 2,700 to 4,000 g (6 to 9 lb).

Newborns will lose up to 10% of their birth weight by 3 to 4 days of age. This is due to fluid shifts, loss of meconium, and limited intake, especially in infants who are breastfed. The birth weight is usually regained by the tenth to fourteenth day of life, depending on the feeding method used. ⓠEBP

PHYSICAL DEVELOPMENT

Fontanel
- Posterior fontanel closes by 6 to 8 weeks of age.
- Anterior fontanel closes by 12 to 18 months of age.

Infant size is tracked using weight, height, and head circumference measurements.
- **Weight**: Infants gain approximately 680 g (1.5 lb) per month during the first 5 months of life. The average weight of a 6 month old infant is 7.26 kg (16 lb). Birth weight is at least doubled by the age of 5 months, and tripled by the age of 12 months to an average of 9.75 kg (21.5 lb).
- **Height**: Infants grow approximately 2.5 cm (1 in) per month the first 6 months of life. Growth occurs in spurts after the age of 6 months, and the birth length increases by 50% by the age of 12 months.
- **Head circumference**: The circumference of infants' heads increases approximately 2 cm (0.75 in) per month during the first 3 months, 1 cm (0.4 in) per month from 4 to 6 months, and then approximately 0.5 cm (0.2 in) per month during the second 6 months.

Dentition
- Six to eight teeth should erupt in infants' mouths by the end of the first year of age. The first teeth typically erupt between the ages of 6 and 10 months (average age 8 months).
- Some children show minimal indications of teething (sucking or biting on their fingers or hard objects and drooling). Others are irritable, have difficulty sleeping, have a mild fever, rub their ears, and have decreased appetite for solid foods.

3.1 Motor skill development by age

	GROSS MOTOR SKILLS	FINE MOTOR SKILLS
1 month	Demonstrates head lag	Has a strong grasp reflex
2 months	Lifts head off mattress when prone	Holds hands in an open position Grasp reflex fading
3 months	Raises head and shoulders off mattress when prone Only slight head lag	No longer has a grasp reflex Keeps hands loosely open
4 months	Rolls from back to side	Grasps objects with both hands
5 months	Rolls from front to back	Uses palmar grasp dominantly
6 months	Rolls from back to front	Holds bottle
7 months	Bears full weight on feet Sits, leaning forward on both hands	Moves objects from hand to hand
8 months	Sits unsupported	Begins using pincer grasp
9 months	Pulls to a standing position Creeps on hands and knees	Has a crude pincer grasp
10 months	Changes from a prone to a sitting position	Grasps rattle by its handle
11 months	Cruises or walks while holding onto something	Places objects into a container Neat pincer grasp
12 months	Sits down from a standing position without assistance Walks with one hand held	Tries to build a two-block tower without success Can turn pages in a book

- Teething pain can be eased using frozen teething rings or an ice cube wrapped in a wash cloth and over-the-counter teething gels. With topical anesthetic ointments, topical anesthetic ointments need to be used under direct supervision of a health care provider. Acetaminophen and/or ibuprofen are appropriate if irritability interferes with sleeping and feeding, but should not be used for more than 3 days. Ibuprofen should be used only in infants over the age of 6 months. Q**s**
- Clean infants' teeth using cool, wet washcloths.
- Bottles should not be given to infants when they are falling asleep because prolonged exposure to milk or juice can cause early childhood dental caries.

COGNITIVE DEVELOPMENT

Piaget: Sensorimotor stage (birth to 24 months) Q**EBP**
- Infants progress from reflexive to simple repetitive to imitative activities.
- Separation, object permanence, and mental representation are the three important tasks accomplished in this stage.
  - **Separation**: Infants learn to separate themselves from other objects in the environment.
  - **Object permanence**: The process by which infants learn that an object still exists when it is out of view. This occurs at approximately 9 to 10 months of age.
  - **Mental representation**: The ability to recognize and use symbols.

Language development

- Crying is the first form of verbal communication.
- Infants cry for 1 to 1 1/2 hr each day up to 3 weeks of age and build up to 2 to 4 hr by 6 weeks.
- Crying decreases by 12 weeks of age.
- Vocalizes with cooing noises by 3 to 4 months.
- Shows considerable interest in the environment by 3 months.
- Turns head to the sound of a rattle by 3 months.
- Laughs and squeals by 4 months.
- Makes single vowel sounds by 2 months.
- By 3 to 4 months the consonants are added.
- Begins speaking two-word phrases and progresses to speaking three-word phrases.
- Says three to five words by the age of 1 year.
- Comprehends the word "no" by 9 to 10 months and obeys single commands accompanied by gestures.

PSYCHOSOCIAL DEVELOPMENT

Erikson: trust vs. mistrust (birth to 1 year) Q**EBP**
- Achieving this task is based on the quality of the caregiver-infant relationship and the care received by the infant.
- The infant begins to learn delayed gratification. Failure to learn delayed gratification leads to mistrust.
- Trust is developed by meeting comfort, feeding, stimulation, and caring needs.
- Mistrust develops if needs are inadequately or inconsistently met, or if needs are continuously met before being vocalized by the infant.

Social development

- Social development is initially influenced by infants' reflexive behaviors and includes attachment, separation, recognition/anxiety, and stranger fear.
- Attachment is seen when infants begin to bond with their parents. This development is seen within the first month, but it actually begins before birth. The process is enhanced when infants and parents are in good health, have positive feeding experiences, and receive adequate rest.
- Separation-individuation occurs during the first year of life as infants first distinguish themselves and their primary caregiver as separate individuals at the same time that object permanence is developing.
- Separation anxiety begins around 4 to 8 months of age. Infants will protest when separated from parents, which can cause considerable anxiety for parents. By 11 to 12 months, infants are able to anticipate the mother's imminent departure by watching the behaviors.
- Stranger fear becomes evident between 6 and 8 months of age, when infants have the ability to discriminate between familiar and unfamiliar people.
- Reactive attachment disorder results from maladaptive or absent attachment between the infant and primary caregiver and continues through childhood and adulthood.

Body-image changes

- Infants discover that mouths are pleasure producers.
- Hands and feet are seen as objects of play.
- Infants discover that smiling causes others to react.

AGE-APPROPRIATE ACTIVITIES Q PCC

- Play should provide interpersonal contact and educational stimulation.
- Infants have short attention spans and will not interact with other children during play (solitary play). Appropriate toys and activities that stimulate the senses and encourage development include the following.
  - Rattles
  - Soft stuffed toys
  - Teething toys
  - Nesting toys
  - Playing pat-a-cake
  - Playing with balls
  - Reading books
  - Mirrors
  - Brightly colored toys
  - Playing with blocks

HEALTH PROMOTION

CARE OF THE NEWBORN AFTER DISCHARGE

- Newborn infants should be placed in an federally approved car seat at a 45 degree angle to prevent slumping and airway obstruction. The car seat is placed rear facing in the rear seat of the vehicle and secured using the safety belt. The shoulder harnesses are placed in the slots at or below the level of the infant's shoulder. The harness should be snug and the retainer clip placed at the level of the infant's armpits.
- Instruct parents that their newborn will require a checkup by a provider. Infants discharged sooner than 48 hours after birth should be examined within 48 hours after discharge from the hospital. Q PCC

IMMUNIZATIONS Q EBP

The Centers for Disease Control and Prevention (CDC) immunization recommendations for healthy infants less than 12 months of age include:
- Birth: hepatitis B (Hep B)
- 2 months: diphtheria and tetanus toxoids and pertussis (DTaP), rotavirus vaccine (RV), inactivated poliovirus (IPV), Haemophilus influenzae type B (Hib), pneumococcal vaccine (PCV), and Hep B
- 4 months: DTaP, RV, IPV, Hib, PCV
- 6 months: DTaP, IPV (6 to 18 months), PCV, and Hep B (6 to 18 months); RV; Hib
- 6 to 12 months: seasonal influenza vaccination yearly (the inactivated influenza vaccine is available as an intramuscular injection)

NUTRITION

- Feeding alternatives
  - Breastfeeding provides a complete diet for infants during the first 6 months.
  - Iron-fortified formula is an acceptable alternative to breast milk. Cow's milk is not recommended.
  - It is recommended to begin vitamin D supplements within the first few days of life to prevent rickets and vitamin D deficiency. Q EBP
  - Iron supplements are recommended for infants who are being exclusively breastfed after the age of 4 months.
  - Alternative sources of fluids (juice or water) are not needed during the first 4 months of life. Excessive intake of water could result in hyponatremia and water intoxication.
  - After the age of 6 months, 100% fruit juice should be limited to 4 to 6 oz per day.
- Solids are introduced around 6 months of age.
  - Indicators for readiness include interest in solid foods, voluntary control of the head and trunk, and disappearance of the extrusion reflex.
  - Iron-fortified cereal is typically introduced first due to its high iron content.
  - New foods should be introduced one at a time, over a 5- to 7-day period, to observe for manifestations of allergy or intolerance, which might include fussiness, rash, vomiting, diarrhea, and constipation.
  - Vegetables or fruits are started first between 6 and 8 months of age. After both have been introduced, meats may be added.
  - Citrus fruits, meat, and eggs are not started until after 6 months of age.
  - Breast milk/formula should be decreased as intake of solid foods increases, but should remain the primary source of nutrition through the first year.
  - Table foods that are well-cooked, chopped, and unseasoned are appropriate by 1 year of age.
  - Appropriate finger foods include ripe bananas, toast strips, graham crackers, cheese cubes, noodles, firmly-cooked vegetables, and raw pieces of fruit (except grapes).
- Weaning can be accomplished when infants show signs of readiness and are able to drink from a cup (sometime in the second 6 months).
  - Gradually replace one bottle or breastfeeding at a time with breast milk or formula in a cup with handles.
  - Bedtime feedings are the last to be stopped.

SLEEP AND REST

- Nocturnal sleep pattern is established by 3 to 4 months of age.
- Infants sleep 14 to 15 hr daily and 9 to 11 hr at night around the age of 4 months.
- Infants sleep through the night and take one to two naps during the day by the age of 12 months.

INJURY PREVENTION Qs

Aspiration of foreign objects
- Hold the infant for feedings; do not prop bottles.
- Small objects that can become lodged in the throat (grapes, coins, candy) should be avoided.
- Age-appropriate toys should be provided.
- Clothing should be checked for safety hazards (loose buttons).

Bodily harm
- Sharp objects should be kept out of reach.
- Anchor heavy objects and furniture so they cannot be overturned on top of the infant.
- Infants should not be left unattended with any animals present.

Burns
- Avoid warming formula in a microwave; check temperature of liquid before feeding.
- The temperature of bath water should be checked.
- Hot water thermostats should be set at or below 49° C (120° F).
- Working smoke detectors should be kept in the home.
- Handles of pots and pans should be kept turned to the back of stoves.
- Sunscreen should be used when infants are exposed to the sun.
- Electrical outlets should be covered.

Drowning
- Infants should not be left unattended in bathtubs or around water sources (toilets, cleaning buckets, or drainage areas).
- Secure fencing around swimming pools.
- Close bathroom doors.

Falls
- Crib mattresses should be kept in the lowest position possible with the rails all the way up.
- Restraints should be used in infant seats.
- Infant seats should be placed on the ground or floor if used outside of the car, and they should not be left unattended or on elevated surfaces.
- Place safety gates at the top and bottom of stairs.

Poisoning
- Exposure to lead paint should be avoided.
- Toxins and plants should be kept out of reach.
- Safety locks should be kept on cabinets that contain cleaners and other household chemicals.
- The phone number for a poison control center should be kept near the phone.
- Medications should be kept in childproof containers, away from the reach of infants.
- A working carbon monoxide detector should be kept in the home.

Motor-vehicle injuries
- Infant-only and convertible infant-toddler car seats are available.
- Infants and toddlers remain in a rear-facing car seat until the age of 2 years or the height recommended by the manufacturer.
- The safest area for infants and children is the backseat of the car.
- Do not place rear-facing car seats in the front seat of vehicles with passenger airbags.
- Infants should not be left in parked cars.

Suffocation
- Plastic bags should be avoided.
- Balloons should be kept away from infants.
- Crib mattresses should fit snugly.
- Crib slats should be no farther apart than 6 cm (2.375 in).
- Crib mobiles and/or crib gyms should be removed by 4 to 5 months of age.
- Pillows should be kept out of the crib.
- Infants should be placed on their backs for sleep.
- Toys with small parts should be kept out of reach.

Application Exercises

1. A nurse is assisting with collecting data from 12-month-old infant during a well-child visit. Which of the following findings should the nurse report to the provider?

   A. Closed anterior fontanel

   B. Eruption of six teeth

   C. Birth weight doubled

   D. Birth length increased by 50%

2. A nurse is collecting data during a developmental screening on a 10-month-old infant. Which of the following fine motor skills should the nurse expect the infant to perform? (Select all that apply.)

   A. Grasp a rattle by the handle

   B. Try building a two-block tower

   C. Use a crude pincer grasp

   D. Place objects into a container

   E. Walks with one hand held

3. A nurse is collecting data during a well-baby visit with a 4-month-old infant. Which of the following immunizations should the nurse plan to administer to the infant? (Select all that apply.)

   A. Measles, mumps, rubella (MMR)

   B. Polio (IPV)

   C. Pneumococcal vaccine (PCV)

   D. Varicella

   E. Rotavirus vaccine (RV)

4. A nurse is reinforcing teaching about when introducing new foods to the guardians of a 4-month-old infant. The nurse should recommend that the caregiver introduce which of the following foods first?

   A. Strained yellow vegetables

   B. Iron-fortified cereals

   C. Pureed fruits

   D. Whole milk

5. A nurse is reinforcing teaching about dental care and teething to the caregiver of a 9-month-old infant. Which of the following statements by the caregiver suggests an understanding of the teaching?

   A. "I can give my baby a warm teething ring to relieve discomfort."

   B. "I should clean my baby's teeth with a cool, wet wash cloth."

   C. "I can give Advil for up to 5 days while my baby is teething."

   D. "I should place diluted juice in the bottle my baby drinks while falling asleep."

Active Learning Scenario

A nurse is assisting with preparing an educational program for a group of caregivers of infants. Use the ATI Active Learning Template: Growth and Development to complete this item.

DEVELOPMENTAL STAGE: Identify the infant's developmental stage according to Piaget and Erikson.

COGNITIVE DEVELOPMENT: List two cognitive developmental tasks the infant should accomplish in the first year of life.

AGE-APPROPRIATE ACTIVITIES: List five activities appropriate for infants.

INJURY PREVENTION: Identify two injury prevention methods in each of the following categories.

- Aspiration
- Poisoning
- Drowning
- Suffocation

Application Exercises Key

1. A. By the age of 12 to 18 months, the infant's anterior fontanel should close.
   B. By the age of 12 months, the infant should have six to eight teeth erupted.
   C. **CORRECT:** By the age of 12 months, the infant's birth weight should have tripled. Therefore, report this finding to the provider.
   D. By the age of 12 months, the infant's birth length should increase by 50%.

   Ⓝ *NCLEX® Connection: Health Promotion and Maintenance, Data Collection Techniques*

2. A. **CORRECT:** The infant should be able to grasp a rattle by the handle at the age of 10 months.
   B. The infant should try building a two-block tower at the age of 12 months.
   C. **CORRECT:** The infant should be able to use a crude pincer grasp at the age of 9 months.
   D. The infant should be able to place objects into a container at the age of 11 months.
   E. The infant should be able to walk with one hand held at the age of 12 months.

   Ⓝ *NCLEX® Connection: Health Promotion and Maintenance, Developmental Stages and Transitions*

3. A. The first MMR vaccine is given between the ages of 12 and 15 months.
   B. **CORRECT:** Administer an IPV vaccine to a 4-month-old infant.
   C. **CORRECT:** Administer a PCV vaccine to a 4-month-old infant.
   D. The first varicella vaccine is given at a minimum age of 12 months.
   E. **CORRECT:** Administer an RV vaccine to a 4-month-old infant.

   Ⓝ *NCLEX® Connection: Health Promotion and Maintenance, Health Promotion/Disease Prevention*

4. A. Strained yellow vegetables are not the best source of needed nutrients and should not be the first food introduced.
   B. **CORRECT:** Iron-fortified cereals are the first solid food introduced due to the high iron content. The order of introducing solid foods after this is variable.
   C. Pureed fruits are not the best source of needed nutrients and should not be the first food introduced.
   D. Whole milk is not the best source of needed nutrients and should not be the first food introduced.

   Ⓝ *NCLEX® Connection: Basic Care and Comfort, Nutrition and Oral Hydration*

5. A. Teething pain can be relieved using frozen teething rings or an ice cube wrapped in a wash cloth.
   B. **CORRECT:** It is appropriate to use a cool, wet wash cloth for cleaning the infant's teeth.
   C. Ibuprofen (Advil) should not be used for more than 3 days.
   D. To prevent early childhood caries, infants should not be given bottles while falling asleep.

   Ⓝ *NCLEX® Connection: Health Promotion and Maintenance, Aging Process*

Active Learning Scenario Key

Using the ATI Active Learning Template: Growth and Development

DEVELOPMENTAL STAGE
- Piaget: Sensorimotor stage
- Erikson: Trust vs. mistrust

COGNITIVE DEVELOPMENT
- Infants progress from reflexive to simple repetitive to imitative activities.
- Separation: Learning to separate themselves from other objects in the environment.
- Object permanence: Understanding that an object still exists when it is out of view.
- Mental representation: Ability to recognize and use symbols.

AGE-APPROPRIATE ACTIVITIES
- Rattles
- Soft stuffed toys
- Teething toys
- Nesting toys
- Playing pat-a-cake
- Playing with balls
- Reading books
- Mirrors
- Brightly colored toys
- Playing with blocks

INJURY PREVENTION
- Aspiration
  - Avoid small objects.
  - Hold infant for feedings; do not prop bottles.
  - Provide age-appropriate toys.
  - Check clothing for hazards (loose buttons).
- Poisoning
  - Keep toxins and plants out of reach.
  - Place safety locks on cabinets where cleaners/chemicals are stored.
  - Use a carbon monoxide detector in the home.
  - Keep medications in childproof containers and out of reach.
- Drowning
  - Do not leave unattended around any water source.
  - Secure fencing around swimming pool.
  - Keep bathroom door closed.
- Suffocation
  - Avoid plastic bags.
  - Ensure crib mattress fits snugly.
  - Remove crib mobiles by 4 to 5 months of age.
  - Keep pillows out of the crib.
  - Place on back to sleep.

Ⓝ *NCLEX® Connection: Health Promotion and Maintenance, Health Promotion/Disease Prevention*

UNIT 1   FOUNDATIONS OF NURSING CARE OF CHILDREN
SECTION: PERSPECTIVES OF NURSING CARE OF CHILDREN

CHAPTER 4 *Health Promotion of Toddlers (1 to 3 Years)*

EXPECTED GROWTH AND DEVELOPMENT

PHYSICAL DEVELOPMENT

- Anterior fontanels close by 18 months of age.
- **Weight**: At 30 months of age, toddlers should weigh four times their birth weight. Toddlers gain approximately 1.8 to 2.7 kg (4 to 6 lb) per year.
- **Height**: Toddlers grow about 7.5 cm (3 in) per year.
- **Head circumference** and chest circumference are usually equal by 1 to 2 years of age.

COGNITIVE DEVELOPMENT

Piaget: Sensorimotor phase transitions to the preoperational phase around 2 years of age. Q EBP
- The concept of object permanence increases.
- Toddlers have and demonstrate memories of events that they relate to.
- Domestic mimicry (playing house) is evident.
- Preoperational thought does not allow for toddlers to understand other viewpoints, but it does allow them to symbolize objects and people to imitate previously seen activities.

Language development

- Language increases to between 50 and 300 words by the age of 2 years.
- 1 year: has a three to five word vocabulary; understands simple commands.
- 2 to 3 years: using multiword sentences by combining two to three words; language increases to about 300 words; imitates animal sounds; refers to self by name; begins to use verbs in past tense.

PSYCHOSOCIAL DEVELOPMENT

Erikson: autonomy versus shame and doubt Q EBP
- Independence is paramount for toddlers, who are attempting to do everything for themselves.
- Toddlers often use negativism, or negative responses, as they begin to express their independence.

- Ritualism, or maintaining routines and reliability, provides a sense of comfort for toddlers as they begin to explore the environment beyond those most familiar to them.

Moral development

- Moral development is closely associated with cognitive development.
- Egocentric: Toddlers are unable to see things from the perspectives of others; they can only view things from their personal points of view.
- Punishment and obedience orientation begin with a sense that good behavior is rewarded and bad behavior is punished.

Social development

Toddlers begin to develop feelings of concern for others and progressively see themselves as separate from their guardians and increase their explorations away from them.

Body-image changes

- Toddlers appreciate the usefulness of various body parts.
- Toddlers develop gender identity and recognize gender differences by 3 years of age.

AGE-APPROPRIATE ACTIVITIES Q PCC

- Solitary play evolves into parallel play, in which toddlers observe other children and then might engage in activities nearby.
- Appropriate activities
  - Filling and emptying containers
  - Water toys and clay
  - Playing with blocks
  - Looking at books
  - Push-pull toys
  - Tossing balls
  - Finger paints
  - Large-piece puzzles
  - Thick crayons
- Temper tantrums result when toddlers are frustrated with restrictions on independence. Providing consistent, age-appropriate expectations helps toddlers to work through frustration.

4.1 Motor skill development by age

	GROSS MOTOR SKILLS	FINE MOTOR SKILLS
15 months	Walks without help Creeps up stairs	Uses a cup well Builds a tower of two blocks
18 months	Runs clumsily; falls often Throws a ball overhand Jumps in place with both feet Pulls and pushes toys	Manages a spoon without rotation Turns pages in a book, two or three at a time Builds tower of three or four blocks
2 years	Walks up and down stairs by placing both feet on each step	Builds a tower of six or seven blocks Turns pages of books one at a time
2.5 years	Jumps across the floor and off a chair or step using both feet Stands on one foot momentarily Takes a few steps on tiptoe	Draws circles Has good hand-finger coordination Builds a tower of eight blocks

- Toilet training can begin when toddlers have the sensation of needing to urinate or defecate. Guardians should demonstrate patience and consistency in toilet training. Nighttime control might develop last.
- Discipline should be consistent with well-defined boundaries that are established to develop acceptable social and emotional behavior. Time-out, redirection, and positive reinforcement are effective methods for toddlers.

HEALTH PROMOTION

IMMUNIZATIONS

The Centers for Disease Control and Prevention immunization recommendations for healthy toddlers 12 months to 3 years of age include: Q EBP

- 12 to 15 months: inactivated poliovirus (third dose between 6 to 18 months); *Haemophilus influenzae* type B; pneumococcal conjugate vaccine; measles, mumps, and rubella; and varicella
- 12 to 23 months: hepatitis A (Hep A), given in two doses at least 6 months apart
- 15 to 18 months: diphtheria, tetanus, and acellular pertussis
- 12 to 36 months: yearly seasonal inactivated influenza vaccine; live attenuated influenza vaccine by nasal spray (must be 2 years or older)

NUTRITION

- Children might establish lifetime eating habits during early childhood.
- Toddlers begin developing taste preferences and are generally picky eaters who repeatedly request their favorite foods.
- Physiologic anorexia occurs, resulting in toddlers becoming fussy eaters because of a decreased appetite.
- Toddlers should consume 24 to 28 oz of milk per day, and can switch from drinking whole milk to drinking low-fat milk after 2 years of age.
- Juice consumption should be limited to 4 to 6 oz per day.
- Trans fatty acids and saturated fats should be avoided.
- Diet should include 1 cup of fruit daily.
- Food serving size should be 1 tbsp for each year of age, or ¼ to 1/3 of an adult portion.
- Toddlers generally prefer finger foods because of increasing autonomy.
- Regular meal times and nutritious snacks best meet nutrient needs.
- Snacks or desserts that are high in sugar, fat, or sodium should be avoided.
- Foods that are potential choking hazards (nuts, grapes, hot dogs, peanut butter, raw carrots, dried beans, tough meats, popcorn) should be avoided.
- Adult supervision should always be provided during snack and mealtimes.
- Foods should be cut into small, bite-size pieces to make them easier to swallow and to prevent choking.
- Toddlers should not be allowed to engage in drinking or eating during play activities or while lying down.

- Parents and guardians should follow the U.S. Department of Agriculture's guidelines. Probiotics are classified as an alternative therapy. Other alternative therapy treatments are not recommended in this age group.

SLEEP AND REST

- Toddlers typically average 11 to 12 hr of sleep per day, including one nap.
- Naps often are eliminated in older toddlerhood.
- Resistance to bedtime and expression of fears are common in this age group.
- Maintaining a regular bedtime and bedtime routines are helpful to promote sleep.

DENTAL HEALTH

- Children should have an established dental provider by the age of 1 year.
- Flossing and brushing should be performed by the adult caregiver and are the best methods of removing plaque.
- Brushing should occur after meals and at bedtime. Nothing to eat or drink, except water, is given to the child after the bedtime cleaning.
- Fluoride is supplemented for children living in areas without adequate levels in drinking water.
- Early childhood caries is a form a tooth decay that develops in toddlers and is more common in children who are put to bed with a bottle of juice or milk.
- Consumption of cariogenic foods should be eliminated if possible. If not, the frequency of consumption should be limited.

INJURY PREVENTION Q S

Aspiration of foreign objects
- Small objects (grapes, coins, colored beads, candy) that can become lodged in the throat should be avoided.
- Toys that have small parts should be kept out of reach.
- Age-appropriate toys should be provided.
- Clothing should be checked for safety hazards (loose buttons).
- Balloons should be kept away from toddlers.
- Guardians should know emergency procedures for choking.

Bodily harm
- Sharp objects should be kept out of reach.
- Firearms should be kept in locked boxes or cabinets.
- Toddlers should not be left unattended with any animals present.
- Toddlers should be taught stranger safety.

Burns
- The temperature of bath water should be checked.
- Thermostats on hot water heaters should be turned down to less than 49° C (120° F).
- Working smoke detectors should be kept in the home.
- Pot handles should be turned toward the back of the stove.
- Electrical outlets should be covered.
- Toddlers should wear sunscreen when outside.

Drowning

- Toddlers should not be left unattended in bathtubs.
- Toilet lids should be kept closed.
- Toddlers should be closely supervised when near pools or any other body of water.
- Toddlers should be taught to swim.

Falls
- Doors and windows should be kept locked.
- Crib mattresses should be kept in the lowest position with the rails all the way up.
- Safety gates should be used across the top and bottom of stairs.

Motor-vehicle injuries
- Infants and toddlers remain in a rear-facing safety seat until the age of 2 years or until they exceed the height and weight recommended by the manufacturer.
- Toddlers over the age of 2 years, or who exceed the height and weight recommendations for rear-facing safety seats, are moved to a forward-facing safety seat with a harness.
- Safest area for infants and children is the backseat of the car.
- Do not place rear-facing safety seats in the front seat of vehicles with deployable passenger airbags.

Poisoning
- Exposure to lead paint should be avoided.
- Safety locks should be placed on cabinets that contain cleaners and other chemicals.
- The phone number for a poison control center should be kept near the phone.
- Medications should be kept in childproof containers, away from the reach of toddlers.
- A working carbon monoxide detector should be placed in the home.

Suffocation
- Plastic bags should be avoided.
- Crib mattresses should fit tightly.
- Crib slats should be no farther apart than 6 cm (2.375 in).
- Pillows should be kept out of cribs.
- Drawstrings should be removed from jackets and other clothing.

Application Exercises

1. A nurse is collecting data from a 2½-year-old toddler at a well-child visit. Which of the following findings should the nurse report to the provider?
   - A. Height increased by 7.5 cm (3 in) in the past year.
   - B. Head circumference exceeds chest circumference.
   - C. Anterior and posterior fontanels are closed.
   - D. Current weight equals four times the birth weight.

2. A nurse is assisting with a developmental screening on an 18 month old. Which of the following skills should the toddler be able to perform? (Select all that apply.)
   - A. Build a tower with six blocks
   - B. Throw a ball overhand
   - C. Walk up and down stairs
   - D. Stand on one foot for a few seconds
   - E. Use a spoon without rotation

3. A nurse is reinforcing teaching about growth and development characteristics to the guardian of a 2-year-old toddler. Which of the following statements by the guardian indicates an understanding of the teaching?
   - A. "My child should be able to turn the pages of a book one at a time."
   - B. "My child should be able to walk on their tiptoes for several steps."
   - C. "My child should be able to cut out an outline using scissors."
   - D. "My child should be able to put the toys away after using them."

4. A nurse is providing anticipatory guidance to the adoptive parents of a toddler. Which of the following information should the nurse include? (Select all that apply.)
   - A. Develop food habits that will prevent dental caries.
   - B. Meeting caloric needs results in an increased appetite.
   - C. Expression of bedtime fears is common.
   - D. Expect behaviors associated with negativism and ritualism.
   - E. Annual screenings for phenylketonuria are important.

Application Exercises Key

1. A. Toddler height should increase by 7.5 cm (3 in) each year. Therefore, do not report this finding to the provider.
   B. **CORRECT:** The head and chest circumference should be equal by 1 to 2 years of age, with the chest circumference continuing to increase in size until it exceeds the head circumference. Therefore, report this finding to the provider.
   C. The posterior fontanel closes by the age of 6 to 8 weeks, and the anterior fontanel closes by 12 to 18 months. Therefore, do not report this finding to the provider.
   D. The current weight should be four times the birth weight at the age of 2½ years. Therefore, do not report this finding to the provider.
   Ⓝ *NCLEX® Connection: Health Promotion and Maintenance, Data Collection Techniques*

2. A. The toddler should build a tower with six blocks at the age of 2 years.
   B. **CORRECT:** An 18 month old should be able to throw a ball overhand.
   C. The toddler should be able to walk up and down stairs by placing both feet on each step at the age of 2 years.
   D. The toddler should be able to stand on one foot momentarily at the age of 2½ years.
   E. **CORRECT:** An 18 month old should be able to use a spoon without rotation.
   Ⓝ *NCLEX® Connection: Health Promotion and Maintenance, Developmental Stages and Transitions*

3. A. **CORRECT:** This statement by the guardian indicates an understanding of the expected growth and development information provided by the nurse. A 2-year-old toddler should be able to turn pages in a book one at a time.
   B. Walking on tiptoes for several steps is an age-appropriate activity for a 2½-year-old child.
   C. Cutting out an outline using scissors is an age-appropriate activity for a 3-year-old child.
   D. Putting away toys after using them is an age-appropriate activity for a 3-year-old child.
   Ⓝ *NCLEX® Connection: Health Promotion and Maintenance, Developmental Stages and Transitions*

4. A. **CORRECT:** Because the toddler is developing taste preferences, the development of food habits that will prevent dental caries should be included in the anticipatory guidance.
   B. Toddlers often experience physiologic anorexia and become fussy eaters because of a decreased appetite.
   C. **CORRECT:** Expression of bedtime fears is common for toddlers and should be included in the anticipatory guidance.
   D. **CORRECT:** Negativism and ritualism are exhibited by toddlers as they seek autonomy, and associated behaviors should be included in the anticipatory guidance.
   E. Screening for phenylketonuria occurs in the newborn, not the toddler.
   Ⓝ *NCLEX® Connection: Health Promotion and Maintenance, Aging Process*

Active Learning Scenario

A nurse is conducting a well-child visit with a 2-year-old toddler. Use the ATI Active Learning Template: Growth and Development to complete this item.

DEVELOPMENTAL STAGE: Identify the toddler's developmental stage according to Piaget and Erikson.

NUTRITION: List three concepts to include in the teaching with the family.

INJURY PREVENTION: Identify two injury prevention methods to include when reinforcing teaching with the family for each of the following categories.

- Bodily harm
- Drowning
- Burns
- Falls

Active Learning Scenario Key

Using the ATI Active Learning Template: Growth and Development

DEVELOPMENTAL STAGE
- Piaget: Preoperational stage
- Erikson: Autonomy vs. shame and doubt

NUTRITION
- Can switch from whole milk to low fat milk after the age of 2 years.
- Trans fatty acids and saturated fats should be avoided.
- Diet should include 1 cup of fruit daily.
- Limit fruit juice to 4 to 6 oz per day.
- Cut food into small, bite-size pieces to prevent choking.
- Do not allow drinking or eating during play activities or while lying down.

INJURY PREVENTION
- Bodily harm
  - Keep sharp objects out of reach.
  - Lock firearms in a cabinet or box.
  - Reinforce toddler stranger safety.
  - Do not leave toddler unattended with animals.
- Drowning
  - Do not leave toddler unattended in bathtub.
  - Keep toilet lids closed.
  - Begin reinforcing toddler water safety and to swim.
  - Keep bathroom doors closed.
- Burns
  - Check bath water temperature prior to toddler contact with water.
  - Set hot water heaters to less than 49° C (120° F) .
  - Keep pot handles pointed to back of stove when cooking.
  - Cover electrical outlets.
  - Keep working smoke detectors in the home.
  - Apply sunscreen when toddler will be outside.
- Falls
  - Keep doors and windows locked.
  - Place crib mattresses in lowest position with rails all the way up.
  - Use safety gates at the top and bottom of stairs.
Ⓝ *NCLEX® Connection: Health Promotion and Maintenance, Aging Process*

CHAPTER 5 *Health Promotion of Preschoolers (3 to 6 Years)*

EXPECTED GROWTH AND DEVELOPMENT

PHYSICAL DEVELOPMENT

WEIGHT: Preschoolers should gain about 2 to 3 kg (4.5 to 6.5 lb) per year.

HEIGHT: Preschoolers should grow about 6.2 to 9 cm (2.4 to 3.5 in) per year.

5.1 Average height and weight by age

	3-YEAR-OLD	4-YEAR-OLD	5-YEAR-OLD
Weight	14.5 kg (32 lb)	16.5 kg (36.5 lb)	18.5 kg (41 lb)
Height	95 cm (37.5 in)	103 cm (40.5 in)	110 cm (43.5 in)

Preschoolers' bodies evolve from an unsteady wide stance and protruding abdomen of the toddler, into a more graceful, erect posture, and physical stance.

FINE AND GROSS MOTOR SKILLS

Preschoolers show improvement in fine motor skills, which will be displayed by activities like copying figures on paper and dressing independently. (5.2)

COGNITIVE DEVELOPMENT QEBP

Piaget: preoperational phase
The preconceptual thought transitions to the phase of intuitive thought around the age of 4 years. The phase of intuitive thought lasts until the age of 7 years.
- The preschooler moves from totally egocentric thoughts to social awareness and the ability to consider the viewpoints of others.

- Preschoolers make judgments based on visual appearances. Variations in thinking during this age include:
  - **Magical thinking:** Thoughts are all powerful and can cause events to occur.
  - **Animism:** Ascribing lifelike qualities to inanimate objects.
  - **Centration:** Focus on one aspect instead of considering all possible alternatives.
  - **Time:** Preschoolers begin to understand the sequence of daily events. Time is best explained to them in relation to an event. By the end of the preschool years, children have a better comprehension of time-oriented words.

Language development

- The vocabulary of preschoolers increases to more than 2,100 words by the end of the fifth year.
- Preschoolers speak in sentences of three to four words at the ages of 3 and 4 years, and four to five words at the age of 4 to 5 years.
- This age group talks incessantly, asks many questions, and language becomes a major method of communication and social interaction.
- Names familiar objects, body parts, animals and family members. Imitates new words proficiently.

PSYCHOSOCIAL DEVELOPMENT QEBP

Erikson: initiative vs. guilt
- Preschoolers become energetic learners, despite not having all of the physical abilities necessary to be successful at everything.
- Guilt can occur when preschoolers believe they have misbehaved or when they are unable to accomplish a task.
- Guiding preschoolers to attempt activities within their capabilities while setting limits is pertinent.

Kohlberg: moral development
- Preschoolers at 2 to 4 years old have a basic understanding of moral judgment, and actions are taken based on whether or not it will result in a reward or punishment.
- Preschoolers at 4 to 6 years old primarily take actions based on satisfying personal needs, yet understand the concepts of justice and fairness.

5.2 Motor skill development by age

	GROSS MOTOR SKILLS	FINE MOTOR SKILLS
3 years	Rides a tricycle Jumps off bottom step Stands on one foot for a few seconds	Builds tower of 9-10 blocks Copies a circle Imitates a cross when drawing
4 years	Skips and hops on one foot Throws ball overhead Catches ball reliably	Laces shoes Uses scissors to cut out a picture
5 years	Jumps rope Walks backward with heel to toe Throws and catches a ball with ease	Uses a pencil and small tools well Prints simple words and first name

Body-image changes

- Preschoolers begin to recognize differences in appearances and identify what is considered acceptable and unacceptable.
- By the age of 5 years, preschoolers begin comparing themselves with peers.
- Poor understanding of anatomy makes intrusive experiences (injections or tooth extraction), frightening to preschoolers.

Social development

- Preschoolers generally do not exhibit stranger anxiety and have less separation anxiety.
- Changes in daily routine are tolerated, but they can develop more imaginary fears.
- Prolonged separation (during hospitalization) can provoke anxiety. Favorite toys and appropriate play should be used to help ease preschoolers' fears.
- Pretend play is healthy and allows preschoolers to determine the difference between reality and fantasy.

AGE-APPROPRIATE ACTIVITIES Q͏PCC

Parallel play shifts to associative play during the preschool years. Play is not highly organized, but cooperation does exist between children. Appropriate activities include:
- Playing ball
- Putting puzzles together
- Riding tricycles
- Playing pretend and dress-up activities
- Role playing
- Hand puppets
- Painting
- Simple sewing
- Reading books
- Wading pools
- Sand boxes
- Skating
- Computer programs
- Musical toys
- Electronic games

HEALTH PROMOTION

IMMUNIZATIONS

The Centers for Disease Control and Prevention (CDC) immunization recommendations for healthy preschoolers 3 to 6 years of age include: Q͏EBP

4 TO 6 YEARS: Diphtheria and tetanus toxoids and pertussis (DTaP); measles, mumps, and rubella (MMR); varicella; and inactivated poliovirus (IPV)

3 TO 6 YEARS: Yearly seasonal influenza vaccine; inactivated influenza vaccine; or live attenuated influenza vaccine by nasal spray

NUTRITION

- Preschoolers who are moderately active require an estimated caloric intake range from 1200 to 1400 kcal/day.
- Finicky eating can remain a behavior in preschoolers, but often by 5 years of age they become more willing to sample different foods.
- Preschoolers need 13 to 19 g/day of protein (2- to 4-oz equivalents), in addition to 700 to 1000 mg/day of calcium, 19 to 25 g/day of fiber, as well as adequate intake of iron, folate, and vitamins A and C.
- Saturated fats should be less than 10% of preschoolers' total caloric intake, and total fat should be 30% of total caloric intake over several days.
- With obesity rates in young children increasing, the American Academy of Pediatrics recommends a 5-2-1-0 framework, which includes that preschoolers have 5 servings of fruits and vegetables per day, 2 hr or less of screen time, 0 servings of sugar-sweetened beverages, and 1 hr of physical activity per day.

Guardians should follow the American Academy of Pediatrics' healthy diet recommendations.

SLEEP AND REST

- On average, preschoolers need about 12 hr of sleep per day, and infrequently take daytime naps.
- Sleep disturbances frequently occur during early childhood, and problems range from difficulty going to bed to night terrors. Recommended interventions vary, but can include the following.
  - Keep a consistent bedtime routine.
  - Use a night-light in the room.
  - Provide the child with a favorite toy.
  - Leave a drink of water by the bed.
  - Reassure preschoolers who are frightened, but discourage sleeping with parents.
  - Ignore attention-seeking behaviors.

DENTAL HEALTH

- Eruption of deciduous (primary) teeth is finalized by the beginning of the preschool years.
- To prevent dental caries, parents and guardians should assist and supervise brushing and flossing to ensure it is performed correctly.
- Trauma to teeth is common in preschoolers and should be immediately evaluated by a dentist.

INJURY PREVENTION Q͏S

Bodily harm
- Firearms should be kept in locked cabinets or containers.
- Preschoolers should be taught stranger safety.
- Preschoolers should be taught to wear protective equipment (helmet, pads).
- Preschoolers are less prone to falls due to improved fine and gross motor skills, coordination, and balance.

Burns

- Hot water thermostats should be set at or below 49° C (120° F).
- Working smoke detectors should be kept in the home.
- Preschoolers should have sunscreen applied when outside.

Drowning

- Preschoolers should not be left unattended in bathtubs.
- Preschoolers should be closely supervised when near the pool or any other body of water.
- Preschoolers should be taught to swim.

Motor-vehicle injuries

- Preschoolers should use a federally approved car restraint according to the manufacturer recommendations.
- When the forward-facing car seat is outgrown, the preschooler transitions to a booster seat.
- It is recommended that children use an approved car restraint system until they achieve a height of 145 cm (4 feet, 9 in) or 8 to 12 years old. Ⓠ**EBP**
- Safest area for children is the backseat of the car.
- Supervise preschool-age children when playing outside, and do not allow them to play near a curb or parked cars.
- Reinforce pedestrian safety rules to preschool-age children.
  - Stand back from curb while waiting to cross the street.
  - Before crossing the street, look left, then right, then left again.
  - Walk on the left, facing traffic, when there are no sidewalks.
  - At night, wear light-colored clothing with fluorescent materials attached.

Active Learning Scenario

A nurse is providing anticipatory guidance to the guardians of a preschooler. Use the ATI Active Learning Template: Growth and Development to complete this item.

PHYSICAL DEVELOPMENT: Identify general expectations for height and weight during the preschool years.

COGNITIVE DEVELOPMENT: List two concepts related to language development in preschoolers.

AGE-APPROPRIATE ACTIVITIES: List five activities appropriate for preschoolers.

INJURY PREVENTION: Identify two pedestrian safety rules guardians should teach children.

Application Exercises

1. A nurse is reinforcing teaching to the guardian of a preschooler about methods to promote sleep. Which of the following statements by the guardian indicates an understanding of the teaching?
   - A. "I will sleep in the bed with my child if she wakes up during the night."
   - B. "I will let my child stay up an additional 2 hours on weekend nights."
   - C. "I will let my child watch television for 30 minutes just before bedtime each night."
   - D. "I will keep a dim lamp on in my child's room during the night."

2. A nurse is conducting a well-child visit with a 5-year-old child who is up to date with current immunizations. Which of the following immunizations should the nurse plan to administer to the child? (Select all that apply.)
   - A. Diphtheria, tetanus, pertussis (DTaP)
   - B. Inactivated poliovirus (IPV)
   - C. Measles, mumps, rubella (MMR)
   - D. Pneumococcal (PCV)
   - E. Haemophilus influenzae type B (Hib)

3. A nurse is assisting an education program for a group of caregivers of preschooler about promoting optimum nutrition. Which of the following information should the nurse include in the program?
   - A. Saturated fats should equal 20% of total daily caloric intake.
   - B. Average calorie intake should be 1,800 calories per day.
   - C. Daily intake of fruits and vegetables should total 2 servings.
   - D. Healthy diets include a total of 8 g protein each day.

4. A nurse is collecting data from a 3-year-old child during a well-child visit. Which of the following gross-motor skills should the nurse expect the child to perform?
   - A. Ride a tricycle
   - B. Hop on one foot
   - C. Jump rope
   - D. Throw a ball overhead

5. A nurse is caring for a preschooler who expresses the need to leave because their doll is scared to be at home alone. Which of the following characteristics of preoperational thought is the child exhibiting?
   - A. Egocentrism
   - B. Centration
   - C. Animism
   - D. Magical thinking

Application Exercises Key

1. A. The child should not be allowed to sleep in the same bed as the guardian.
   B. The guardian should maintain a consistent bedtime routine and avoid allowing the child to stay up past a reasonable hour.
   C. Watching television prior to bed can cause the child to resist and delay sleep.
   D. **CORRECT:** Leaving a light on in the child's room is an appropriate method to promote sleep for a preschool-age child.

   Ⓝ *NCLEX® Connection: Basic Care and Comfort, Rest and Sleep*

2. A. **CORRECT:** DTaP is a recommended immunization for 4- to 6-year-olds, and should be administered by the nurse.
   B. **CORRECT:** IPV is a recommended immunization for 4- to 6-year-olds, and should be administered by the nurse.
   C. **CORRECT:** MMR is a recommended immunization for 4- to 6-year-olds, and should be administered by the nurse.
   D. PCV is given as a series of immunizations in the first 15 months of life, and is not recommended for 4- to 6-year-olds.
   E. Hib is given as a series of immunizations in the first 15 months of life, and is not recommended for 4- to 6-year-olds.

   Ⓝ *NCLEX® Connection: Health Promotion and Maintenance, Health Promotion/Disease Prevention*

3. A. Saturated fats should be less than 10% of total caloric intake.
   B. **CORRECT:** Preschool-age children should consume an average of 1,800 calories/day.
   C. Preschoolers should consume a total of 5 servings of fruits and vegetables per day.
   D. Healthy diets include 13 to 19 g protein each day.

   Ⓝ *NCLEX® Connection: Basic Care and Comfort, Nutrition and Oral Hydration*

4. A. **CORRECT:** A 3-year-old child should be able to ride a tricycle.
   B. A 4-year-old child should be able to hop on one foot.
   C. A 5-year-old child should be able to jump rope.
   D. A 4-year-old child should be able to throw a ball overhead.

   Ⓝ *NCLEX® Connection: Health Promotion and Maintenance, Developmental Stages and Transitions*

5. A. Egocentrism occurs when the child is unable to see another person's perspective.
   B. Centration occurs when the child focuses on one aspect of something instead of considering the whole.
   C. **CORRECT:** Animism occurs when the child gives living qualities to inanimate objects (a doll feeling scared).
   D. Magical thinking occurs when the child believes their thoughts cause an event to occur.

   Ⓝ *NCLEX® Connection: Health Promotion and Maintenance, Developmental Stages and Transitions*

Active Learning Scenario Key

Using the ATI Active Learning Template: Growth and Development

PHYSICAL DEVELOPMENT
- Weight: Preschoolers should gain about 2 to 3 kg (4.5 to 6.5 lb) per year.
- Height: Preschoolers should grow about 6.2 to 9 cm (2.4 to 3.5 in) per year.

COGNITIVE DEVELOPMENT
- Vocabulary increases to more than 2,100 words by the end of the fifth year.
- Speak in sentences of three to four words at the ages of 3 and 4 years.
- Speak in sentences of four to five words at the age of 4 to 5 years.
- Talks incessantly, and language becomes a major method of communication.

AGE-APPROPRIATE ACTIVITIES
- Putting puzzles together
- Playing ball
- Playing pretend and dress-up activities
- Painting
- Role playing
- Riding tricycles
- Simple sewing
- Reading books
- Sandboxes
- Wading pools
- Skating
- Computer programs
- Musical toys
- Electronic games

INJURY PREVENTION
- Stand back from curb while waiting to cross the street.
- Before crossing the street, look left, then right, then left again.
- Walk on the left, facing traffic, when there are no sidewalks.
- At night, wear light-colored clothing with fluorescent materials attached.

Ⓝ *NCLEX® Connection: Health Promotion and Maintenance, Aging Process*

CHAPTER 6 *Health Promotion of School-Age Children (6 to 12 Years)*

EXPECTED GROWTH AND DEVELOPMENT

PHYSICAL DEVELOPMENT

Weight: School-age children will gain about 2 to 3 kg (4.4 to 6.6 lb) per year.

Height: School-age children will grow about 5 cm (2 inches) per year.

Prepubescence
- Preadolescence is typically when prepubescence occurs.
- Onset of physiologic changes begins around the age of 9 years, particularly in girls.
- Rapid growth in height and weight occurs.
- Differences in the rate of growth and maturation between boys and girls becomes apparent.
- Visible sexual maturation is minimal in boys during preadolescence.
- Permanent teeth erupt.
- Bladder capacity differs, but remains greater in girls than boys.
- Immune system improves.
- Bones continue to ossify.

COGNITIVE DEVELOPMENT

Piaget: concrete operations ○EBP
- Transitions from perceptual to conceptual thinking
- Masters the concept of conservation:
  ○ Conservation of mass is understood first, followed by weight, and then volume
- Learns to tell time
- Classifies more complex information
- Able to see the perspective of others
- Able to solve problems

PSYCHOSOCIAL DEVELOPMENT

Erikson: industry vs. inferiority
- A sense of industry is achieved through the development of skills and knowledge that allows the child to provide meaningful contributions to society.
- A sense of accomplishment is gained through the ability to cooperate and compete with others.
- Children should be challenged with tasks that need to be accomplished, and be allowed to work through individual differences in order to complete the tasks.
- Creating systems that reward successful mastery of skills and tasks can create a sense of inferiority in children unable to complete the tasks or acquire the skills.
- Children should be taught that not everyone will master every skill.

Moral development

EARLY SCHOOL-AGE YEARS
- Do not understand the reasoning behind rules and expectations for behavior.
- Believe what they think is wrong, and what others tell them is right.
- Judgment is guided by rewards and punishment.
- Sometimes interpret accidents as punishment.

LATER SCHOOL-AGE YEARS
- Able to judge the intentions of an act rather than just its consequences.
- Understand different points of view instead of just whether or not an act is right or wrong.
- Conceptualizes treating others as they like to be treated.

Self-concept development

- School-age children develop an awareness of themselves in relation to others, as well as an understanding of personal values, abilities, and physical characteristics.
- Confidence is gained through establishing a positive self-concept, which leads to feelings of worthiness and the ability to provide significant contributions.
- Parents continue to influence the school-age child's self-ideals, but by middle childhood the opinions of peers and teachers become more valuable.

Body-image changes

- Solidification of body image occurs.
- Curiosity about sexuality should be addressed with education regarding sexual development and the reproductive process.
- School-age children are more modest than preschoolers and place more emphasis on privacy issues.

Social development

- Peer groups play an important part in social development. Peer pressure begins to take effect.
- Clubs and best friends are popular.
- Bullying actions are intended to cause harm or to control someone, and are sometimes attributed to poor relationships with peers and difficulty identifying with a group.
- During early school-age years, children often prefer the company of same-sex companions, but begin developing an interest in others toward the end of the school-age years.
- Most relationships come from school associations.
- Conformity becomes evident.

AGE-APPROPRIATE ACTIVITIES ○PCC

Competitive and cooperative play is predominant.

CHILDREN FROM 6 TO 9 YEARS OF AGE
- Play simple board and number games.
- Play hopscotch.
- Jump rope.
- Collect rocks, stamps, cards, coins, or stuffed animals.
- Ride bicycles.
- Build simple models.
- Join organized sports (for skill building).

CHILDREN FROM 9 TO 12 YEARS OF AGE
- Make crafts.
- Build models.
- Collect things/engage in hobbies.
- Solve jigsaw puzzles.
- Play board and card games.
- Join organized competitive sports.

HEALTH PROMOTION

IMMUNIZATIONS

The Centers for Disease Control and Prevention (CDC) immunization recommendations for healthy school-age children 6 to 12 years of age include: ◯EBP
- If not given between 4 and 5 years of age, children should receive the following vaccines by 6 years of age: diphtheria and tetanus toxoids and pertussis (DTaP); inactivated poliovirus; measles, mumps, and rubella (MMR); and varicella.
- Yearly seasonal influenza vaccine: inactivated influenza vaccine (IIV) or live, attenuated influenza vaccine (LAIV) by nasal spray.
- 11 to 12 years: tetanus and diphtheria toxoids and pertussis vaccine (Tdap); human papillomavirus (HPV) vaccine, and meningococcal vaccine.

HEALTH SCREENINGS

Scoliosis: School-age children should be screened for scoliosis by examining for a lateral curvature of the spine before and during growth spurts. Screening can take place at schools or at health care facilities.

NUTRITION

- By the end of the school-age years, children should eat adult portions of food. They need quality nutritious snacks.
- Obesity is an increasing concern of this age group that predisposes children to low self-esteem, diabetes, heart disease, and high blood pressure. Advise parents to: ◯EBP
  ○ Avoid using food as a reward.
  ○ Emphasize physical activity.
  ○ Ensure that a balanced diet is consumed by following the U.S. Department of Agriculture's healthy diet recommendations.
  ○ Reinforce to children to make healthy food selections for meals and snacks.
  ○ Avoid eating fast-food frequently.
  ○ Avoid skipping meals.
  ○ Model healthy behaviors.

SLEEP AND REST

- Required sleep is highly variable in the school-age years, and is dependent on the following:
  ○ Age
  ○ Level of activity
  ○ Health status
- Approximately 9 hr of sleep is needed each night at the age of 11 years.
- Resistance to bedtime is sometimes experienced around the age of 8 and 9 years, and again around the age of 11 years, but is typically resolved by the age of 12 years.

DENTAL HEALTH

- The first permanent teeth erupt around 6 years of age.
- Children should brush after meals and snacks, and at bedtime.
- Children should floss daily.
- Children should have regular checkups.
- If necessary, children should have regular fluoride treatments.

INJURY PREVENTION ◯s

Bodily harm
- Keep firearms in locked cabinets or boxes.
- Identify safe play areas.
- Teach stranger safety to children.
- Teach children to wear helmets and/or pads when roller skating, skateboarding, bicycling, riding scooters, skiing, and snowboarding.

Burns
- Teach fire safety and potential burn hazards.
- Keep working smoke detectors in the home.
- Children should use sunscreen when outside.
- Teach safety precautions for children to take while cooking.

Drowning
- Children should be supervised when swimming or when near a body of water.
- Children should be taught to swim.
- Check depth of water before allowing children to dive.
- Encourage breaks to prevent children from becoming over-tired.

Motor-vehicle injuries
- Children should use an approved car restraint system until they achieve a height of 145 cm (4 feet, 9 inches). ◯s
- Teach children appropriate seat belt use when no longer using a car restraint system or booster seat.
- Safest area for children is the backseat of the car.
- Never let children ride in the bed of a pickup truck.
- Reinforce safe pedestrian behaviors.

Poisoning/substance misuse ◯s
- Cleaners and chemicals should be kept in locked cabinets or out of reach of younger children.
- Children should be taught to say "no" to substance misuse.

Application Exercises

1. A nurse is participating in a discussion about prepubescence and preadolescence with a group of guardians of school-age children. Which of the following information should the nurse include in the discussion?

   A. Initial physiologic changes appear during early childhood.

   B. Changes in height and weight occur slowly during this period.

   C. Growth differences between boys and girls become evident.

   D. Sexual maturation becomes highly visible in boys.

2. A nurse is assisting with conducting a well-child visit with a child who is scheduled to receive the recommended immunizations for 11- to 12-year-olds. Which of the following immunizations should the nurse administer? (Select all that apply.)

   A. Inactivated influenza (IIV)

   B. Pneumococcal (PCV)

   C. Meningococcal (MenB-4C)

   D. Tetanus and diphtheria toxoids and pertussis (Tdap)

   E. Rotavirus (RV)

3. A nurse is assisting with providing education about age-appropriate activities for the caregivers of a 6-year-old child. Which of the following activities should the nurse include in teaching?

   A. Jumping rope

   B. Playing table games

   C. Solving jigsaw puzzles

   D. Joining competitive sports

4. A nurse is assisting with teaching a course about safety during the school-age. Which of the following information should the nurse include in the course? (Select all that apply.)

   A. Gating stairs at the top and bottom

   B. Wearing helmets when riding bicycles or skateboarding

   C. Riding safely in bed of pickup trucks

   D. Implementing firearm safety

   E. Wearing seat belts

Active Learning Scenario

A nurse is assisting with providing anticipatory guidance to the guardians of a school-age child. Use the ATI Active Learning Template: Growth and Development to complete this item.

DEVELOPMENTAL STAGE: Identify the child's developmental stage according to Piaget and Erikson.

PHYSICAL DEVELOPMENT: Identify three facts relevant to the child's physical development.

NUTRITION: List three strategies the family can implement to reduce the risk of obesity.

Application Exercises Key

1. A. Initial physiologic changes appear toward the end of middle childhood, around the age of 9 years.
   B. Changes in height and weight occur rapidly during this time period.
   C. **CORRECT:** Plan to include in the discussion that growth differences between boys and girls become evident.
   D. Visible sexual maturation is minimal in boys.

   Ⓝ *NCLEX® Connection: Health Promotion and Maintenance, Developmental Stages and Transitions*

2. A. **CORRECT:** IIV is a recommended immunization for 11- to 12-year-olds, and should be administered by the nurse.
   B. PCV is recommended as a series of immunizations in the first 15 months of life.
   C. **CORRECT:** Meningococcal vaccine is recommended for 11 to 12 year olds, and should be administered by the nurse.
   D. **CORRECT:** Tdap is a recommended immunization for 11- to 12-year-olds, and should be administered by the nurse.
   E. RV is recommended as a series of immunizations in the first 6 months of life.

   Ⓝ *NCLEX® Connection: Health Promotion and Maintenance, Health Promotion/Disease Prevention*

3. A. **CORRECT:** Recommend activities (playing hopscotch, jumping rope, riding bicycles, and joining organized sports).
   B. Playing table games is not an appropriate activity for a 6-year-old child.
   C. Solving jigsaw puzzles is not an appropriate activity for a 6-year-old child.
   D. Joining an organized competitive sport is an appropriate activity for a child who is 9 to 12 years old.

   Ⓝ *NCLEX® Connection: Health Promotion and Maintenance, Developmental Stages and Transitions*

4. A. Gating stairs at the top and bottom should not be included in the teaching. This is appropriate information to include when teaching about safety during infant and toddler years.
   B. **CORRECT:** When assisting with teaching about safety in the school-age years, include information about wearing helmets when riding bicycles or skateboarding.
   C. The nurse should reinforce that it is never safe to ride in the bed of a pickup truck.
   D. **CORRECT:** Include information about implementing firearm safety when assisting with teaching about safety in the school-age years.
   E. **CORRECT:** Include information about wearing seat belts when assisting with teaching about safety in the school-age years.

   Ⓝ *NCLEX® Connection: Safety and Infection Control, Accident/Error/Injury Prevention*

Active Learning Scenario Key

Using the ATI Active Learning Template: Growth and Development

DEVELOPMENTAL STAGE
- Piaget: concrete operations
- Erikson: industry vs. inferiority

PHYSICAL DEVELOPMENT
- Will gain about 2 to 3 kg (4.4 to 6.6 lb) per year.
- Will grow about 5 cm (2 in) per year.
- Bladder capacity is variable with each child.
- Immune system improves.
- Bones continue to ossify.

NUTRITION
- Avoid using food as a reward.
- Emphasize physical activity.
- Ensure a balanced diet is consumed.
- Reinforce to children to select healthy foods and snacks.
- Avoid eating fast foods frequently.
- Avoid skipping meals.
- Model healthy behaviors.

Ⓝ *NCLEX® Connection: Health Promotion and Maintenance, Developmental Stages and Transitions*

CHAPTER 7 *Health Promotion of Adolescents (12 to 20 Years)*

EXPECTED GROWTH AND DEVELOPMENT

PHYSICAL DEVELOPMENT

- The final 20% to 25% of height is achieved during puberty.
- Acne can appear during adolescence.
- Girls stop growing at about 2 to 2.5 years after the onset of menarche. They grow 5 to 20 cm (2 to 8 in) and gain 7 to 25 kg (15.5 to 55 lb).
- Boys stop growing at around 18 to 20 years of age. They grow 10 to 30 cm (4 to 12 in) and gain 7 to 30 kg (15.5 to 66 lb).
- In females, sexual maturation occurs in the following order.
  - Breast development
  - Pubic hair growth (some girls experience hair growth before breast development)
  - Axillary hair growth
  - Menstruation
- In males, sexual maturation occurs in the following order.
  - Testicular enlargement
  - Pubic hair growth
  - Penile enlargement
  - Growth of axillary hair
  - Facial hair growth
  - Vocal changes

COGNITIVE DEVELOPMENT

Piaget: formal operations
- Able to think through more than two categories of variables concurrently
- Capable of evaluating the quality of their own thinking
- Able to maintain attention for longer periods of time
- Highly imaginative and idealistic
- Increasingly capable of using formal logic to make decisions
- Think beyond current circumstances
- Able to understand how the actions of an individual influence others
- Able to think in terms of abstract possibilities and hypothetical situations

PSYCHOSOCIAL DEVELOPMENT

Erikson: identity vs. role confusion
- Adolescents often try different roles and experiences to develop a sense of personal identity, and come to view themselves as unique individuals.
- Group identity: Adolescents become part of a peer group that greatly influences behavior.

Psychological health

- Swings or variations in emotions are common during early adolescence, with outward expressions of emotions.
- During middle adolescence, introspection is increased.
- Stability of emotions and anger management are usually developed by the later adolescent years.

Sexual identity

- Begins with close, same-sex friendships during early adolescence, which sometimes involve sexual experimentation driven by curiosity.
- Self-exploration occurs through masturbation.
- Transition from friendships to intimate relationships during adolescence.
- In late adolescence, sexual identity typically is formed through the integration of sexual experiences, feelings, and knowledge.

Health perceptions

Adolescents can view themselves as invincible to bad outcomes of risky behaviors.

Moral development

- Solve moral dilemma using internalized moral principles
- Question relevance of existing moral values to society and individuals

Religion and spirituality

- Adolescents' views regarding religion and spirituality become more personalized, with decreased focus on religious tradition.
- Beliefs are influenced primarily by peers and can influence self-identity.

Self-concept development

- View themselves in relation to similarities with peers during early adolescence
- View themselves according to their unique characteristics as the adolescent years progress

Body-image changes

- Base their own normality on comparisons with peers.
- The image established during adolescence is retained throughout life.

Social development

- Peer relationships develop. These relationships act as a support system for adolescents.
- Best-friend relationships are more stable and longer-lasting than they were in previous years.
- Parent–child relationships change to allow a greater sense of independence.

AGE-APPROPRIATE ACTIVITIES Qpcc

- Nonviolent video games
- Nonviolent music
- Sports
- Caring for a pet
- Career-training programs
- Reading
- Social interaction (going to movies, school dances, electronic messaging, and social media)

HEALTH PROMOTION

IMMUNIZATIONS

Centers for Disease Control and Prevention (CDC) recommendations for healthy adolescents 13 to 18 years old include catch-up doses of any recommended immunizations not received at 11 to 12 years old. QEBP

- Yearly seasonal influenza vaccine: inactivated influenza vaccine or live attenuated influenza vaccine by nasal spray. Recommendation can be season-specific.
- 16 to 18 years: Meningococcal (MCV4) booster is recommended if first dose was received between the ages of 13 and 15 years. A booster dose is not needed if the first dose is received at age 16 or older.

HEALTH SCREENINGS

- Screenings for scoliosis should continue during the adolescent years. These screenings should include an examination for a lateral curvature of the spine before and during growth spurts. Screenings can take place at school or at a health care facility.
- Annual height and weights for BMI calculations should be obtained.
- Hemoglobin and hematocrit.
- Universal lipid screenings.
- Screenings for STIs if sexually active.

NUTRITION

- Rapid growth and high metabolism require increases in quality nutrients and make adolescents unable to tolerate caloric restrictions.
  - During times of rapid growth, additional calcium, iron, protein, and zinc are needed.
  - Inadequate intake of folic acid, vitamin B_6, vitamin A, iron, calcium, and zinc is common.

- Overeating and undereating present challenges during the adolescent years.
  - Yearly assessments of height, weight, and BMI for age are needed in order to identify nutritional issues and intervene early.
- Overweight and obesity rates are of particular concern; anorexia and bulimia are common in this age group as well.
- Advise guardians to:
  - Avoid using food as a reward.
  - Reinforce physical activity.
  - Reinforce that a balanced diet is consumed by following the U.S. Department of Agriculture's healthy diet recommendations.
  - Encourage adolescents to make healthy food selections for meals and snacks.

SLEEP AND REST

- Adolescents should get about 9 hours of sleep each night.
- Sleep habits change with puberty due to increased metabolism and rapid growth.
- Adolescents tend to stay up late, sleep in later in the morning, and can sleep more than during the school-age years.
- During periods of active growth, the need for sleep increases. Sleep habits can change with puberty due to increased metabolism and rapid growth during the adolescent years.
- Sleep deprivation is a concern with many adolescents; discuss the importance of sleep and encourage adequate rest.

DENTAL HEALTH

- Corrective appliances are most common with this age group.
- Adolescents should brush after meals and snacks, and at bedtime.
- Adolescents should floss daily.
- Adolescents should have regular checkups.
- If necessary, adolescents should have regular fluoride treatments.

SEXUALITY

- Provide adolescents with accurate information, and discuss what is heard from peers.
- Emphasize abstinence and safe sexual behaviors (oral, vaginal, or anal).
- Provide information about preventing sexually transmitted infections and pregnancy, and perform STI screenings for at-risk adolescents.
- Promote an atmosphere where adolescents are comfortable asking questions.
- Assist adolescents with problem-solving and decision-making skills.
- Ask adolescents about risky sexual behaviors and discuss the need for mutual consent prior to sexual contact.

INJURY PREVENTION Qs

Bodily harm
- Keep firearms unloaded and in a locked cabinet or box.
- Reinforce teaching about the proper use of sporting equipment prior to use.
- Insist on helmet use and/or pads when roller skating, skateboarding, bicycling, riding scooters, skiing, and snowboarding.
- Be aware of changes in mood. Monitor for self-harm in adolescents who are at risk. Watch for the following.
  - Poor school performance
  - Lack of interest in things that were of interest to the adolescent in the past
  - Social isolation
  - Disturbances in sleep or appetite
  - Expression of suicidal thoughts
- Discuss non-violent conflict resolution strategies.
- Discuss bullying, including cyberbullying.
- Warn about the risk of sexual predators, who often communicate through electronic interactions.

Burns
- Reinforce teaching about fire safety.
- Adolescents should apply sunscreen when outside.
- Adolescents should avoid tanning beds.

Drowning
- Encourage adolescents to learn how to swim.
- Advise adolescents not to swim alone.

Motor-vehicle injuries
- Encourage attendance at drivers' education courses. Emphasize the need for adherence to seat belt use.
- Insist on helmet use with bicycles, motorcycles, skateboards, roller skates, and snowboards.
- Discuss the dangers of using cell phones or texting while driving and enforce laws regarding use.
- Reinforce the dangers of combining substance use with driving.
- Role model desired behavior.

Substance use disorder
- Monitor for indications of substance use disorder in adolescents who are at risk. Ask adolescents while collecting health data about alcohol, tobacco, and marijuana use, including the frequency of use.
- Reinforce the risks of smoking and using smokeless tobacco or nicotine-containing products, including electronic cigarettes.
- Reinforce the short-term effects of substance use on school or work performance.

Application Exercises

1. A nurse is reinforcing teaching about expected changes during puberty to a group of guardians of early adolescent girls. Which of the following statements by one of the guardians indicates an understanding of the information?
   - A. "Girls usually stop growing about 2 years after menarche."
   - B. "Girls are expected to gain about 65 pounds during puberty."
   - C. "Girls experience menstruation prior to breast development."
   - D. "Girls typically grow more than 10 inches during puberty."

2. A nurse is assisting with providing anticipatory guidance to the caregiver of a 13-year-old adolescent. Which of the following screenings should the nurse recommend for the adolescent? (Select all that apply.)
   - A. Body mass index
   - B. Blood lead level
   - C. 24-hr dietary recall
   - D. Weight
   - E. Scoliosis

3. A nurse is caring for an adolescent whose guardian expresses concerns about the child sleeping such long hours. Which of the following conditions should the nurse inform the guardian as requiring additional sleep during adolescence?
   - A. Sleep terrors
   - B. Rapid growth
   - C. Elevated zinc levels
   - D. Slowed metabolism

4. A nurse is assisting teaching a class about puberty in boys. Which of the following should the nurse include as the first manifestation of sexual maturation?
   - A. Pubic hair growth
   - B. Vocal changes
   - C. Testicular enlargement
   - D. Facial hair growth

Application Exercises Key

1. A. **CORRECT:** Girls usually stop growing about 2 years after menarche. This statement by the guardian indicates and understanding of the teaching.
   B. Girls are expected to gain 7 to 25 kg (15.5 to 55 lb) during puberty. This statement by the guardian does not indicate an understanding of the teaching.
   C. Breast development is usually the first manifestation of sexual maturity in girls and appears before menstruation. This statement by the guardian does not indicate an understanding of the teaching.
   D. Girls typically grow 5 to 20 cm (2 to 8 in) during puberty. This statement by the guardian does not indicate an understanding of the teaching.

   Ⓝ *NCLEX® Connection: Health Promotion and Maintenance, Developmental Stages and Transitions*

2. A. **CORRECT:** Recommend that the adolescent have a body mass index screening annually.
   B. Blood lead level screenings are recommended for children at the age of 1 and 2 years and for children between the ages of 3 and 6 years who have not previously been screened.
   C. A 24-hr dietary recall is not a routine screening for an adolescent.
   D. **CORRECT:** Recommend that the adolescent have a weight screening annually.
   E. **CORRECT:** Recommend that the adolescent have a scoliosis screening annually.

   Ⓝ *NCLEX® Connection: Health Promotion and Maintenance, Health Promotion and Disease Prevention*

3. A. Sleep terrors occur most often in preschool-age children and do not contribute to the adolescent's need for additional sleep.
   B. **CORRECT:** Rapid growth during the adolescent years results in the need for additional sleep.
   C. Zinc levels do not typically elevate during the adolescent years, and do not contribute to the adolescent's need for additional sleep. Zinc is often identified as deficient due to inadequate dietary intake during adolescence.
   D. An increased metabolism contributes to the adolescent's need for additional sleep.

   Ⓝ *NCLEX® Connection: Health Promotion and Maintenance, Aging Process*

4. A. Pubic hair appears during early puberty, but is not the first manifestation of sexual maturation in males.
   B. Vocal changes occur after the appearance of pubic hair, typically in early to midpuberty, and are not the first manifestation of sexual maturation in males.
   C. **CORRECT:** Testicular enlargement is the first manifestation of sexual maturation in males.
   D. Facial hair growth typically appears about 2 years after pubic hair, and is not the first manifestation of sexual maturation in males.

   Ⓝ *NCLEX® Connection: Health Promotion and Maintenance, Developmental Stages and Transitions*

Active Learning Scenario

A nurse is assisting with preparing an educational program for a group of caregivers of adolescents. Use the ATI Active Learning Template: Growth and Development to complete this item.

DEVELOPMENTAL STAGE: Identify adolescent developmental stages according to Piaget and Erikson.

COGNITIVE DEVELOPMENT: List five cognitive developmental tasks the adolescent should accomplish.

INJURY PREVENTION: Identify three injury prevention methods in each of the following categories.

- Bodily harm
- Motor vehicle injuries

Active Learning Scenario Key

Using the ATI Active Learning Template: Growth and Development

DEVELOPMENTAL STAGE
- Piaget: formal operations
- Erikson: identity vs. role confusion

COGNITIVE DEVELOPMENT
- Able to think through more than two categories of variables concurrently
- Capable of evaluating the quality of own thinking
- Able to maintain attention for longer periods of time
- Highly imaginative and idealistic
- Increasingly capable of using formal logic to make decisions
- Think beyond current circumstances
- Understand how the actions of an individual influence others

INJURY PREVENTION
- Bodily injury
  - Keep firearms unloaded and in a locked cabinet or box.
  - Reinforce proper use of sporting equipment prior to use.
  - Insist on helmet use and/or pads when roller skating, skateboarding, bicycling, riding scooters, skiing, and snowboarding.
  - Be aware of changes in mood. Continuously monitor adolescents at risk for self-harm.
- Motor vehicle injuries
  - Encourage attendance at drivers' education courses.
  - Emphasize the need for adherence to seat belt use.
  - Discourage use of cell phones while driving and enforce laws regarding use.
  - Reinforce the dangers of combining substance use with driving.
- Role model desired behavior.

Ⓝ *NCLEX® Connection: Health Promotion and Maintenance, Aging Process s*

ⓝ NCLEX® Connections

When reviewing the following chapters, keep in mind the relevant topics and tasks of the NCLEX outline, in particular:

Health Promotion and Maintenance

AGING PROCESS: Provide care that meets the needs of the preschool, school-age, and adolescent client ages 3 through 17 years.

DEVELOPMENTAL STAGES AND TRANSITIONS
Identify occurrence of expected body image changes.

Compare client developmental milestones.

Modify approaches to care in accordance with client developmental stage.

HEALTH PROMOTION/DISEASE PREVENTION
Provide assistance for screening examinations.

Assist client in disease prevention activities.

Psychosocial Integrity

CULTURAL AWARENESS: Identify importance of client culture/ethnicity when planning/providing/monitoring care.

END-OF-LIFE CONCEPTS
Provide care or support for the client/family at end-of-life.

Provide end-of-life care and education to clients.

Basic Care and Comfort

NONPHARMACOLOGICAL COMFORT INTERVENTIONS
Assist in planning comfort interventions for client with impaired comfort.

Monitor client nonverbal signs of pain/discomfort.

Evaluate pain using standardized rating scales.

Pharmacological Therapies

EXPECTED ACTIONS/OUTCOMES: Apply knowledge of pathophysiology when addressing client pharmacological agents.

MEDICATION ADMINISTRATION
Identify client need for PRN medications.

Administer medication by oral route.

Administer a subcutaneous, intradermal, or intramuscular medication.

Administer medication by ear, eye, nose, inhalation, rectum, vagina, or skin route.

CHAPTER 8 **Safe Administration of Medication**

Growth and organ system maturity affect the metabolism and excretion of medications in infants and children.

Administration of medications to the pediatric population can be challenging, and requires nursing patience and creativity.

Pediatric dosages are based on age, body weight, and body surface area.

DATA COLLECTION

- Medication and food allergies
- Appropriateness of medication dose for the child's age and weight
- Child's developmental age
- Child's physiological and psychological condition
- Tissue and skin integrity when administering intramuscular (IM), subcutaneous, and topical medications
- IV patency when administering intravenous (IV) medications

NURSING INTERVENTIONS

MEDICATION ADMINISTRATION

- Calculate the safe dosage for medication. Qs
- Notify the provider if medication dosage is determined to be outside the safe dosage range and for any questions about medication preparation or route.
- Double-check high-alert and facility-regulated medications with another nurse.
- Use two client identifiers prior to administration: client name and date of birth. Use guardian(s) for verification of infants or nonverbal children. Two of the following identifiers from the ID band must be confirmed: client name, date of birth, or hospital identification number. Computers can also be used to scan the child's ID band for electronic record updating.
- Determine parental involvement with administration.
- Allow the child to make appropriate choices regarding administration (choosing the left or right leg, whether the guardian or nurse will administer the medication).
- Prepare the child according to age and developmental stage.

Oral

This route of medication administration is preferred for children. Available in preparations (liquids, chewables, and meltaways).
- Determine the child's ability to swallow pills.
- Use the smallest measuring device for doses of liquid medication. Use an oral medication syringe for smaller amounts, and a medication cup for larger amounts.
- Avoid measuring liquid medication in a teaspoon or tablespoon.
- Use rigid plastic cups instead of paper cups for liquid medications.
- Avoid mixing medication with formula or putting it in a bottle of formula because the infant might not take the entire feeding, and the medication can alter the taste of the formula.
- Hold the infant in a semi-reclining position similar to a feeding position.
- Hold the small child in an upright position to prevent aspiration.
- Administer the medication in the side of the mouth in small amounts. This allows the infant or child to swallow.
- Only use the droppers that come with the medication for measurement.
- Stroke the infant under the chin to promote swallowing while holding cheeks together.
- Reinforce teaching with the child to swallow tablets that aren't available in liquid form and can't be crushed. Instruct in short sessions using verbal instruction, demonstration, and positive reinforcement.
- Provide atraumatic care.
  ○ Mix the medication in a small amount of sweet nonessential food (applesauce or sherbet).
  ○ Offer juice, a soft drink, or snack after administration.
  ○ Add flavoring to medications as available.
  ○ Use a nipple to allow the infant to suck the medication.
  ○ Reward small child with a prize or sticker afterwards.
- Administer medications via a feeding tube.
  ○ Confirm placement.
  ○ Use liquid formulation.
  ○ Do not add medication to the formula bag.
  ○ If administering several medications, flush tubing with water after the administration of each medication to clear tubing of residual medication.

Optic

- Place the child in a supine or sitting position.
- Extend the child's head and ask the child to look up.
- Pull the lower eye lid downward and apply medication in the conjunctiva pocket.
- Administer ointments from the inner to outer canthus of the eye preferably before nap or bedtime.
- Provide atraumatic care.
  ○ If infants clench their eyes closed, place the drops in the nasal corner. When the infant opens their eyes, the medication will enter the eye.
  ○ Apply light pressure to the lacrimal conjunctiva of the eye for 1 min to prevent unpleasant taste.
  ○ Play games with younger children.

Otic

- Place the child in a prone or supine position with the affected ear upward.
- Children younger than 3 years: pull the pinna downward and straight back.
- Children older than 3 years: pull the pinna upward and back.
- Provide atraumatic care.
  - Allow refrigerated medications to warm to room temperature prior to administration.
  - Massage the outer area for a few minutes following administration.
  - Play games with younger children.
  - Praise child after procedure.

Nasal

- Remove mucus prior to administration.
- Position the child with the head hyperextended.
- Use a football hold position for infants.
- Provide atraumatic care.
  - Insert the tip into the naris vertically, then angle it prior to administration.
  - Play games with younger children.

Aerosol

- Use a mask for younger children.
- Provide atraumatic care.
  - Allow guardians to hold the child during treatment.
  - Use distraction.

Rectal

- Provide lubrication to the medication by using warm water or other lubricant, if the medication is not pre-lubricated.
- Insert beyond both rectal sphincters (small child less than 0.5 inches, older child 1 inch).
- Hold the buttocks gently together for 5 to 10 min.
- If necessary to half the dose, cut the medication lengthwise.
- Provide atraumatic care.
  - Perform the procedure quickly.
  - Use distraction.

Transdermal/topical

- Ensure the skin is dry and intact.
- Apply to the body or major muscle (try to hide from smaller children).
- Monitor skin site of administration regularly.
- Rotate sites frequently.

Injection

- Change needle if it pierced a rubber stopper on a vial.
- Secure the infant or child prior to injections.
- Determine the need for assistance.
- Avoid tracking of medication.
- When selecting sites, consider the following.
  - Medication amount, viscosity, and type
  - Muscle mass, condition, access of site, and potential for contamination
  - Treatment course and number of injections
  - Age and size of child

Intradermal

- Administer on the inside surface of the forearm.
- Use a TB syringe with 26- to 30-gauge needle with an intradermal bevel.
- Insert needle at 15° angle.
- Do not aspirate.

Subcutaneous

Give anywhere there is adequate subcutaneous tissue. Common sites are the lateral aspect of the upper arm, abdomen, and anterior thigh.
- Inject volumes of less than 0.5 mL.
- Use a 1 mL syringe with a 26- to 30-gauge needle.
- Insert at a 90° angle. Use a 45° angle for children who are thin.
- Check policy for aspiration practices.

Intramuscular

- Use a 22- to 25-gauge, ½- to 1-inch needle.

Vastus lateralis
- This is the recommended site in infants and small children.
- Position the child supine, side-lying, or sitting.
- Inject up to 0.5 mL for infants.
- Inject up to 2 mL for children.

Ventrogluteal
- Position the child supine, side-lying, or prone.
- Inject 0.5 to 1 mL, depending on muscle size of infant.
- Inject up to 2 mL in children.

Deltoid
- Explain the procedure to the child and guardians.
- Position the child sitting or standing.
- Inject up to 1 mL.
- Provide atraumatic care.
  - Apply lidocaine and prilocaine topical ointment to the site for 60 min prior to injection.
  - Change needle after puncturing a rubber stopper.
  - Use the smallest gauge of needle possible. Q︎PCC
  - Use therapeutic hugging.
  - Secure the child firmly to decrease movement of the needle while injecting.
  - Use distraction.
  - Encourage guardians to hold the child after.
  - Offer praise.
  - Use play therapy.
  - Offer sucrose pacifiers to infants.

Intravenous

Monitor venipuncture site per facility protocol and prior to administration of medications.

Peripheral venous access devices (also called intermittent infusion devices, peripheral/saline/heparin locks)
- Use a 24- to 22-gauge catheter.
- Use for continuous and intermittent IV medication administration.
- Short-term IV therapy can be completed at home with the assistance of a home health nurse.

Central venous access devices (CVADS)
- Short term: non-tunneled catheter or peripherally-inserted central catheters (PICC) require an x-ray to verify placement prior to use.
- Long term: tunneled catheter or implanted infusion ports.
- Provide atraumatic care.
  - Insert a PICC before multiple peripheral attempts.
  - Use a transilluminator to assist in vein location.
  - Avoid terminology such as a "bee sting" or "stick".
  - Attach an extension tubing to decrease movement of the catheter.
  - Use play therapy.
  - Apply lidocaine and prilocaine topical ointment to the site for 60 min prior to attempt.
  - Keep equipment out of site until procedure begins.
  - Perform procedure in a treatment room. Q̶PCC
  - Use nonpharmacological therapies.
  - Allow guardians to stay if they prefer.
  - Use therapeutic holding.
  - Avoid using the dominant or sucking hand.
  - Cover site with a protective cover that allows visibility of the IV site.
  - Swaddle infants.
  - Offer nonnutritive sucking to infants before, during, and after the procedure.
  - Reinforce with guardians how to properly care for device.

Intraosseous

- A temporary route of administration for use in an emergent situation in which venous access cannot be obtained.
- Use an intraosseous or large bore needle that is inserted into the tibia.
- Monitor site for infection, leakage of fluid.
- Monitor distal pulses, temperature of leg, and color frequently.
- Risk for compartment syndrome.

Application Exercises

1. A nurse is planning to administer the influenza vaccine to a toddler. Which of the following actions should the nurse take?
   - A. Administer subcutaneously in the abdomen.
   - B. Use a 20-gauge needle.
   - C. Divide the medication into two injections.
   - D. Place the child in the supine position.

2. A nurse is preparing to administer an intramuscular (IM) injection to a child. Which of the following muscle groups is contraindicated?
   - A. Deltoid
   - B. Ventrogluteal
   - C. Vastus lateralis
   - D. Dorsogluteal

3. A nurse is reinforcing teaching with the guardian of an infant about administration of oral medications. Which of the following should the nurse include in the teaching? (Select all that apply.)
   - A. Use a universal dropper for medication administration.
   - B. Ask the pharmacy to add flavoring to the medication.
   - C. Add the medication to a formula bottle before feeding.
   - D. Use the nipple of a bottle to administer the medication.
   - E. Hold the infant in an semi-reclining position.

4. A nurse is preparing to administer medication to a toddler. Which of the following actions should the nurse take? (Select all that apply.)
   - A. Identify the toddler by asking the caregiver.
   - B. Tell the caregiver to administer the medication.
   - C. Calculate the safe dosage.
   - D. Ask the toddler to pick a toy to hold during administration.
   - E. Offer juice after the medication.

5. A nurse is caring for an infant who needs otic medication. Which of the following is an appropriate action for the nurse to take?
   - A. Hold the infant in an upright position.
   - B. Pull the pinna downward and straight back.
   - C. Hyperextend the infant's neck.
   - D. Ensure that the medication is cool.

Application Exercises Key

1. A. The influenza vaccination is administered IM.
   B. A 22- to 25-gauge needle is recommended for IM injections.
   C. The total volume of the influenza vaccination is 0.5 mL, which can be administered in the vastus lateralis.
   D. **CORRECT:** The vastus lateralis is recommended for administering IM medications. Placing the toddler in a supine position is the appropriate action for the nurse to take.

   Ⓝ *NCLEX® Connection: Pharmacological Therapies, Medication Administration*

2. A. The deltoid muscle can be used once developed for IM injections in children for medication containing up to 1 mL fluid.
   B. The ventrogluteal muscle can be used for IM injections in children for medication containing up to 2 mL fluid.
   C. The vastus lateralis muscle can be used for intramuscular injections in children for medication containing up to 2 mL fluid.
   D. **CORRECT:** The dorsogluteal site has major nerves and blood vessels and is not a recommended site for IM injections for children.

   Ⓝ *NCLEX® Connection: Pharmacological Therapies, Medication Administration*

3. A. Medication has different viscosities, and droppers do not have a standard opening. A universal dropper is not an accurate way to measure medications.
   B. **CORRECT:** Multiple flavorings are available to add to medications and can assist in masking the taste.
   C. Because an infant might not finish an entire bottle of formula, it is not recommended to add medication to the bottle.
   D. **CORRECT:** Administering medications through an empty nipple can assist with successful administration of the medication.
   E. **CORRECT:** For successful medication administration, the infant should be held in a semireclining position, similar to feeding.

   Ⓝ *NCLEX® Connection: Pharmacological Therapies, Medication Administration*

4. A. For safe medication administration, confirm two identifiers by looking at the identification band or having the toddler state their name and date of birth.
   B. Determine the preferred level of involvement of the caregivers prior to medication administration.
   C. **CORRECT:** For safe medication administration, calculate safe dosage prior to administering medication.
   D. **CORRECT:** Offering choices to the toddler is an example of atraumatic care.
   E. **CORRECT:** Offering juice after the medication is an example of atraumatic care.

   Ⓝ *NCLEX® Connection: Pharmacological Therapies, Medication Administration*

5. A. Position the infant supine or prone for administration of otic medication.
   B. **CORRECT:** Pulling the pinna downward and straight back will straighten the ear canal to allow medication to flow into the ear.
   C. Hyperextending the infant's neck could occlude the airway and should not be performed during otic medication administration.
   D. Allowing the otic medication to warm up to room temperature is recommended to provide atraumatic care.

   Ⓝ *NCLEX® Connection: Pharmacological Therapies, Medication Administration*

Active Learning Scenario

A nurse is assisting with initiating IV access for a toddler. What actions should the nurse plan to take? Use the ATI Active Learning Template: Basic Concept to complete this item.

NURSING INTERVENTIONS: Describe 10 atraumatic care interventions.

Active Learning Scenario Key

Using the ATI Active Learning Template: Basic Concept

NURSING INTERVENTIONS

- Decide to insert a peripherally inserted catheter before multiple peripheral attempts.
- Use a transilluminator to assist in vein location.
- Avoid terminology such as a "bee sting" or "stick."
- Attach extension tubing to decrease movement of the catheter.
- Use play therapy.
- Apply lidocaine and prilocaine topical ointment to the site for 60 min prior to attempts.
- Keep equipment out of sight until procedure begins.
- Perform the procedure in a treatment room.
- Use nonpharmacologic therapies.
- Allow caregivers to stay if they prefer.
- Use therapeutic holding.
- Avoid using the dominant or sucking hand.
- Cover site with a colorful wrap.
- Swaddle infants.
- Offer nonnutritive sucking to infants before, during, and after the procedure.

Ⓝ *NCLEX® Connection: Basic Care and Comfort, Non–Pharmacological Comfort Interventions*

CHAPTER 9 *Pain Management*

Determination of pain depends on the child's cognitive, emotional, and physical development.

Atraumatic care is the use of interventions that minimize or eliminate physical and psychological distress. Pain is managed by atraumatic, nonpharmacological, and pharmacological interventions.

INFLUENTIAL FACTORS

Influential factors that can have a positive or negative effect on pain perception
- Age
- Development stage
- Chronic or acute disease
- Prior experiences with pain
- Personality
- Family dynamics
- Culture
- Socioeconomic status

DATA COLLECTION

EXPECTED FINDINGS

Developmental characteristics

Young infant
- Loud cry
- Rigid body or thrashing
- Local reflex withdrawal from pain stimulus
- Expressions of pain (eyes tightly closed, mouth open in a squarish shape, eyebrows lowered and drawn together)
- Lack of association between stimulus and pain

Older infant
- Loud cry
- Deliberate withdrawal from pain
- Facial expression of pain

Toddler
- Loud cry or screaming
- Verbal expressions of pain
- Thrashing of extremities
- Attempt to push away or avoid stimulus
- Noncooperation
- Clinging to a significant person
- Behaviors occur in anticipation of painful stimulus
- Requests physical comfort

School-age child
- Stalling behavior
- Muscular rigidity
- Any behaviors of the toddler, but less intense in the anticipatory phase and more intense with painful stimulus

Adolescent
- More verbal expressions of pain with less protest
- Muscle tension with body control

Pain intensity (9.1)

- Data collection includes behavioral measures, multidimensional, and self-report.
- Self-report is used for children 4 years or older. Children under 4 are unable to accurately report their pain.
- Multiple tools have been developed and researched as reliable.
- Choose an appropriate pain tool that will adequately evaluate the infant or child's pain.
- Include the caregiver in rating the child's pain.
- Determine the location, quality, and severity of pain.

PATIENT-CENTERED CARE

NURSING CARE

- Recheck the child's pain level frequently.
- Use nonpharmacological, pharmacological, or both approaches to manage pain.
- Ask parent or caregiver to monitor their child's pain level.
- Ask the parent or caregiver their satisfaction of the pain management.
- Monitor the child for adverse reactions to pain medications.
- Review laboratory reports.
- Monitor the child's physical functioning following pain management intervention.
- Monitor for negative effects or distress the child might experience related to pain (anxiety, withdrawal, sleep disruption, fear, depression, or unhappiness).

ATRAUMATIC MEASURES

- Use a treatment room for painful procedures.
- Avoid procedures in "safe places" (the play room or the child's bed).
- Use developmentally appropriate terminology when explaining procedures.
- Offer choices to the child.
- Allow parents to stay with the child during painful procedures.
- Use play therapy to explain procedures, allowing the child to perform the procedure on a doll or toy.

PHARMACOLOGICAL MEASURES

- The World Health Organization (2012) recommends a two-step approach for pharmacological management of pain in children.
  - For children above 3 months of age with mild pain, the first step is to administer a non-opioid. Nonsteroidal anti-inflammatory drugs (NSAIDs) are frequently used for mild pain.
  - The second step for children who have moderate or severe pain is to administer a strong opioid. Morphine is the drug of choice.
- Optimal dosage of medications control pain without causing severe adverse effects.
- Select the least traumatic route for medication administration.
- Give medications routinely, vs. PRN (as needed), to manage pain that is expected to last for an extended period of time.
- Combine adjuvant medications (steroids, antidepressants, sedatives, antianxiety medications, muscle relaxants, anticonvulsants) with other analgesics.

- Use non-opioid and opioid medications.
  - Acetaminophen and NSAIDs are acceptable for mild to moderate pain.
  - Opioids are acceptable for moderate to severe pain. Medications used include morphine sulfate, hydromorphone, and fentanyl.
  - Combining a non-opioid and an opioid medication treats pain peripherally and centrally. This offers greater analgesia with fewer adverse effects (respiratory depression, constipation, nausea).

APPROPRIATE ROUTES Qs

- IM injections are not recommended for pain control in children.
- Intranasal medications are not recommended for children younger than 18 years.
- Intradermal medications are used for skin anesthesia prior to procedures.

Oral

NURSING ACTIONS

- Route is preferred due to convenience, cost, and ability to maintain steady blood levels.
- Take 1 to 2 hr to reach peak analgesic effects. Oral medications are not suited for children experiencing pain that requires rapid relief or pain that is fluctuating in nature.

9.1 Pain data collection tool for evaluation by age

FLACC: 2 months to 7 years
Pain rated on a scale of 0 to 10.
Observe behaviors of the child.

FACE (F)
LEGS (L)
ACTIVITY (A)
CRY (C)
CONSOLABILITY (C)

Numeric scale: 5 years and older
Pain rated on a scale of 0 to 10.
Explain to the child that 0 means "no pain" and 10 means "worst pain."
Have the child verbally report a number or point to their level of pain on a visual scale.

FACES: 3 years and older
Pain rated on a scale of 0 to 5 using a diagram of six faces.
Substitute 0, 2, 4, 6, 8, 10 for 0 to 5 to convert to the 0 to 10 scale.
Explain each face to the child; ask the child to choose a face that best describes how they are feeling.

0: No hurt	2: Hurts a little more	4: Hurts a whole lot
1: Hurts a bit	3: Hurts even more	5: Hurts worst

Oucher: 3 to 13 years
Pain rated on a scale of 0 to 5 using six photographs.
Substitute 0, 2, 4, 6, 8, 10 for 0 to 5 to convert to the 0 to 10 scale.
Have the child organize the photographs in order of no pain to the worst pain; ask the child to choose a picture that best describes how they are feeling.

0: No hurt	2: Hurts a little more	4: Hurts a whole lot
1: Hurts a bit	3: Hurts even more	5: Hurts worst

AGE: 0   3   5   7   10   13   15   18

FLACC
FACES
OUCHER
NUMERIC SCALE

Topical/transdermal

NURSING ACTIONS

Lidocaine and prilocaine is available in a cream or gel.

- Used for any procedure in which the skin will be punctured (IV insertion, biopsy) 60 min prior to a superficial puncture.
- Place an occlusive dressing over the cream after application.
- Prior to procedure, remove the dressing and clean the skin. Indication of an adequate response is reddened or blanched skin.
- Demonstrate to the child that the skin is not sensitive by tapping or scratching lightly.
- Reinforce to parents to apply medication at home prior to the procedure.

Fentanyl PATCH

- Use for children older than 12 years of age.
- Use to provide continuous pain control. Onset of 12 to 24 hr and a duration of 72 hr.
- Use an immediate-release opioid for breakthrough pain.
- Treat respiratory depression with naloxone.

Intravenous

NURSING ACTIONS

Bolus

- Rapid pain control in approximately 5 min
- Use for medications (morphine, hydromorphone)
- Continuous: provides steady blood levels

Patient-controlled analgesia (PCA)

- Self-administration of pain medication
- Can be basal, bolus, or combination
- Has lockouts to prevent overdosing

Family-controlled analgesia

- Same concept as PCA
- Parent or caregiver manages the child's pain

NONPHARMACOLOGICAL MEASURES Qpcc

Distraction
- Use play, radio, a computer game, or a movie.
- Tell jokes or a story to the child.

Relaxation
- Hold or rock the infant or young child.
- Assist older children into a comfortable position.
- Assist with breathing techniques.

Guided imagery
- Assist the child in an imaginary experience.
- Have the child describe the details.

Positive self-talk: Have the child say positive things during a procedure or painful episode.

Behavioral contracting
- Use stickers or tokens as rewards.
- Give time limits for the child to cooperate.
- Reinforce cooperation with a reward.

Containment
- Swaddle the infant.
- Place rolled blankets around the child.
- Maintain proper positioning.

Nonnutritive sucking
- Offer pacifier with sucrose before, during, and after painful procedures.
- Offer nonnutritive sucking during episodes of pain.

Kangaroo care: skin-to-skin contact between infants and parents

Complementary and alternative medicine
- Offer foods, vitamins, or supplements.
- Offer massage or chiropractic options.
- Review energy-based treatments (magnets).
- Discuss mind-body techniques (hypnosis, homeopathy, or naturopathy).

COMPLICATIONS

Opioid adverse effects
- Administer stool softeners for constipation.
- Monitor child for respiratory depression and sedation.

Application Exercises

1. A nurse is collecting data from an infant about pain. Which of the following pain scales should the nurse use?

   A. FACES

   B. FLACC

   C. Oucher

   D. Numeric scale

2. A nurse is contributing to the plan of care for a child following a surgical procedure. Which of the following interventions should the nurse include in the plan of care?

   A. Administer NSAIDs for pain greater than 7 on a scale of 0 to 10.

   B. Administer intranasal analgesics PRN.

   C. Administer IM analgesics for pain.

   D. Administer IV analgesics on a schedule.

3. A nurse is collecting data from an infant. Which of the following are findings of pain in an infant? (Select all that apply.)

   A. Pursed lips

   B. Loud cry

   C. Lowered eyebrows

   D. Rigid body

   E. Pushes away stimulus

4. A nurse is contributing to the plan of care for an infant who is experiencing pain. Which of the following interventions should the nurse include the plan of care? (Select all that apply.)

   A. Offer a pacifier.

   B. Use guided imagery.

   C. Use swaddling.

   D. Initiate a behavioral contract.

   E. Encourage kangaroo care.

5. A nurse is assisting with preparing a toddler for an intravenous catheter insertion using atraumatic care. Which of the following actions should the nurse take? (Select all that apply.)

   A. Reinforce the procedure using the child's favorite toy.

   B. Ask the guardians to leave during the procedure.

   C. Assist with performing the procedure with the child in his bed.

   D. Allow the child to make one choice regarding the procedure.

   E. Apply lidocaine and prilocaine cream to three potential insertion sites.

Active Learning Scenario

A nurse is reviewing pain evaluation tools with a group of newly licensed nurses. What should the nurse include in the discussion? Use the ATI Active Learning Template: Basic Concept to complete this item.

DESCRIPTION OF SKILL: Describe four pain tools used with pediatric clients.

Application Exercises Key

1. A. The FACES pain evaluation scale is recommended for children 3 years or older.
   B. **CORRECT:** The FLACC pain evaluation scale is recommended for infants and children between 2 months and 7 years of age.
   C. The Oucher pain evaluation scale is recommended for children between the ages of 3 and 13 years.
   D. The Numeric pain evaluation scale is recommended for children 5 years or older.

   Ⓝ *NCLEX® Connection: Pharmacological Therapies, Pharmacological Pain Management*

2. A. NSAIDs are used for mild to moderate pain.
   B. Intranasal analgesics are used for clients older than 18 years.
   C. IM analgesics are not recommended for pain management in children.
   D. **CORRECT:** IV analgesics should be administered on a schedule to achieve optimal pain management.

   Ⓝ *NCLEX® Connection: Pharmacological Therapies, Pharmacological Pain Management*

3. A. Infants who experience pain have their mouth open in a squarish shape.
   B. **CORRECT:** Infants who experience pain exhibit a loud cry.
   C. **CORRECT:** Infants who experience pain lower and draw together their eyebrows.
   D. **CORRECT:** Infants who experience pain exhibit a rigid body.
   E. Infants who experience pain exhibit a local reflex to withdraw from the stimulus.

   Ⓝ *NCLEX® Connection: Pharmacological Therapies, Pharmacological Pain Management*

4. A. **CORRECT:** Nonnutritive sucking is a therapeutic nonpharmacological strategy for pain management with infants.
   B. Guided imagery is a nonpharmacological strategy used with children.
   C. **CORRECT:** Swaddling the infant is a therapeutic nonpharmacological strategy for pain management.
   D. Behavioral contracts are a nonpharmacological strategy used with children.
   E. **CORRECT:** Skin-to-skin touch is a relaxation technique and should be encouraged for infants who have pain.

   Ⓝ *NCLEX® Connection: Basic Care and Comfort, Non-Pharmacological Comfort Interventions*

5. A. **CORRECT:** Explaining the procedure using the child's favorite toy can assist the child to manage fears and provides atraumatic care.
   B. The guardians should be allowed to remain for procedures to offer comfort to the child.
   C. Safe places (the child's bed) should be avoided.
   D. **CORRECT:** Allowing the child to make choices offers a sense of control over the situation and should be used to provide atraumatic care.
   E. **CORRECT:** A topical analgesic (lidocaine and prilocaine cream) decreases pain and should be used to provide atraumatic care.

   Ⓝ *NCLEX® Connection: Basic Care and Comfort, Non-Pharmacological Comfort Interventions*

Active Learning Scenario Key

Using the ATI Active Learning Template: Basic Concept

DESCRIPTION OF SKILL

FLACC (2 months to 7 years)
- Pain rated on a scale of 0 to 10.
- Observe behaviors of the child.
- Face (F)
- Legs (L)
- Activity (A)
- Cry (C)
- Consolability (C)

FACES (3 years and older)
- Pain rated on a scale of 0 to 5 using a diagram of six faces.
- Substitute 0, 2, 4, 6, 8, 10 for 0 to 5 to convert to the 0 to 10 scale.
- Explain each face to the child.
  - 0: No hurt
  - 1: Hurts a bit
  - 2: Hurts a little more
  - 3: Hurts even more
  - 4: Hurts a whole lot
  - 5: Hurts worst
- Ask the child to choose a face that best describes how they are feeling

Oucher (3 to 13 years)
- Pain rated on a scale of 0 to 5 using six photographs.
- Substitute 0, 2, 4, 6, 8, 10 for 0 to 5 to convert to the 0 to 10 scale.
- Have the child organize the photographs in order of no pain to the worst pain.
  - 0: No hurt
  - 1: Hurts a bit
  - 2: Hurts a little more
  - 3: Hurts even more
  - 4: Hurts a whole lot
  - 5: Hurts worst
- Ask the child to choose a picture that best describes how they are feeling.

Numeric scale (5 years and older)
- Pain rated on a scale of 0 to 10.
- Explain to the child that 0 means "no pain" and 10 means "worst pain."
- Have the child verbally report a number or point on a visual scale their pain level.

Ⓝ *NCLEX® Connection: Basic Care and Comfort*

UNIT 1   FOUNDATIONS OF NURSING CARE OF CHILDREN
SECTION: SPECIFIC CONSIDERATIONS OF
NURSING CARE OF CHILDREN

CHAPTER 10 *Hospitalization, Illness, and Play*

A nurse is likely to encounter children who are ill or hospitalized. When caring for these children, it is important for the nurse to understand how these events can affect the child and incorporate interventions to help the child cope.

Hospitalization and illness

- Families and children can experience major stress related to hospitalization. The nurse should monitor for evidence of stress and intervene as appropriate.
- Families should be considered clients when children are ill.
- Separation anxiety during hospitalization manifests in three behavioral responses.
  ○ **Protest:** screaming, clinging to parents, verbal and physical aggression toward strangers
  ○ **Despair:** withdrawal from others, depression, decreased communication, developmental regression
  ○ **Detachment:** interacting with strangers, forming new relationships, happy appearance
- Each child's understanding of illnesses and hospitalization is dependent on the child's stage of development and cognitive ability.

IMPACT BASED ON DEVELOPMENT

Infant

LEVEL OF UNDERSTANDING
- Inability to describe illness and follow directions
- Lack of understanding of the need of therapeutic procedures

IMPACT OF HOSPITALIZATION
- Experiences stranger anxiety between 6 to 8 months of age
- Displays physical behaviors as expressions of discomfort due to inability to verbalize
- Can experience sleep deprivation due to strange noises, monitoring devices, and procedures
- Can experience anxiety due to the unfamiliar environment and fear of the unknown

Toddler

LEVEL OF UNDERSTANDING
- Limited ability to describe illness
- Poorly developed sense of body image and boundaries
- Limited understanding of the need for therapeutic procedures
- Limited ability to follow directions

IMPACT OF HOSPITALIZATION
- Experiences separation anxiety
- Can exhibit an intense reaction to any type of procedure due to the intrusion of boundaries
- Behavior can regress

Preschooler

LEVEL OF UNDERSTANDING
- Limited understanding of the cause of illness but knows what illness feels like
- Limited ability to describe manifestations
- Fears related to magical thinking
- Ability to understand cause and effect inhibited by concrete thinking

IMPACT OF HOSPITALIZATION
- Can experience separation anxiety
- Can harbor fears of bodily harm
- Might believe illness and hospitalization are a punishment

School-age child

LEVEL OF UNDERSTANDING
- Beginning awareness of body functioning
- Ability to describe pain
- Increasing ability to understand cause and effect

IMPACT OF HOSPITALIZATION
- Fears loss of control
- Seeks information as a way to maintain a sense of control
- Can sense when not being told the truth
- Can experience stress related to separation from peers and regular routine

Adolescent

LEVEL OF UNDERSTANDING
- Increasing ability to understand cause and effect
- Perceptions of illness severity are based on the degree of body image changes

IMPACT OF HOSPITALIZATION
- Develops body image disturbance
- Attempts to maintain composure but is embarrassed about losing control
- Experiences feelings of isolation from peers
- Worries about outcome and impact on school/activities
- Might not adhere to treatments/medication regimen due to peer influence

Family responses

- Fear and guilt regarding not bringing the child in for care earlier
- Frustration due to the perceived inability to care for the child
- Altered family roles
- Worry regarding finances if work is missed
- Worry regarding care of other children within the household
- Fear related to lack of knowledge regarding illness or treatments
- Siblings experiencing loneliness, jealousy, guilt, fear, or anger
- Caregiver role strain, related to the impact of hospitalization on family processes

DATA COLLECTION

- Child's and family's understanding of the illness or the reason for hospitalization
- Stressors unique to the child and family (needs of other children in the family, socioeconomic situation, health of other extended family members)
- Past experiences with hospitalization and illness
- Developmental level and needs of child/family
- Parenting role and the family's perception of role changes
- Support available to the child/family
- Coping strategies for periods of crisis

NURSING INTERVENTIONS

- Reinforce with the child and family about what to expect during hospitalization. ◯PCC
- Encourage family members to stay with the child during the hospital experience to reduce the stress.
- Maintain routine as much as possible.
- Encourage independence and choices.
- Explain treatments, procedures, and cares to the child.
- Provide developmentally appropriate activities.

Infants

- Place infants whose parents are not in attendance close to nurses' stations so that their needs can be quickly met.
- Provide consistency in assigning caregivers.

Toddlers

- Encourage parents to provide routine care for the child (changing diapers and feeding).
- Encourage the child's autonomy by offering appropriate choices.
- Provide consistency in assigning caregivers.

Preschoolers

- Explain procedures using simple, clear language. Avoid medical jargon and terms that can be misinterpreted.
- Encourage independence by letting the child provide self-care.
- Encourage the child to express feelings.

- Validate the child's fears and concerns.
- Provide toys that allow for emotional expression (a pounding board to release feelings of protest).
- Provide consistency in assigning caregivers.
- Give choices when possible ("Do you want your medicine in a cup or a spoon?").
- Allow younger children to handle equipment if it is safe.

School-age children

- Provide factual information.
- Encourage the child to express feelings.
- Try to maintain a normal routine for long hospitalizations, including time for school work.
- Encourage contact with peer group.

Adolescents

- Provide factual information.
- Include the adolescent in the planning of care to relieve feelings of powerlessness and lack of control.
- Encourage contact with peer group.

Play

- Allows children to express feelings and fears.
- Facilitates mastery of developmental stages and assists in the development of problem solving abilities.
- Allows children to learn socially acceptable behaviors.
- Activities should be specific to each child's stage of development.
- Can be used to teach children.
- A means of protection from everyday stressors.

CONTENT OF PLAY

Social affective: taking pleasure in relationships

Sense-pleasure: objects in the environment catching the child's attention

Skill: demonstrating new abilities

Unoccupied behavior: focusing attention on something of interest

Dramatic: pretending and fantasizing ◯EBP

Games: imitative, formal, or competitive

SOCIAL CHARACTER OF PLAY

Onlooker: the child observing others

Solitary: the child playing alone

Parallel: children playing independently but among other children, which is characteristic of toddlers

Associative: children playing together without organization, which is characteristic of preschoolers

Team play: organized playing in groups, which is characteristic of school-age children

FUNCTIONS OF PLAY

Play helps in the development of various types of skills.
- Intellectual
- Sensorimotor
- Social
- Self-awareness
- Creativity
- Therapeutic and moral values

PLAY ACTIVITIES RELATED TO AGE

Infants
- Birth to 3 months: colorful moving mobiles, music/sound boxes
- 3 to 6 months: noise-making objects, soft toys
- 6 to 9 months: teething toys, social interaction
- 9 to 12 months: large blocks, toys that pop apart, push-and-pull toys

Toddlers
- Cloth books, puzzles with large pieces
- Large crayons and paper
- Push-and-pull toys, balls
- Tricycles
- Educational and child-appropriate shows and videos

Preschoolers
- Imitative and imaginative play
- Drawing, painting, riding a tricycle, jumping, running
- Educational and child-appropriate shows and videos

School-age children
- Games that can be played alone or with another person
- Team sports
- Musical instruments
- Arts and crafts
- Collections

Adolescents
- Team sports
- School activities
- Reading, listening to music
- Peer interactions

THERAPEUTIC PLAY

- Makes use of dolls and/or stuffed animals
- Encourages the acting out of feelings of fear, anger, hostility, and sadness
- Enables the child to learn coping strategies in a safe environment
- Assists in gaining cooperation for medical treatment

DATA COLLECTION

- Developmental level of the child
- Motor skills
- Level of activity tolerance
- Child's preferences

NURSING INTERVENTIONS

- Select toys that are safe for the child.
- Consider isolation precautions and the child's illness in relation to toy selection.
- Select activities that enhance development.
- Observe the child's play for clues to the child's fears or anxieties.
- Encourage parents to bring one favorite toy from home.
- Use dolls or stuffed animals to demonstrate a procedure before it is performed.
- Provide play opportunities that meet the child's level of activity tolerance.
- Allow the child to go to the play room if able.
- Encourage the adolescent's peers to visit.
- Involve a child life specialist in planning activities.

Application Exercises

1. A nurse is caring for a preschooler. Which of the following is an expected behavior of a preschool-age child?
   - A. Describing manifestations of illness
   - B. Relating fears to magical thinking
   - C. Understanding cause of illness
   - D. Awareness of body functioning

2. A nurse on a pediatric unit is caring for a toddler. Which of the following behaviors is an effect of hospitalization? (Select all that apply.)
   - A. Believes the experience is a punishment
   - B. Experiences separation anxiety
   - C. Displays intense emotions
   - D. Exhibits regressive behaviors
   - E. Manifests disturbance in body image

3. A nurse is reinforcing teaching with a guardian about parallel play in children. Which of the following statements should the nurse include?
   - A. "Children sit and observe others playing."
   - B. "Children exhibit organized play when in a group."
   - C. "The child plays alone."
   - D. "The child plays independently when in a group."

4. A nurse is reinforcing teaching with a group of caregivers about separation anxiety. Which of the following information should the nurse include?
   - A. It is often observed in the school-age child.
   - B. Detachment is the stage exhibited in the hospital.
   - C. It results in prolonged issues of adaptability.
   - D. Kicking a stranger is an example.

Application Exercises Key

1. A. Preschool-age children have limited ability to describe manifestations of illness.
   B. **CORRECT:** Preschool-age children are egocentric and relate fears to magical thinking.
   C. Preschool-age children have limited understanding of cause-and-effect relationship, but understand what illness feels like.
   D. Awareness of body functioning is a behavior of an adolescent.

   Ⓝ *NCLEX® Connection: Health Promotion and Maintenance, Developmental Stages and Transitions*

2. A. Preschool children believe hospitalization is a punishment.
   B. **CORRECT:** Separation anxiety is a potential effect of hospitalization in a toddler.
   C. **CORRECT:** Intense emotions are a potential effect of hospitalization in a toddler.
   D. **CORRECT:** Behavior regression is a potential effect of hospitalization in a toddler.
   E. Body image disturbances can be seen in adolescents who are hospitalized.

   Ⓝ *NCLEX® Connection: Health Promotion and Maintenance, Developmental Stages and Transitions*

3. A. Onlooker play is when a child sits and observes others playing.
   B. Team play is when a child exhibits organized play in a group.
   C. Solitary play is when a child plays alone.
   D. **CORRECT:** Parallel play is when the toddler plays independently but is among other children in a group.

   Ⓝ *NCLEX® Connection: Health Promotion and Maintenance, Aging Process*

4. A. Separation anxiety is commonly observed in the toddler.
   B. The detachment stage is rarely seen in the hospital setting.
   C. Children are adaptable and permanent issues are rare.
   D. **CORRECT:** Physical aggression toward strangers is a behavior seen in the protest stage of separation anxiety.

   Ⓝ *NCLEX® Connection: Health Promotion and Maintenance, Aging Process*

Active Learning Scenario

A nurse working in a pediatric unit is assisting planning play activities for a group of children of different ages. What activities should the nurse recommend? Use the ATI Active Learning Template: Basic Concept to complete this item.

RELATED CONTENT: Identify appropriate toys and activities for children in three age groups.

Active Learning Scenario Key

Using the ATI Active Learning Template: Basic Concept
RELATED CONTENT

Infants
- Birth to 3 months: colorful moving mobiles, music/sound boxes
- 3 to 6 months: noise-making objects, soft toys
- 6 to 9 months: teething toys, social interaction
- 9 to 12 months: large blocks, toys that pop apart, push-and-pull toys

Toddlers
- Cloth books
- Large crayons and paper
- Push-and-pull toys
- Tricycles
- Balls
- Puzzles with large pieces
- Educational and child-appropriate shows and videos

Preschoolers
- Imitative and imaginative play
- Drawing, painting, riding a tricycle, swimming, jumping, running
- Educational and child-appropriate shows and videos

School-age children
- Games that can be played alone or with another person
- Team sports
- Musical instruments
- Arts and crafts
- Collections

Adolescents
- Team sports
- School activities
- Reading, listening to music
- Peer interactions

Ⓝ *NCLEX® Connection: Health Promotion and Maintenance, Developmental Stages and Transitions*

CHAPTER 11 # Death and Dying

A nurse must meet the physical, psychological, spiritual, and emotional needs of a client and the family during illness and at the time of death.

Palliative care is a interprofessional approach that focuses on the improving quality of life rather than prolonging life when cures are not possible. Focus is on control of managing the client's manifestations and offering supportive care.

Hospice care specializes in the care of a client who is dying. Family members are often the primary caregivers. Nursing focus is on pain control, comfort, and allowing the client to die with dignity. Family and client needs are equal. Provide support for the family's grieving process, which can continue after the client's death.

End-of-life decisions require honest information regarding prognosis, disease progression, treatment options, and effects of treatments. These decisions are made during a highly stressful time. It is important that all health care personnel be aware of the child's and family's decisions.

Nurses can experience personal grief when caring for children with whom they have developed rapport and intimacy.

FACTORS INFLUENCING LOSS, GRIEF, AND COPING ABILITY

- Interpersonal relationships and social support networks
- Type and significance of loss
- Culture and ethnicity
- Spiritual and religious beliefs and practices
- Prior experience with loss
- Socioeconomic status

GRIEF AND MOURNING

Anticipatory grief: when death is expected or a possible outcome

Complicated grief: extensive or prolonged grief
- Intense thoughts
- Distressing yearning
- Feelings of loneliness
- Distressing emotions and feelings
- Disturbances in personal activities (sleep)
- Can require referral to an expert in grief counseling

Parental grief
- Intense, long-lasting, and complex
- Secondary losses related to the death of the child (absence of hope and dreams, disruption of the family) unit, loss of identity as a parent
- Parents can experience and express grief differently based on their role in the family.

Sibling grief
- Differs from adult/parental grief
- Reactions depend on age and developmental stage

CURRENT STAGE OF DEVELOPMENT

INFANTS/TODDLERS (BIRTH TO 3 YEARS)
- Have little to no concept of death.
- Egocentric thinking prevents their understanding death (toddlers).
- Mirror parental emotions (sadness, anger, depression, anxiety).
- React in response to the changes brought about by being in the hospital (change of routine, painful procedures, immobilization, less independence, separation from family).
- Can regress to an earlier stage of behavior.

PRESCHOOL CHILDREN (3 TO 6 YEARS)
- Egocentric thinking.
- Magical thinking allows for the belief that thoughts can cause an event such as death. As a result, the child can feel guilt and shame.
- Interpret separation from parents as punishment for bad behavior.
- View dying as temporary because of the lack of a concept of time and because the dead person can still have attributes of the living (sleeping, eating, breathing).

SCHOOL-AGE CHILDREN (6 TO 12 YEARS)
- Start to respond to logical or factual explanations.
- Begin to have an adult concept of death (inevitable, irreversible, universal), which generally applies to older school-age children (9 to 12 years).
- Experience fear of the disease process, death process, the unknown, and loss of control.
- Fear often displayed through uncooperative behavior.
- Can be curious about funeral services and what happens to the body after death.

ADOLESCENTS (12 TO 20 YEARS)

- Can have an adult-like concept of death.
- Can have difficulty accepting death because they are discovering who they are, establishing an identity, and dealing with issues of puberty.
- Rely more on peers than the influence of parents, which can result in the reality of a serious illness causing adolescents to feel isolated.
- Can be unable to relate to peers and communicate with parents.
- Can become increasingly stressed by changes in physical appearance due to medications or illness than the prospect of death.
- Can experience guilt and shame.

Factors that can increase the family's potential for dysfunctional grieving following the death of a child

- Lack of a support system
- Presence of inadequate coping skills
- Association of violence or suicide with the death of a child
- Sudden and unexpected death of a child
- Lack of hope or presence of preexisting mental health issues

DATA COLLECTION

- Knowledge regarding diagnosis, prognosis, and care
- Perceptions and desires regarding diagnosis, prognosis, and care
- Nutritional status, as well as growth and development patterns
- Activity and energy level of the child
- Parents' wishes regarding the child's end-of-life care
- Presence of advance directives
- Family coping and available support
- Stage of grief the child and family are experiencing

PHYSICAL MANIFESTATIONS OF DEATH

- Sensation of heat when the body feels cool
- Decreased sensation and movement in lower extremities
- Loss of senses (hearing is the last to be lost)
- Confusion or loss of consciousness
- Decreased appetite and thirst
- Swallowing difficulties
- Loss of bowel and bladder control
- Bradycardia, hypotension
- Cheyne-Stokes respirations
- Pooling pulmonary and pharyngeal secretions can cause the "death rattle"

NURSING INTERVENTIONS

- Allow an opportunity for anticipatory grieving, which impacts the way a family will cope with the death of a child.
- Provide consistency among nursing personnel who are caring for the client/family.
- Encourage guardians to remain with the client.
- Attempt to maintain a normal environment.
- Communicate with the client honestly and respectfully.
- Encourage independence.

- Stay with the client as much as possible.
- Administer analgesics to control pain.
- Provide privacy.
- Soften lights.
- Offer soft music if desired.
- Assist with arranging religious or cultural rituals desired by the client and family.
- Assist the client with unfinished tasks.
- Provide support for the family and client.

PALLIATIVE CARE

- Plan care for the entire family and its individuals, in addition to the client.
- Provide an environment that is as close to being like home as possible.
- Consult with the client and family for desired measures.
- Respect the family's cultural and religious preferences and rituals. Qpcc
- Provide and clarify information and explanations.
- Encourage physical contact; address feelings; and show concern, empathy, and support.
- Provide comfort measures (warmth, quiet, noise control, dry linens).
- Provide frequent mouth care and oral hygiene.
- Provide adequate nutrition and hydration.
- Collaborate with the RN and provider to control the client's pain.
  - Give medications on a regular schedule.
  - Treat breakthrough pain.
  - Increase doses as necessary to control pain.
  - Encourage use of relaxation, imagery, and distraction to help manage pain.

CARE FOR GRIEVING FAMILIES DURING THE DYING PROCESS

- Reinforce information to the client and family about the disease, medications, procedures, and expected events.
- Encourage and support loved ones to participate in caring for the client.
- Encourage family to remain near the child as much as possible or desired.
- Encourage the client's independence and control as developmentally and physically appropriate.
- Allow for visitation of family and friends as desired.
- Emphasize open, honest communication among the client, family, and health care team.
- Provide support to the client and family with decision-making.
- Provide opportunities for the client and family to ask questions.
- Assist caregivers to cope with their feelings and help them to understand the client's behaviors.
- Use books, movies, art, music, and play therapy to stimulate discussions and provide an outlet for emotions.
- Provide and encourage professional support and guidance from a trusted member of the health care team.
- Remain neutral and accepting.

- Give reassurance that the client is not in pain and that all efforts are being made to maintain comfort and support of the client's life.
- Recognize and support the individual differences of grieving. Advise families that each member can react differently on any given day.
- Give families privacy, unlimited time, and opportunities for any cultural or religious rituals. Respect the family's decisions regarding care of the client.
- Encourage discussion of special memories and people, reading of favorite books, providing favorite toys/objects, physical contact, sibling visits, and continued verbal communication, even if the client seems unconscious.

AFTER DEATH

- Allow family to stay with the body as long as they desire.
- Allow family to rock the infant/toddler, if desired.
- Remove tubes and equipment.
- Offer to allow family to assist with preparation of the body.
- Assist with preparations involving the death ritual.
- Encourage family to prepare siblings for the funeral and related death rituals.
- Remain with the family and offer support.
- Allow family to share stories about the client's life.
- Refer to the client by name.
- Allow all family members to communicate feelings.

SELF-CARE FOR NURSES

- Express personal feelings of loss to someone who can offer support.
- Maintain good general health.
- Develop the ability for empathy.
- Take time off from work as needed.
- Develop well-rounded interests.
- Develop professional and social support systems.
- Focus on the positive aspects of caring for children who are dying.
- Attend funeral services if desired.
- Maintain contact with the family.
- Other useful techniques include:
  - Mindfulness meditation
  - Focus on positive and rewarding aspects of nursing

Active Learning Scenario

A nurse is assisting with planning care for a client who is nearing the end of life. What interventions should the nurse's plan include? Use the ATI Active Learning Template: Basic Concept to complete this item.

NURSING INTERVENTIONS: Describe at least eight nursing interventions to be used.

Application Exercises

1. A nurse is caring for a child who is dying. Which of the following are findings of impending death? (Select all that apply.)
   - A. Heightened sense of hearing
   - B. Tachycardia
   - C. Difficulty swallowing
   - D. Sensation of being cold
   - E. Cheyne-Stokes respirations

2. A nurse is reinforcing teaching with a guardian about complicated grief. Which of the following statements should the nurse make?
   - A. "Complicated grief occurs when little time is spent thinking about the loss."
   - B. "Personal activities are rarely affected when experiencing complicated grief."
   - C. "Guardians will experience complicated grief together."
   - D. "Counseling can be helpful in resolving complicated grief."

3. A nurse is reinforcing teaching with a caregiver of a preschool child about factors that affect the child's perception of death. Which of the following factors should the nurse include?
   - A. Preschool children have no concept of death.
   - B. Preschool children perceive death as temporary.
   - C. Preschool children often regress to an earlier stage of behavior.
   - D. Preschool children experience fear related to the disease process.

4. A nurse often cares for children who are dying. Which of the following are actions for the nurse to take to maintain professional effectiveness? (Select all that apply.)
   - A. Remain in contact with the family after their loss.
   - B. Develop a professional support system.
   - C. Take time off from work.
   - D. Suggest that a hospital representative attend the funeral.
   - E. Demonstrate feelings of sympathy toward the family.

5. A nurse is caring for a child who has a terminal illness and reviews palliative care with an assistive personnel (AP). Which of the following statements by the AP indicates understanding of this review?
   - A. "I'm sure the family is hopeful that the new medication will stop the illness."
   - B. "I'll miss working with this client now that only nurses will be caring for the child."
   - C. "I will get all the client's personal objects out of the room."
   - D. "I will listen and respond as the family talks about their child's life."

Application Exercises Key

1. A. A decrease in the senses of smell, sight, and hearing are physical manifestations of approaching death.
   B. Bradycardia is a physical manifestation of approaching death.
   C. **CORRECT:** Difficulty swallowing is a physical finding of approaching death.
   D. A client's sensation of heat when the body feels cool is a physical manifestation of approaching death.
   E. **CORRECT:** Cheyne-Stokes respirations are an abnormal breathing pattern with periods of apnea that is a physical finding of impending death.

   Ⓝ NCLEX® Connection: Psychosocial Integrity, End-of-Life Concepts

2. A. Counseling can be helpful in resolving complicated grief.
   B. A guardian who is experiencing complicated grief experiences intense emotions that affect personal activities.
   C. Guardians grieve differently, and not all will experience complicated grief.
   D. **CORRECT:** Refer the guardian to an expert in grief counseling if complicated grief is identified.

   Ⓝ NCLEX® Connection: Psychosocial Integrity, Grief and Loss

3. A. Toddlers have no concept of death.
   B. **CORRECT:** Preschool children perceive death as temporary because they have no concept of time.
   C. Toddlers often regress to an earlier stage of behavior.
   D. School-age children experience fear related to the disease process.

   Ⓝ NCLEX® Connection: Psychosocial Integrity, End-of-Life Concepts

4. A. **CORRECT:** Maintaining contact with the family after their loss is an act of support for the family.
   B. **CORRECT:** Developing professional support systems is a strategy that can be used to maintain effectiveness when working with the client who is dying and their family.
   C. **CORRECT:** Taking time off from work is a strategy that can be used to maintain effectiveness when working with the client who is dying.
   D. Participate in funeral rituals as an act of support for the family.
   E. Develop the ability for empathy when dealing with dying clients.

   Ⓝ NCLEX® Connection: Psychosocial Integrity, End-of- Life Concepts

5. A. Palliative care is provided when there is no longer hope for a disease cure.
   B. Palliative care focuses on providing consistency among the interprofessional team to offer supportive care and a normal environment.
   C. Palliative care focuses on offering support and a normal environment as the dying process occurs.
   D. **CORRECT:** Palliative care focuses on the process of dying and grieving, which includes using therapeutic communication.

   Ⓝ NCLEX® Connection: Psychosocial Integrity, End-of-Life Concepts

Active Learning Scenario Key

Using the ATI Active Learning Template: Basic Concept

NURSING INTERVENTIONS
- Allow an opportunity for anticipatory grieving, which affects the way a family will cope with the death of a child.
- Provide consistency among nursing staff caring for the client and family.
- Encourage loved ones to remain with the client.
- Attempt to maintain a normal environment.
- Communicate with the client honestly and respectfully.
- Encourage independence.
- Stay with the client as much as possible.
- Administer analgesics to control pain.
- Provide privacy.
- Soften lights.
- Offer soft music if desired.
- Assist with arranging religious or cultural rituals desired by the client and family.
- Assist the client with unfinished tasks.
- Assist with providing support for the family and client.

Ⓝ NCLEX® Connection: Psychosocial Integrity, Grief and Loss

NCLEX® Connections

When reviewing the following chapters, keep in mind the relevant topics and tasks of the NCLEX outline, in particular:

Health Promotion and Maintenance

DEVELOPMENTAL STAGES AND TRANSITIONS
Identify and report client deviations from expected growth and development.

Identify barriers to communication.

Reduction of Risk Potential

LABORATORY VALUES: Monitor diagnostic or laboratory test results.

POTENTIAL FOR ALTERATIONS IN BODY SYSTEMS
Compare current client clinical data to baseline information.

Perform focused data collection based on client condition.

Reinforce client teaching on methods to prevent complications associated with activity level/diagnosed illness/disease.

THERAPEUTIC PROCEDURES: Reinforce client teaching on treatments and procedures.

POTENTIAL FOR COMPLICATIONS OF DIAGNOSTIC TESTS/ TREATMENTS/PROCEDURES: Use precautions to prevent injury and/or complications associated with a procedure or diagnosis

Physiological Adaptation

ALTERATIONS IN BODY SYSTEMS
Provide care to client who has experienced a seizure.

Reinforce education to client regarding care and condition

MEDICAL EMERGENCIES: Notify primary health care provider about client unexpected response/emergency situation.

CHAPTER 12   Acute Neurologic Disorders

Meningitis is an inflammation of the meninges, which are the connective tissues that cover the brain and spinal cord. Meningitis is caused by bacteria, a virus, or fungus in the cerebrospinal fluid (CSF).

Reye syndrome is a life-threatening disorder that involves acute encephalopathy and fatty changes of the liver.

Meningitis and Reye syndrome have similar manifestations and are both sometimes preceded by viral infections. Testing is necessary to differentiate between the two.

Meningitis

Viral (aseptic) meningitis usually requires supportive care for recovery.

Bacterial (septic) meningitis is a contagious infection. Prognosis depends on how quickly care is initiated.

DATA COLLECTION

RISK FACTORS

VIRAL MENINGITIS: Many viral illnesses (cytomegalovirus, herpes simplex virus, enterovirus, HIV, and arbovirus)

BACTERIAL MENINGITIS
- Infections caused by bacterial agents: *Neisseria meningitidis* (meningococcal), *Streptococcus pneumoniae* (pneumococcal), *Haemophilus influenzae* type B (Hib), *Escherichia coli*
  - Incidence of bacterial meningitis has decreased in all age groups except infants under the age of 2 months since the introduction of the Hib and pneumococcal conjugate vaccines (PCV). Q̇EBP
- Injuries that provide direct access to CSF (skull fracture, penetrating head wound)
- Crowded living conditions

EXPECTED FINDINGS
- Photophobia
- Vomiting
- Irritability
- Headache

PHYSICAL FINDINGS
Manifestations of viral and bacterial meningitis are similar.

Newborns
- No illness is present at birth, but it progresses within a few days.
- Manifestations are vague and difficult to diagnose.
  - Poor muscle tone, weak cry, poor suck, refuses feeding, and vomiting or diarrhea
  - Possible fever or hypothermia
- Neck is supple without nuchal rigidity.
- Bulging fontanels are a late finding.

3 months to 2 years
- Seizures with a high-pitched cry
- Fever and irritability
- Bulging fontanels
- Possible nuchal rigidity
- Poor feeding
- Vomiting
- Brudzinski's and Kernig's signs not reliable for diagnosis

2 years through adolescence
- Seizures (often initial finding)
- Nuchal rigidity
- Positive Brudzinski's sign (flexion of extremities occurring with deliberate flexion of the child's neck)
- Positive Kernig's sign (resistance to extension of the child's leg from a flexed position)
- Fever and chills
- Headache
- Vomiting
- Irritability and restlessness that can progress to drowsiness, delirium, stupor, and coma
- Petechiae or purpuric-type rash (with meningococcal infection)
- Involvement of joints (with meningococcal and *Hib*)
- Chronic draining ear (with pneumococcal infection)

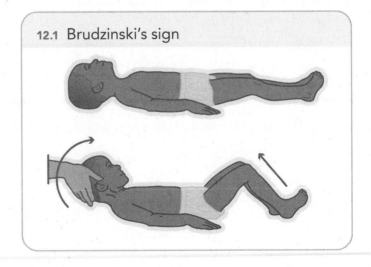

12.1 Brudzinski's sign

LABORATORY TESTS

- Blood cultures are sometimes positive when the CSF culture is negative.
- Collect complete blood counts.
- CSF analysis indicative of meningitis.
  - BACTERIAL
    - Cloudy color
    - Elevated WBC count
    - Elevated protein content
    - Decreased glucose content
    - Positive Gram stain
  - VIRAL
    - Clear color
    - Slightly elevated WBC count
    - Normal or slightly elevated protein content
    - Normal glucose content
    - Negative Gram stain

DIAGNOSTIC PROCEDURES

Lumbar puncture

This is the definitive diagnostic test for meningitis.
- The provider inserts a spinal needle into the subarachnoid space between L3 and L4, or L4 and L5 vertebral spaces.
- The provider measures spinal fluid pressure and collects CSF for analysis.

NURSING ACTIONS
- Have the client void prior to the procedure.
- Assist the provider with the procedure.
- A topical anesthetic cream (lidocaine and prilocaine) can be applied over the biopsy area 45 min to 1 hr prior to the procedure. Qᴘᴄᴄ
- Place the client in the side-lying position with the head flexed and knees drawn up toward the chest, and assist in maintaining the position. Use distraction methods as necessary.
- The provider can sedate the client with fentanyl and midazolam.
- The provider cleans the skin and injects a local anesthetic.
- The provider takes pressure readings and collects three to five test tubes of CSF.
- Pressure and an elastic bandage are applied to the puncture site after the needle is removed.
- Label specimens appropriately, and deliver them to the laboratory.
- Monitor the site for bleeding, hematoma, or infection.

CLIENT EDUCATION: Remain in bed in a flat position to prevent leakage and a resulting spinal headache. This might not be possible for an infant, toddler, or preschooler. Time required for bed rest depends on facility protocol and amount of fluid collected. Qᴘᴄᴄ

CT scan or MRI

Performed to identify increased intracranial pressure (ICP) or an abscess

NURSING ACTIONS
- Assist with positioning.
- Administer sedatives as prescribed.

PATIENT-CENTERED CARE

NURSING CARE

- The presence of petechiae or a purpuric-type rash requires immediate medical attention. Qᴇʙᴘ
- Isolate the client as soon as meningitis is suspected, and maintain droplet precautions per facility protocol.
  - Droplet precautions require a private room or a room with clients who have an infection from the same infectious disease, and ensuring that each client has designated equipment.
  - Providers and visitors should wear a mask.
  - Maintain respiratory isolation for a minimum of 24 hr after initiation of antibiotic therapy.
- Monitor vital signs, urine output, fluid status, pain level, and neurologic status.
- Monitor and treat fever.
- Correct fluid volume deficits and then restrict fluids until no evidence of increased ICP and blood sodium levels are within the expected range.
- Maintain NPO status if the client has a decreased level of consciousness. As the client's condition improves, advance to clear liquids and then a diet the client can tolerate.
- Decrease environmental stimuli.
  - Provide a quiet environment.
  - Minimize exposure to bright light (natural and electric).
- Provide comfort measures.
  - Keep the room cool.
  - Position the client without a pillow, and slightly elevate the head of the bed. The client can also be positioned side-lying to reduce neck discomfort.
- Maintain safety (keep the bed in a low position, implement seizure precautions). Qs
- Keep the family informed of the client's condition.

MEDICATIONS

Antibiotics

Assist with administering IV antibiotics for bacterial infections. Length of therapy is determined by the client's condition and CSF results (normal blood glucose levels, negative culture). Therapy can last up to 10 days.

NURSING ACTIONS
- Check for allergies.
- Provide support for the client and family.
- Reinforce with the family about the need to complete the entire course of medication.

Corticosteroids: dexamethasone

- Not indicated for viral meningitis
- Assists with initial management of increased ICP, but might not be effective for long-term complications
- Most effective for reducing neurologic complications in children who have infections caused by Hib

NURSING ACTIONS
- Monitor for effectiveness of medication.
- Provide support for the client and family.
- Reinforce teaching about the administration and possible adverse effects of the medication.

CLIENT EDUCATION

- Early and complete treatment is necessary for upper respiratory infections.
- Maintain appropriate immunizations for the client. Children should receive the Hib and PCV vaccines at 2, 4, and 6 months of age, then again between 12 and 15 months of age.

COMPLICATIONS

Increased intracranial pressure

Could lead to neurologic dysfunction

NURSING ACTIONS
- Monitor for manifestations of increased ICP. Q**s**
  - **Newborns and infants:** bulging or tense fontanels, increased head circumference, high-pitched cry, distended scalp veins, irritability, bradycardia, and respiratory changes
  - **Children:** increased irritability, headache, nausea, vomiting, diplopia, seizures, bradycardia, and respiratory changes
- Provide interventions to reduce ICP (positioning; avoidance of coughing, straining, and bright lights; minimizing environmental stimuli).

Reye syndrome

- Reye syndrome primarily affects the liver and brain, causing liver dysfunction and cerebral edema.
- The cause of Reye syndrome is not understood.
- Peak incidence of Reye syndrome occurs when influenza is most common.
- The prognosis for the client who has Reye syndrome is best with early recognition and treatment which includes ruling out other illnesses that have manifestations similar to Reye syndrome.

DATA COLLECTION

RISK FACTORS

- There is a potential association between using aspirin (salicylate) products for treating fevers caused by viral infections and the development of Reye syndrome. Q**EBP**
- Reye syndrome typically follows a viral illness (influenza, gastroenteritis, varicella).

12.2 Kernig's sign

EXPECTED FINDINGS

Recent viral illness or use of aspirin or aspirin-containing products.

PHYSICAL FINDINGS
Reye syndrome presents in clinical stages based on the severity of liver and neurologic findings.
- Lethargy
- Irritability
- Combativeness
- Confusion
- Delirium
- Profuse vomiting
- Seizures
- Loss of consciousness

LABORATORY TESTS

- Liver enzymes (alanine aminotransferase [ALT], aspartate aminotransferase [AST]): elevated.
- Blood ammonia level: elevated.
- Blood electrolytes: altered due to cerebral edema and liver changes.
- Coagulation times can be extended.

DIAGNOSTIC PROCEDURES

Liver biopsy

A liver biopsy consists of taking a piece of liver tissue via a large-bore needle and sending this tissue to the pathology department. Ensure that clotting studies are within normal limits prior to the procedure.

NURSING ACTIONS
- Maintain NPO status prior to the procedure.
- Monitor for hemorrhage postprocedure.
- Monitor vital signs frequently postprocedure.

CLIENT EDUCATION: Limit the client's postprocedure activities to decrease the risk of hemorrhage.

CSF analysis

A lumbar puncture should be performed to collect CSF and rule out meningitis.

PATIENT-CENTERED CARE

NURSING CARE

- Maintain hydration while preventing cerebral edema.
  - Assist with the administration of IV fluids as prescribed.
  - Maintain accurate I&O.
  - Insert indwelling urinary catheter as ordered.
- Position the client. Qs
  - Avoid extreme flexion, extension, or rotation.
  - Maintain the head in a midline neutral position.
  - Keep the head of the bed elevated 30°.
- Monitor coagulation and prevent hemorrhage.
  - Note unexplained or prolonged bleeding.
  - Apply pressure after procedures that cause bleeding.
- Monitor pain status and response to painful stimuli. Administer pain medications when appropriate.
- Monitor respiratory status. Intubation and mechanical ventilation can be necessary.
- Implement seizure precautions.
- Keep the family informed of the client's status.
- Provide private time for the family to be with the client if death is imminent.
- Assist with making referrals for resources to support the family.

MEDICATIONS

Osmotic diuretic: mannitol

To decrease cerebral swelling

NURSING ACTIONS: Monitor for increased ICP.

INTERPROFESSIONAL CARE

- A client who has neurologic deficits post-Reye syndrome requires interventions from other members of the health care team.
- Occupational therapy and physical therapy can be needed to help the client adapt to neurologic deficits.
- A dietitian can be needed to assist in maintaining adequate nutrition.

CLIENT EDUCATION

- Children should not receive salicylates for pain or fever.
- Caregiver should read labels of over-the-counter medications to check for the presence of salicylates.
- Liver function is usually regained but neurologic deficits might persist.

COMPLICATIONS

Neurologic sequelae

Neurologic complications vary by degree of severity, and sometimes include speech or hearing impairment, and developmental delays based on the length and severity of illness.

NURSING ACTIONS
- Explain the client's condition and needs to the family.
- Help the family identify support services for home care.

Death

NURSING ACTIONS
- Support the family in grief.
- Assist with making referrals to provide spiritual support as appropriate.

Application Exercises

1. A nurse is assisting with the care of a client who has suspected meningitis and a decreased level of consciousness. Which of the following actions should the nurse take?

   A. Place the client on NPO status.

   B. Prepare the client for a liver biopsy.

   C. Position the client dorsal recumbent.

   D. Put the client in a protective environment.

2. A nurse is reviewing cerebrospinal fluid analysis for a client who has suspected meningitis. Which of the following findings should the nurse identify as indicating viral meningitis? (Select all that apply.)

   A. Negative Gram stain

   B. Normal glucose content

   C. Turbid and cloudy color

   D. Decreased WBC count

   E. Normal protein content

3. A nurse is collecting data from a 4-month-old infant who has meningitis. Which of the following manifestations should the nurse expect?

   A. Depressed anterior fontanel

   B. Constipation

   C. Presence of the rooting reflex

   D. High-pitched cry

4. A nurse is reviewing the medical record of a client who has Reye syndrome. Which of the following findings should the nurse identify as a risk factor for Reye syndrome?

   A. Recent history of infectious cystitis caused by *Candida*

   B. Recent history of bacterial otitis media

   C. Recent episode of gastroenteritis

   D. Recent episode of *Haemophilus influenzae* meningitis

5. A nurse is assisting with the development of an in-service about viral and bacterial meningitis. The nurse should include that the introduction of which of the following immunizations decreased the incidence of bacterial meningitis in children? (Select all that apply.)

   A. Inactivated polio vaccine (IPV)

   B. Pneumococcal conjugate vaccine (PCV)

   C. Diphtheria and tetanus toxoids and acellular pertussis vaccine (DTaP)

   D. *Haemophilus influenzae* type B (Hib) vaccine

   E. Inactivated influenza vaccine (IIV)

Active Learning Scenario

A nurse is assisting with the admission of a client who has Reye Syndrome. Use the ATI Active Learning Template: System Disorder to complete this item.

ALTERATION IN HEALTH (DIAGNOSIS)

EXPECTED FINDINGS: Identify five.

LABORATORY TESTS: List two results indicative of Reye syndrome.

Application Exercises Key

1. A. **CORRECT:** Place the client on NPO status due to the client's decreased level of consciousness to prevent aspiration.
   B. Expect a client who has Reye syndrome to require a liver biopsy.
   C. Position the client without a pillow and slightly elevate the head of the bed to prevent increasing intracranial pressure.
   D. Clients who are immunocompromised require a protective environment. Place a client who has suspected meningitis should be placed on droplet precautions for at least 24 hr after the initiation of antibiotic therapy.

   Ⓝ *NCLEX® Connection: Physiological Adaptation, Alterations in Body Systems*

2. A. **CORRECT:** Expect a client who has viral meningitis to have a negative Gram stain.
   B. **CORRECT:** Expect a client who has viral meningitis to have a glucose level within the expected reference range.
   C. Expect a clear color for a client who has viral meningitis.
   D. Expect a slightly elevated WBC count for a client who has viral meningitis.
   E. **CORRECT:** Expect a client who has viral meningitis to have a protein level within the expected reference range.

   Ⓝ *NCLEX® Connection: Reduction of Risk Potential, Laboratory Values*

3. A. Expect a 4-month-old infant who has meningitis to have a bulging anterior fontanel.
   B. Identify vomiting as an expected finding of meningitis.
   C. Identify the rooting reflex as an expected finding in infants until the age of 3 to 4 months, which can remain until the age of 12 months.
   D. **CORRECT:** Identify a high-pitched cry as a finding associated with meningitis between ages 3 months to 2 years.

   Ⓝ *NCLEX® Connection: Physiological Adaptation, Basic Pathophysiology*

4. A. Identify that *Candida* is a fungus and is therefore not a risk factor for Reye syndrome.
   B. Identify that a bacterial infection is not a risk factor for Reye syndrome.
   C. **CORRECT:** Identify that gastroenteritis is a viral illness, which is a risk factor for developing Reye syndrome. Reye syndrome typically follows a viral illness (influenza, gastroenteritis, or varicella).
   D. Identify that *Haemophilus influenzae* is a bacteria and is therefore not a risk factor for Reye syndrome.

   Ⓝ *NCLEX® Connection: Physiological Adaptation, Basic Pathophysiology*

5. A. Include the IPV because it does not decrease the incidence of bacterial meningitis.
   B. **CORRECT:** The introduction of the PCV decreased the incidence of bacterial meningitis in children, as it provides immunity against bacteria that causes the illness.
   C. Do not include the DTaP vaccine because it does not decrease the incidence of bacterial meningitis.
   D. **CORRECT:** The introduction of the Hib vaccine decreased the incidence of bacterial meningitis in children, as it provides immunity against bacterium that cause the illness.
   E. Do not include the TIV because it does not decrease the incidence of bacterial meningitis.

   Ⓝ *NCLEX® Connection: Health Promotion and Maintenance, Health Promotion/Disease Prevention*

Active Learning Scenario Key

Using the ATI Active Learning Template: System Disorder

ALTERATION IN HEALTH (DIAGNOSIS): Reye syndrome is a life-threatening disorder involving acute encephalopathy and fatty changes of the liver.

EXPECTED FINDINGS
- Recent viral illness
- Recent use of aspirin-containing medicine
- Lethargy
- Irritability
- Combativeness
- Confusion
- Delirium
- Profuse vomiting
- Seizures
- Loss of consciousness

LABORATORY TESTS
- Altered blood electrolytes due to cerebral edema and liver changes
- Possibly extended coagulation times
- Elevated liver enzymes
- Elevated blood ammonia levels

Ⓝ *NCLEX® Connection: Physiological Adaptation, Basic Pathophysiology*

UNIT 2   SYSTEM DISORDERS
SECTION: NEUROLOGIC DISORDERS

CHAPTER 13 *Seizures*

Seizures are abnormal, involuntary, excessive electrical discharges of neurons within the brain.

Seizures are classified according to their type and etiology. Focal (partial) seizures involve one area of the brain. Generalized seizures involve the entire brain.

A diagnosis of epilepsy is made if a client has two unprovoked seizures at least 24 hr apart, or if a single unprovoked seizure occurs during a time period of 10 years following two unprovoked seizures.

DATA COLLECTION

RISK FACTORS FOR SEIZURES

- Some seizures have no known etiology
- Febrile episode
- Cerebral edema
- Intracranial infection or hemorrhage
- Brain tumors or cysts
- Anoxia
- Toxins or drugs
- Lead poisoning
- Tetanus, *Shigella*, or *Salmonella*
- Metabolic conditions

RISK FACTORS FOR EPILEPSY

- Trauma
- Hemorrhage
- Congenital defects
- Anoxia
- Infection
- Toxins
- Hypoglycemic injury
- Uremia
- Migraine
- Cardiovascular dysfunction

EXPECTED FINDINGS

Generalized

Tonic-clonic seizure (previously referred to as grand mal)
- Onset without warning ⓆEBP
- Most prevalent of all seizure types
- Tonic phase (10 to 30 seconds)
  - Eyes roll upward
  - Loss of consciousness
  - Tonic contraction of entire body, with arms flexed and legs, head and neck extended
  - Mouth snaps shut and tongue can be bitten
  - Thoracic and abdominal muscles contract
  - Possible piercing cry
  - Flushing
  - Loss of swallowing reflex and increased salivation
  - Apnea leading to cyanosis
- Clonic phase (typically 30 to 50 seconds; can last 30 min or longer)
  - Violent jerking movements of the body
  - Trunk and extremities experience rhythmic contraction and relaxation
  - Can having foaming in the mouth
  - Can be incontinent of urine and feces
  - Gradual slowing of movements until cessation
- Postical state (30 min)
  - Remains semiconscious but arouses with difficulty
  - Confused for several hours
  - Impairment of fine motor movements
  - Lack of coordination
  - Possible vomiting, headache, visual or speech difficulties
  - Sleeps for several hours
  - Feels tired and can complain of sore muscles
  - No recollection of the seizure

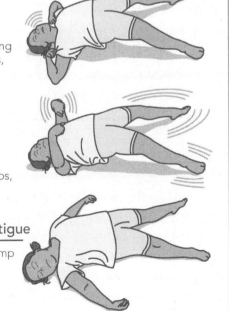

13.1 Tonic-clonic seizure

tonic phase

piercing cry
pallor
generalize stiffening
of body and limbs,
back arched

clonic phase

salivary frothing
eye blinking
pallor
incontinence
clonic jerks of limbs,
body, and head

**postictal
confusional fatigue**

limbs and body limp

Absence seizure (previously referred to petit mal)
- Onset between ages of 4 to 12 years and ceases by the teenage years
- Loss of consciousness lasting 5 to 10 seconds
- Motionless, blank stare
- Affects schoolwork, which is often first indication of a problem
- Minimal or no change in behavior
- Resembles daydreaming or inattentiveness
- Can drop items being held, but the child seldom falls
- Automatisms: Lip smacking, twitching of eyelids or face, or slight hand movements
- Unable to recall episodes, but can be momentarily confused
- Can immediately resume previous activities

Myoclonic seizure
- Variety of seizure episodes
- Symmetric or asymmetric involvement
- Brief contractions of muscle or groups of muscle
- Can involve only the face and trunk or one or more extremities
- No postictal state
- Might not lose consciousness

Atonic or akinetic seizure
- Also known as "drop attacks."
- Onset between 2 and 5 years of age.
- Muscle tone is lost for a few seconds, which often causes a fall.
- A period of confusion follows.
- If seizures are frequent, child should wear a helmet to prevent injury.

Partial (focal/local)

Simple partial seizures with motor manifestations
- Aversive seizure (most common): Eyes and head turn away from the side of focus, with or without loss of consciousness
- Rolandic (Sylvan) seizure: Tonic-clonic movements involving the face, salivation, arrested sleep, and most common during sleep

Simple partial seizure with sensory manifestations
- Tingling, numbness or pain in one area of the body then spreading to other parts, with visual sensations
- Motor development (hypertonia or posturing)

Complex partial seizures (psychomotor seizures)
- Altered behavior
- Inability to respond to the environment
- Impaired consciousness but regains in less than 5 min
- Confusion and inability to recall event
- Aura: warning of onset of seizure activity that can be a strange feeling in the throat, an odor, or taste. It can also produce auditory or visual hallucinations, feelings of fear, distorted sense of time and self

Unclassified

West syndrome (infantile spasms)
Rare disorder of unknown origin with a peak onset between 4 and 8 months of age. Rarely occurs after 2 years of age.
- Sudden, brief, symmetric muscle contractions
- Flexed head, extended arms with legs drawn up
- Possible eye deviation or nystagmus
- Possible cry or irritability during or after seizure spasms
- Can occur as a single event or in a cluster of up to 150 seizures
- Treated with adrenocorticotropic hormone (ACTH)

Lennox-Gastaut syndrome
- Mixture of different seizures in child with cognitive deficits
- Aggressive and hyperactive behavior
- Difficult to treat
- Poor prognosis

Febrile seizures
- Associated with as sudden spike in temperature as high as 38.9° to 40° C (102° to 104° F)
- Duration of 15 to 20 seconds

TREATMENT
- After seizure subsides, take actions to reduce the fever.
  - Administer acetaminophen or ibuprofen when the child has a fever.
  - Dress the child in light clothing.
  - Administer a tepid sponge baths.

LABORATORY TESTS

Depend on age, history, and physical condition
- Lead level
- WBC
- Blood glucose
- Metabolic panel
- Chromosomal analysis
- Toxicology screen

DIAGNOSTIC PROCEDURES

Electroencephalogram (EEG)

Records electrical activity and can identify the origin of seizure activity
- Can be monitored during sleep, when awake, and with stimulation and hyperventilation.
- Test can last 1 hr to multiple periods and days of monitoring.
- Can be performed with video monitoring.
- A normal EEG does not rule out seizures.

CLIENT EDUCATION
- Remain quiet during the procedure.
- If prescribed, withhold sleep from child prior to the test.
- Strobe lights or hyperventilation can be used to induce a seizure.
- Abstain from caffeine for several hours prior to the procedure.
- Wash hair (no oils or sprays) before and after the procedure to remove electrode gel.

Magnetic resonance imaging (MRI)

More detailed and used to detect malformations, cortical dysplasia, or tumors

Lumbar puncture

Measures spinal fluid pressure and detects infection (meningitis)

Computed tomography (CT) scan

Detects hemorrhage, infarction, or malformations

PATIENT-CENTERED CARE

NURSING CARE

Initiate seizure precautions for any child at risk.
- Pad side rails of bed, crib, and wheelchair.
- Keep bed free of objects that could cause injury.
- Have suction and oxygen equipment available.

During a seizure

- Protect from injury. If child is on the floor, place blanket under head.
- Maintain a position to provide a patent airway.
- Be prepared to suction oral secretions.
- Turn child to a side-lying position (decreases risk of aspiration).
- Loosen restrictive clothing.
- Do not attempt to restrain the child.
- Do not attempt to open the jaw or insert an airway during seizure activity. (This can damage teeth, lips, or tongue). Do not put anything in the child's mouth.
- Remove the child's glasses.
- Prepare to administer oxygen.
- Remain with the child.
- Note onset, time, and characteristics of seizure.
- Remain calm and reassure caregivers.

Postseizure

- Maintain the child in a side-lying position to prevent aspiration and to facilitate drainage of oral secretions.
- Check breathing, vital signs, and position of head and tongue.
- Check the head and body for injuries, including the mouth (tongue, teeth).
- Perform neurologic checks.
- Allow for rest if necessary.
- Reorient and calm the child (due to agitation or confusion).
- Maintain seizure precautions, including placing the bed in the lowest position and padding the side rails to prevent future injury.
- Note the time of the postictal period.
- Remain with the child.
- Do not offer food or liquids until completely awake and swallowing reflex has returned.
- Encourage child to describe the period before, during, and after the seizure activity.

- Determine if the child experienced an aura, which can indicate the origin of seizure in the brain.
- Try to determine the possible trigger, (fatigue or stress).
- Document the onset and duration of seizure and client findings/observations prior to, during, and following the seizure (level of consciousness, apnea, cyanosis, motor activity, incontinence).

MEDICATIONS

Antiepileptic drugs (AEDs)

EXPECTED EFFECT: Decrease incidence and severity of seizures
Diazepam, phenytoin, carbamazepine, valproic acid, and fosphenytoin sodium, topiramate, lamotrigine, clonazepam
- Medication selection is based on the client's age, type of seizure, and other medical factors.
- A single medication is initiated at low dosage and gradually increased until seizures are controlled.
- A second medication can be added to achieve seizure control.

NURSING ACTIONS
- Monitor for seizure control.
- Check for allergies.
- Monitor for adverse effects.
- Monitor therapeutic blood medication levels for required medications.

CLIENT EDUCATION
- Take medications at the same time every day to enhance effectiveness.
- Be aware of medication and food interactions that are specific to each medication.
- Observe for adverse effects of the medications.
- Dosage can need to be increased as the child grows.
- Blood cell counts, urinalysis, and liver function tests will need to be obtained at frequent intervals to determine effect on organ function.

INTERPROFESSIONAL CARE

- The school nurse should be involved in providing for the child's safety in the school setting. This can include implementation of an individualized education plan or another specialized program.
- Referral to nutrition services if a ketogenic diet is prescribed.

THERAPEUTIC PROCEDURES

Brain surgery

- Removal of a tumor, lesion, or hematoma
- **Focal resection** of an area of the brain to remove epileptogenic zone
- **Hemispherectomy:** removal of one hemisphere of the brain; procedure is reserved for catastrophic, intractable epilepsy
- **Corpus callosotomy:** separation of the connection between the two hemispheres in the brain

Vagal nerve stimulator

- Under general anesthesia, the stimulator is implanted into the left chest wall and connected to an electrode that is placed at the left vagus nerve. The device is then programmed to administer intermittent vagal nerve stimulation at a rate specific to the client's needs.
- Adjunctive therapy to reduce seizure frequency for partial onset seizures which are unmanageable with antiepileptic medications.
- In addition to routine stimulation, the client can initiate vagal nerve stimulation by holding a magnet over the implantable device at the onset of seizure activity. This will either abort the seizure or lessen its severity.
- Short-term adverse effects include throat discomfort, cough, and dysphonia.

CLIENT EDUCATION

- It is important to undergo periodic laboratory testing to monitor AED levels.
- Do not stop medications without provider authorization.
- Adhere to the medication regimen.
- Possible medication interactions include decreased effectiveness of oral contraceptives.
- Ensure the client wears a medical alert bracelet or necklace at all times.
- Refer to the state's Department of Motor Vehicles to determine laws regarding driving for adolescents who have seizure disorders.
- Children should wear safety devices (helmets) while participating in sport (biking, skiing, horseback riding).
- Do not leave the child unattended in water or permit climbing on objects taller than the child.
- Older children should be encouraged to use a shower, rather than a bathtub, and leave the bathroom door unlocked while showering.
- Avoid triggering factors (emotional stress, sleep deprivation, bright lights, fatigue, physical abuse).
- Not all disorders that cause epilepsy will affect the child's intelligence. The child can attend regular school.
- A ketogenic diet (high-fat, low-carbohydrate, and adequate protein) can be prescribed to promote body use of fat instead of glucose for energy. This can reduce seizure frequency, especially if the child has a metabolic disorder.
  - Monitor for adverse effects of diet therapy (lethargy, kidney or bladder stones, weight loss).
- Apply the same child-rearing techniques for the child as you would for other children (establishing rules, boundaries, consequences, and rewards).

! Call Emergency Medical Service if any of the following occur.
- Apnea
- Seizure lasts more than 5 min
- Status epilepticus
- Pupils are not equal following seizure
- Vomiting continuously for 30 min after the seizure
- Unresponsive to pain or difficult to arouse
- Seizure occurs in water
- First seizure episode

COMPLICATIONS

Status epilepticus

Status epilepticus is prolonged seizure activity lasting 30 min or longer or continuous seizure activity in which the client does not enter a postictal phase. This acute condition requires immediate emergent treatment to prevent loss of brain function, which can become permanent.

NURSING ACTIONS
- Maintain airway, administer oxygen, establish IV access, perform ECG monitoring, and monitor pulse oximetry and ABG results.
- Administer a loading dose of diazepam or lorazepam. Buccal, rectal, or nasal medications can be given until intravenous access is established. If seizures continue after the loading dose is given, fosphenytoin followed by phenobarbital should be administered.
- Adverse effects include throat discomfort, cough, and dysphonia.
- Provide support for the client and family.

Developmental delays

NURSING ACTIONS
- Promote optimal development.
- Make appropriate referrals.
- Provide support for the family.

Application Exercises

1. A nurse is caring for a child who has absence seizures. Which of the following findings should the nurse expect? (Select all that apply.)
   A. Loss of consciousness
   B. Appearance of daydreaming
   C. Dropping held objects
   D. Falling to the floor
   E. Having a piercing cry

2. A nurse is caring for a child who just experienced a generalized seizure. Which of the following is the priority action for the nurse to take?
   A. Position the child in a side-lying position.
   B. Try to determine the seizure trigger.
   C. Reorient the child to the environment.
   D. Note the time of the postictal period.

3. A nurse is reinforcing teaching to the guardians of a child who is to have an electroencephalogram (EEG). Which of the following statements by a guardian indicates teaching was effective?
   A. "My child should remain quiet and still during this procedure."
   B. "I cannot wash my child's hair prior to the procedure."
   C. "I should not give my child anything to eat prior to the procedure."
   D. "This procedure will be very painful for my child."

4. A nurse is reinforcing teaching with a group of caregivers about the risk factors for seizures. Which of the following factors should the nurse include? (Select all that apply.)
   A. Febrile episodes
   B. Hypoglycemia
   C. Sodium imbalances
   D. Low blood lead levels
   E. Presence of diphtheria

5. A nurse is preparing to reinforce treatment options with the guardian of a child who has worsening seizures. Which of the following treatment options should the nurse include in the discussion? (Select all that apply.)
   A. Vagal nerve stimulator
   B. Additional antiepileptic medications
   C. Corpus callosotomy
   D. Focal resection
   E. Radiation therapy

Active Learning Scenario

A nurse is contributing to the plan of care for a child who has tonic-clonic seizures. What actions should the nurse include? Use the ATI Active Learning Template: System Disorder to complete this item.

NURSING CARE: Describe nursing actions during and after a seizure.

Application Exercises Key

1. A. **CORRECT:** Loss of consciousness for 5 to 10 seconds is a manifestation of an absence seizure.
   B. **CORRECT:** Behavior that resembles daydreaming is a manifestation of an absence seizure.
   C. **CORRECT:** A child who is having absence seizures might drop a held object.
   D. Falling to the floor is a manifestation of a tonic-clonic seizure.
   E. A piercing cry is a manifestation of a tonic-clonic seizure.

   Ⓝ *NCLEX® Connection: Physiological Adaptation, Alterations in Body Systems*

2. A. **CORRECT:** Following a seizure, children often experience vomiting. Using the airway, breathing, circulation priority-setting framework, the first action is to take is to place the child in a side-lying position to maintain a patent airway and prevent aspiration of secretions.
   B. Determining the seizure trigger can help prevent future seizure episodes. However, it is not the priority action.
   C. Reorienting the child to the environment following a generalized seizure is an appropriate action. However, it is not the priority action.
   D. Noting the timing of the postictal period can assist with planning seizure management. However, it is not the priority action.

   Ⓝ *NCLEX® Connection: Physiological Adaptation, Alterations in Body Systems*

3. A. **CORRECT:** The child should remain still and quiet during the test. Excessive movements can cause false-positive results.
   B. The child's hair should be washed to remove oils that permit adherence of the EEG electrodes.
   C. Foods are not withheld prior to an EEG.
   D. The procedure is not painful; however, it can cause anxiety for the child.

   Ⓝ *NCLEX® Connection: Reduction of Risk Potential, Diagnostic Tests*

4. A. **CORRECT:** Febrile episodes can cause general tonic-clonic seizures in infants and young children.
   B. **CORRECT:** Seizure activity is a late manifestation of hypoglycemia.
   C. **CORRECT:** Seizure activity is a manifestation of hyponatremia and hypernatremia.
   D. High blood lead levels are a risk factor for seizure activity.
   E. Diphtheria is a respiratory illness causing difficulty breathing and is not a risk factor for seizures.

   Ⓝ *NCLEX® Connection: Health Promotion and Maintenance, Health Promotion/Disease Prevention*

5. A. **CORRECT:** The implantation of a vagal nerve stimulator is an option to provide seizure control.
   B. **CORRECT:** Additional antiepileptic medication can be added to the current medication regime to control seizures.
   C. **CORRECT:** A corpus callosotomy can be performed for uncontrolled seizures.
   D. **CORRECT:** A focal resection can be performed for uncontrolled seizures.
   E. Radiation therapy is used in cancer treatment and is not used to control seizures.

   Ⓝ *NCLEX® Connection: Reduction of Risk Potential, Therapeutic Procedures*

Active Learning Scenario Key

Using the ATI Active Learning Template: System Disorder

NURSING CARE

- During a seizure
  - Protect the child from injury. (Move furniture away, hold the child's head in lap if on the floor.)
  - Position the child to maintain a patent airway.
  - Be prepared to suction oral secretions.
  - Turn the child to the side (decreases risk of aspiration).
  - Loosen restrictive clothing.
  - Do not attempt to restrain the child.
  - Do not attempt to open the jaw or insert an airway during seizure activity. (This can damage teeth, lips, or tongue.) Do not use padded tongue blades.
  - Remove glasses.
  - Administer oxygen if needed.
  - Remain with the child.
  - Note the onset, time, and characteristics of the seizure.
- Postseizure
  - Maintain the child in a side-lying position to prevent aspiration and to facilitate drainage of oral secretions.
  - Check for breathing, check vital signs, and check position of head and tongue.
  - Check for injuries, including the mouth.
  - Perform neurologic checks.
  - Allow the child to rest, if necessary.
  - Reorient and calm the child (they can be agitated or confused).
  - Maintain seizure precautions, including placing the bed in the lowest position and padding the side rails to prevent future injury.
  - Check inside the mouth to see if the lips and tongue have been bitten.
  - Note the time of the postictal period.
  - Remain with the child.
  - Do not offer food or liquids until completely awake and has a swallowing reflex has returned.
  - Encourage the child to describe the period before, during, and after the seizure activity.
  - Determine if the child experienced an aura, which can indicate the origin of seizure in the brain.
  - Try to determine the possible trigger (fatigue or stress).
  - Document the onset and duration of seizure and client findings/observations prior to, during, and following the seizure (level of consciousness, apnea, cyanosis, motor activity, incontinence).

Ⓝ *NCLEX® Connection: Physiological Adaptation, Alterations in Body Systems*

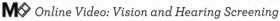

CHAPTER 14

UNIT 2   SYSTEM DISORDERS
SECTION: NEUROLOGIC DISORDERS

CHAPTER 14 *Cognitive and Sensory Impairments*

Sensory impairments in children most commonly affect the eyes and ears. Adequate vision and hearing are necessary for normal growth and development. Therefore, it is important to identify any impairments early in life.

Down syndrome is a common chromosomal abnormality that affects the child's growth and development and results in cognitive and sensory impairments.

Visual impairments

- Visual impairments encompass both partial sight and legal blindness.
- Common visual impairments in children include myopia, hyperopia, astigmatism, anisometropia, amblyopia, strabismus, cataracts, and glaucoma.

HEALTH PROMOTION AND DISEASE PREVENTION

Screen children for visual impairments yearly.

DATA COLLECTION

RISK FACTORS

- Prenatal or postnatal conditions (retinopathy of prematurity, trauma, meningitis, and postnatal infections)
- Perinatal infections (herpes, rubella, syphilis, chlamydia, gonorrhea, and toxoplasmosis)
- Chronic illness (sickle cell disease, rheumatoid arthritis, retinoblastoma, albinism, and Tay–Sachs disease)

EXPECTED FINDINGS

Visual impairment manifestations

Myopia (nearsightedness)
- Sees close objects clearly, but not objects in the distance
- Headaches and vertigo
- Eye rubbing
- Difficulty reading
- Clumsiness (frequently walking into objects)
- Poor school performance

Hyperopia (farsightedness)
- Sees distant objects clearly, but not objects that are close
- Because of accommodation, not usually detected until age 7

Astigmatism
- Uneven refractive curvatures in vision in which only parts of letters on a page can be seen
- Headache and vertigo
- Appearance of normal vision because tilting the head enables all letters to be seen

Anisometropia
- Different refractive strength in each eye
- Headache and vertigo
- Excessive eye rubbing
- Poor school performance

Amblyopia (lazy eye): Reduced visual acuity in one eye

Strabismus: Esotropia (inward deviation of eye); **exotropia** (outward deviation of eye)
- Abnormal corneal light reflex or cover test
- Misaligned eyes
- Frowning or squinting
- Difficulty seeing print clearly
- One eye closed to enable better vision
- Head tilted to one side
- Headache, dizziness, diplopia, photophobia, and crossed eyes

Cataracts
- Gray opacity of the lens which prevents light from entering into the eye
- Decreased ability to see clearly
- Possible loss of peripheral vision
- Nystagmus
- Strabismus
- Absence of red reflex
- Infant: inability to reach and grab objects, such as a toy rattle

Glaucoma
- Increase in ocular pressure in the eye
- Loss of peripheral vision
- Perception of halos around objects
- Red eye
- Excessive tearing (epiphora)
- Photophobia
- Spasmodic winking (blepharospasm)
- Corneal haziness
- Enlargement of the eyeball (buphthalmos)
- Possible pain
- Red reflex of the eye will appear gray to green

DIAGNOSTIC PROCEDURES

Visual screening
- This is completed using the Snellen letter, tumbling E, or picture chart (HOTV test) useful for preschoolers.
  - Place the child 20 feet from the chart with heels on the 20-foot mark.
  - The child should be wearing glasses, if appropriate, and keep both eyes open during the screening.
  - While covering one eye, the child reads each line on the chart, starting at the bottom of the chart, until he can pass a line. The child needs to identify four of the six characters in the line correctly to pass.
  - The child is then asked to start at the top and move down until he can no longer pass a line.
  - The procedure is repeated with the other eye.
- **Partial visual impairment** is classified as visual acuity of 20/70 to 20/200.
- **Legal blindness** is classified as visual acuity of 20/200 or worse or a visual field of 20 degrees or less in the child's better eye. This is a legal definition not diagnosis.

Ocular alignment: Observed using the corneal light reflex test
- A flashlight is shone directly into the client's eye, from a distance of 16 inches.
- Reflected light should be observed in the same location on both pupils.

Cover test: Client is asked to cover each eye and observe an object at a distance of 13 inches. The cover is removed and the eye is observed for movement, which should not occur.

Peripheral vision: Evaluated by having the client fixate on an object
- A pencil is moved from beyond the field of vision into the range of peripheral vision.
- The client is asked to say stop when the object is noted in the peripheral vision. This angle is then measured.
- Each quadrant of peripheral vision is tested. The test is repeated in the other eye.
- Normal findings are 50° upward, 70° downward, 60° nasalward, and 90° temporally.

Color vision: Evaluated using the Ishihara or Hardy–Rand–Rittler test
- The client is shown a set of cards and asked to identify the number embedded in the confusion of colors.
- The client should identify all of the numbers on the cards with correct color vision.

PATIENT-CENTERED CARE

NURSING CARE

- Maintain normal to bright lighting for the child when reading, writing, or participating in any activity that requires close vision.
- Check infants and children for visual impairments, and identify children that are high-risk.
- Observe for behaviors that suggest a decrease or loss of vision.

- Promote child's optimal development and parent-child attachment.
- Identify safety hazards, and prevent injury to the eyes (helmets, safety glasses). Qs
- Reinforce information regarding laser surgery for clients who have myopia, hyperopia, or astigmatism.

CLIENT EDUCATION
- Possible corrective measures include:
  - Myopia: Biconcave lenses, contact lenses (adolescents), laser surgery (adolescents)
  - Hyperopia: Convex lenses, laser surgery
  - Astigmatism: Lenses that compensate for refractive errors, laser surgery
  - Anisometropia: Lenses that compensate for refractive errors, preferably corrective contacts, laser surgery
  - Amblyopia: Treat primary visual defect.
  - Strabismus: Occlusion therapy (patch stronger eye, remove patch 1 hr each day), laser surgery
  - Cataracts and glaucoma: Surgery

CARING FOR A CHILD WHO HAS A VISION IMPAIRMENT
- Reassure the child and family.
- Orient the child to the surroundings and provide a safe environment.
- Promote independence and meeting developmental milestones while assisting with play and socialization. Qpcc
- Assist with making referrals for educational services for visual impairment (Braille, audio tapes, special computers).
- Work with the child's school to make accommodations as needed.

Hearing impairments

Hearing impairments affect speech and the ability to clearly process linguistic sounds.

HEALTH PROMOTION AND DISEASE PREVENTION

- Screen for hearing impairments. Newborns are screened after delivery.
- Avoid hazardous noises, and wear ear protection in loud environments.

DATA COLLECTION

RISK FACTORS

- Exposure to loud environmental sounds
- Pregnancy or labor and delivery factors (anatomic malformation, maternal ingestion of toxic substances during pregnancy, perinatal asphyxia, perinatal infection)
- Chronic ear infection or ototoxic medications
- Chronic conditions (Down syndrome, cerebral palsy)

TYPES OF HEARING IMPAIRMENT

- **Conductive losses** involve interference of sound transmission, which can result from otitis media, external ear infection, foreign bodies, or excessive ear wax.
- **Sensorineural losses** involve interference of the transmission along the nerve pathways, which can result from congenital defects or secondary to acquired conditions (infection, ototoxic medication, exposure to constant noise [as in a NICU]).
- **Central auditory imperception** involves all other hearing losses related to natural causes (aphasia, agnosia [inability to interpret sounds]).

EXPECTED FINDINGS

INFANTS
- Lack of startle reflex
- Failure to respond to noise
- Absence of vocalization by 7 months
- Lack of response to the spoken word
- Failure to localize sound by 6 months

OLDER CHILDREN
- Using gestures rather than talking after 15 months
- Failure to develop understood speech by 24 months
- Yelling to express emotions
- Irritability due to inability to gain attention
- Seeming shy or withdrawn
- Inattentive to surroundings
- Speaking in monotone
- Need for repeated conversation
- Speaking loudly for situation

PATIENT-CENTERED CARE

NURSING CARE

- Check children for hearing impairment.
- Promote speech development, lip reading, and use of cued speech (hand gestures with verbal communication).
- Encourage socialization and use of aids to promote independence (flashing light when the doorbell or phone rings, telecommunication devices, closed captioning on the television).
- Assist with making a referral for child and family to community support groups.
- Use sign language or an interpreter if appropriate when working with a child who has hearing loss. Always talk to the child, not the interpreter.
- Monitor gait/balance for instability.
- Identify safety hazards and adjust environment as needed. Qs
- Assist with the use of hearing aids.
  - Store batteries in safe place.
  - If whistling sound present, turn down the volume or readjust the hearing aid in ear.
- Reinforce with families on methods to prevent further damage to hearing.

THERAPEUTIC PROCEDURES

Cochlear implants: Used for extensive hearing loss. Send impulses to the auditory nerve. Surgically implanted under skin or worn externally.

COMPLICATIONS

Delayed growth and development

Visual and hearing impairments can affect the child's speech and motor development. Identifying the impairment early can minimize this.

NURSING ACTIONS
- Encourage self-care and optimal independence.
- Assist with making interprofessional referrals as needed (social services, speech therapy, physical therapy, occupational therapy, teachers). Qtc

CLIENT EDUCATION: Assist the family to obtain and access appropriate assistive devices.

Down syndrome

- Most common chromosomal abnormality of a generalized syndrome. Trisomy 21 is seen in 92% of cases of Down syndrome.
- Many medical conditions accompany Down syndrome (congenital heart malformation, hypotonicity, dysfunction of the immune system, thyroid dysfunction, leukemia).

DATA COLLECTION

RISK FACTORS

- The cause is unclear but might be multicausal in nature.
- Maternal age greater than 35 years

EXPECTED FINDINGS

- Separated sagittal suture
- Enlarged anterior fontanel
- Small round head
- Occipital area of head flattened
- Upward, outward slant to eyes
- Small nose with depressed nasal bridge (saddle nose)
- Small ears with short pinna
- Epicanthal folds observed in ocular area
- High-arched narrow palate
- Protruding tongue
- Short, broad neck
- Shortened rib cage
- Possible congenital heart defect
- Protruding abdomen
- Incurved fifth finger (clinodactyly)
- Broad, short feet and hands with stubby toes and fingers
- Transverse palmar crease

- Large space between big and second toes with plantar crease
- Short stature
- Hyperflexibility, muscle weakness, and hypotonia
- Dry skin that cracks easily

DIAGNOSTIC PROCEDURES

PRENATAL: Testing for alpha-fetoprotein in maternal blood

INFANT: Chromosome analysis and echocardiography

CHILD: Neck x-rays prior to participation in sports

PATIENT-CENTERED CARE

NURSING CARE

- Swaddle the infant to prevent heat loss due to limp, extended body position.
- Assist family with feeding difficulties, and monitor dietary intake.
- Promote good skin care.
- Monitor developmental progress at regular intervals.
- Support family at the time of diagnosis.
- Assist with making appropriate referrals.
- Assist the parents in holding and bonding with the infant.

THERAPEUTIC PROCEDURES

Surgical interventions depend on the associated congenital anomalies. These can include cardiac defects or strabismus.

INTERPROFESSIONAL CARE

Social work, home health, school early intervention, genetic counseling, speech therapy, physical therapy, occupational therapy

NURSING ACTIONS: Listen to the concerns of the guardians and discuss ethical dilemmas regarding treatment for physical defects. Assist with providing standard postoperative care with emphasis on wound care, respiratory care, and pain management.

CLIENT EDUCATION
- Reinforce postoperative and home-care management.
- Reinforce the therapeutic plan of care.

CLIENT EDUCATION

- Aspirate nasal secretions.
- Change the infant's position frequently.
- Use feeding strategies to accommodate for the protruding tongue. A long handled spoon can be used for feeding to decrease tongue protrusion during feeding.
- Care for skin using moisturizing creams daily.
- A diet high in fiber and fluid can prevent constipation, and monitoring calorie intake can prevent obesity.

- Attend regular health care visits.
- Monitor developmental milestones.
- Monitor height and weight by plotting growth on National Center for Health Statistics or World Health Organization charts.
- Report manifestations of spinal cord compression: neck pain, loss of motor function, bladder incontinence, impaired sensations.
- Prepare for surgery for cardiac problems or strabismus if indicated.
- Evaluate eyesight and hearing frequently.
- Schedule frequent thyroid functioning tests.
- Check for atlantoaxial instability (neck pain, weakness, and torticollis).
- Perform strategies to prevent complications.

COMPLICATIONS

INTELLIGENCE: Mental capacity varies typically from mild to moderate cognitive impairment.

CONGENITAL ANOMALIES: About 40% to 45% have congenital heart disease. Other possible anomalies include hip subluxation, patella dislocation, duodenal atresia, tracheoesophageal fistula, and Hirschsprung's disease.

SENSORY PROBLEMS
- **Ocular problems** include strabismus, nystagmus, astigmatism, myopia, hyperopia, head tilt, excessive tearing, and cataracts.
- **Hearing loss** can occur due to shorter ear canals, otitis media, and impacted cerumen. Frequent otitis media, narrow canals, and impacted cerumen can contribute to the hearing problems.

OTHER PHYSICAL DISORDERS
- Frequent respiratory tract infections
- Increased incidence of leukemia
- Thyroid dysfunctions
- Cardiac deficiencies

GROWTH: Both height and weight are reduced. Weight gain is more rapid than growth in height and can result in excessive weight by 36 months.

SEXUAL DEVELOPMENT: Male (lower fertility rates) and female genitalia can be underdeveloped and delayed.

Respiratory infections

Respiratory infections are common due to decreased muscle tone and impaired drainage of mucus associated underdeveloped nasal bone.

NURSING ACTIONS
- Rinse the child's mouth with water after feeding and at other times of the day when it is dry. Mucous membranes are dry due to constant mouth breathing, which also increases the risk for respiratory infection.
- Provide cool mist humidification to moisten secretions and clearing of the nasal passages with a bulb syringe as needed.

CLIENT EDUCATION

- Increase the oral intake of fluids.
- Rinse the client's mouth after feedings.
- Use cool mist in the room to assist in moistening secretions Practice good hand hygiene. Dispose of contaminated tissues properly.
- Frequently reposition the child to promote respiratory function.
- Keep up to date with routine immunizations.
- Seek health care at the earliest indication of infection.
- Follow the antibiotic schedule if prescribed.

Active Learning Scenario

A nurse is preparing to assist with performing a visual screening test on a child. What nursing actions should the nurse include? Use the ATI Active Learning Template: Nursing Skill to complete this item.

DESCRIPTION OF SKILL: Explain the procedure.

OUTCOMES/EVALUATION: Describe findings that indicate visual impairment.

Application Exercises

1. A nurse is assisting with performing a peripheral vision test on a child. Which of the following actions should the nurse take?

   A. Place the child 10 feet away from a Snellen chart.

   B. Show a set of cards to the child one at a time.

   C. Cover the child's eye while performing the test on the other eye.

   D. Have the child focus on an object while performing the test.

2. A nurse is reinforcing teaching with a group of caregivers about possible manifestations of Down syndrome. Which of the following findings should the nurse include? (Select all that apply.)

   A. A large head with bulging fontanels

   B. Larger ears that are set back

   C. Protruding abdomen

   D. Broad, short feet and hands

   E. Hypotonia

3. A nurse is collecting data from a child who has myopia. Which of the following findings should the nurse expect? (Select all that apply.)

   A. Headaches

   B. Photophobia

   C. Difficulty reading

   D. Difficulty focusing on close objects

   E. Poor school performance

4. A nurse is collecting screening data from a toddler for possible hearing loss. Which of the following findings are indications of a hearing impairment? (Select all that apply.)

   A. Uses monotone speech

   B. Speaks loudly

   C. Repeats sentences

   D. Appears shy

   E. Is overly attentive to the surroundings

5. A nurse is reinforcing teaching with the guardian of an infant who has Down syndrome. Which of the following statements by the guardian indicates an understanding of the teaching?

   A. "I should expect him to have frequent diarrhea."

   B. "I should place a cool mist humidifier in his room."

   C. "I should avoid the use of lotion on his skin."

   D. "I should expect him to grow faster in length than other infants."

Application Exercises Key

1. A. Place the child 20 feet away from a Snellen chart when performing a visual acuity test.
    B. Show a set of cards to the child one at a time when performing a color test.
    C. Cover the child's eye while performing the test on the other eye when performing a cover test.
    D. **CORRECT:** When performing a peripheral vision test, ask the child to focus on an object while bringing a pencil into the child's peripheral vision.

    Ⓝ NCLEX® Connection: Health Promotion and Maintenance, Health Screening

2. A. A child who has hydrocephalus will exhibit a large head with bulging fontanels due to the increased CSF in the head.
    B. A child who has Down syndrome will exhibit small features (small ears with a short pinna).
    C. **CORRECT:** A child who has Down syndrome will exhibit a protruding abdomen.
    D. **CORRECT:** A child who has Down syndrome will exhibit small features (broad, short feet and hands).
    E. **CORRECT:** A child who has Down syndrome will exhibit hyperflexibility and hypotonia.

    Ⓝ NCLEX® Connection: Physiological Adaptation, Basic Pathophysiology

3. A. **CORRECT:** Headaches are a manifestation of myopia.
    B. Photophobia is a manifestation of strabismus.
    C. **CORRECT:** Difficulty reading is a manifestation of myopia.
    D. Difficulty focusing on close objects is a manifestation of hyperopia.
    E. **CORRECT:** Poor school performance is a manifestation of myopia.

    Ⓝ NCLEX® Connection: Physiological Adaptation, Basic Pathophysiology

4. A. **CORRECT:** Monotone speech is a manifestation of a hearing impairment.
    B. **CORRECT:** Speaking loudly is a manifestation of a hearing impairment.
    C. Repeating sentences is an expected developmental task for a toddler.
    D. **CORRECT:** Shyness and withdrawn behavior are manifestations of a hearing impairment.
    E. Inattentiveness to surroundings is a manifestation of a hearing impairment.

    Ⓝ NCLEX® Connection: Reduction of Risk Potential, Potential for Complications of Diagnostic Test/Treatments/Procedures

5. A. Reinforce with the guardian that Down syndrome increases the risk for constipation, resulting in the need for additional fluid and fiber in the diet.
    B. **CORRECT:** Reinforce with the guardian that Down syndrome increases the risk for respiratory infections. Using a cool mist humidifier in the infant's room helps prevent respiratory infections.
    C. Reinforce with the guardian that Down syndrome causes the infant to have dry skin that cracks easily. The guardian should practice good skin care, including the application of lotion.
    D. Reinforce with the guardian that Down syndrome results in reduced growth in length for infants and height for children.

    Ⓝ NCLEX® Connection: Physiological Adaptation, Alterations in Body Systems

Active Learning Scenario Key

Using the ATI Active Learning Template: Nursing Skill

DESCRIPTION OF SKILL
- Choose appropriate chart: Snellen Letter, tumbling E, or picture chart.
- Place child 20 feet from the chart with heels on the 20-foot mark.
- Screen child wearing glasses, if appropriate.
- Child keeps both eyes open and covers one eye.
- First have the child start at the bottom and read each line, continuing up until the child can pass a line.
- Then, have the child start at the top and move down until the child can no longer pass a line.
- To pass, the child needs to identify four of the six characters correctly.
- Repeat the procedure with the other eye.

OUTCOMES/EVALUATION
- Partial visual impairment is classified as visual acuity of 20/70 to 20/200.
- Legal blindness is classified as visual acuity of 20/200 or worse or a visual field of 20 degrees or less in the child's better eye.

Ⓝ NCLEX® Connection: Health Promotion and Maintenance, Health Promotion and Disease Prevention

When reviewing the following chapters, keep in mind the relevant topics and tasks of the NCLEX outline, in particular:

Pharmacological Therapies

EXPECTED ACTIONS/OUTCOMES
Apply knowledge of pathophysiology when addressing client pharmacological agents.

Reinforce education to client regarding medications.

Reduction of Risk Potential

DIAGNOSTIC TESTS: Perform diagnostic testing.

POTENTIAL FOR COMPLICATIONS OF DIAGNOSTIC TESTS/TREATMENTS/PROCEDURES: Evaluate client oxygen (O_2) saturation.

POTENTIAL FOR COMPLICATIONS FROM SURGICAL PROCEDURES AND HEALTH ALTERATIONS: Identify client response to surgery or health alterations.

THERAPEUTIC PROCEDURES: Reinforce client teaching on treatments and procedures.

Physiological Adaptation

ALTERATIONS IN BODY SYSTEMS
Intervene to improve client respiratory status.

Reinforce education to the client regarding care and condition.

BASIC PATHOPHYSIOLOGY
Identify signs and symptoms related to an acute or chronic illness.

Consider general principles of client disease process when providing care.

Apply knowledge of pathophysiology to monitoring client for alterations in body systems.

UNIT 2   SYSTEM DISORDERS
SECTION: RESPIRATORY DISORDERS

CHAPTER 15 *Oxygen and Inhalation Therapy*

Oxygen is used to maintain adequate cellular oxygenation. It is used in the treatment of many acute and chronic respiratory problems (hypoxemia, cystic fibrosis, asthma). Supplemental oxygen can be delivered using a variety of methods, depending on individual circumstances.

Pulse oximetry is used to monitor the effectiveness of inhalation therapies.

Common treatment methods for children who have respiratory issues (acute or chronic) are nebulized aerosol therapy, metered-dose inhaler (MDI), dry powder inhaler (DPI), chest physiotherapy (CPT), oxygen therapy, suctioning, and artificial airway.

Pulse oximetry

- Pulse oximetry is a noninvasive measurement of the oxygen saturation (SaO_2) of arterial blood.
- A pulse oximeter is a device that is operated by battery or electricity and has a sensor probe that is attached securely to the child's fingertip, toe, earlobe, or around the foot with a clip or band.

INDICATIONS

Pulse oximetry is used for a variety of situations in which quick data collection of a child's respiratory status is needed.

CONSIDERATIONS

PREPROCEDURE NURSING ACTIONS

- Find an appropriate probe site. The probe site must be dry and have adequate circulation. Remove polish from nails or remove earrings if using the earlobe.
- Be sure the child is in a comfortable position and that the arm is supported if a finger is used as a probe site.

INTRAPROCEDURE NURSING ACTIONS

- Note the pulse reading and compare it with the child's radial pulse. Any discrepancy between the values warrants further data collection.
- If continuous monitoring is required, make sure the alarms are set for a low and a high limit, the alarms are functioning, and the sound is audible. Move the probe every 4 to 8 hr or per facility policy to prevent pressure necrosis in infants who have disrupted skin integrity or poor perfusion.

POSTPROCEDURE NURSING ACTIONS

Report unexpected findings to the provider.

If a child's SaO_2 is less than the expected range (usually 90% to 92%) Qs

- Confirm that the sensor probe is properly placed with the light-emitting diode (LED) placed on the top of the nail when digits are used.
- Confirm that the oxygen delivery system is functioning and that the child is receiving the prescribed oxygen flow rate. Increase oxygen rate as prescribed.
- Place the child in a semi-Fowler's or Fowler's position to maximize ventilation.
- Encourage deep breathing.
- Report significant findings to the provider.
- Remain with the child and provide emotional support to decrease anxiety.

INTERPRETATION OF FINDINGS

- The expected reference range for SaO_2 is 95% to 100%. Acceptable levels can range from 91% to 100%. Some illnesses can allow for a SaO_2 of 85% to 89%.
- Results less than 91% require nursing intervention to assist the child to regain acceptable SaO_2 levels. A SaO_2 of less than 86% is a life-threatening emergency. The lower the SaO_2 level, the less accurate the value.

Nebulized aerosol therapy

The process of nebulization breaks up medications into minute particles that are then dispersed throughout the respiratory tract. These droplets are much finer than those created by inhalers.

INDICATIONS

Respiratory conditions that necessitate bronchodilators, corticosteroids, mucolytics, or antibiotics

CONSIDERATIONS

PREPARATION OF THE CLIENT

- Instruct the child and family that the treatment can take 10 to 15 min.
- Determine if the child should use a mouthpiece, mask, or blow-by.
- Collect preprocedure collection of data, including vital signs and oxygen saturation.
- Pour the medication into the small container and attach the device to an air or oxygen source.

ONGOING CARE

- Encourage the child to take slow, deep breaths by mouth.
- Monitor the child during the treatment, watching carefully for indications of local tracheal or bronchial effects (spasms, edema).
- Check vital signs, oxygen saturation, and lung sounds at the completion of treatment.
- Assist the family with obtaining a nebulizer for home use if needed.
- Reinforce recommendations for aerosolized medications.
- Monitor for adverse reactions to medications.

CLIENT EDUCATION

- Reinforce with the family how to operate a home nebulizer.
- Reinforce with the family about adverse effects of the prescribed medications.

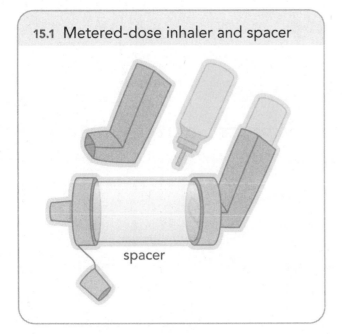

15.1 Metered-dose inhaler and spacer

spacer

Metered-dose inhaler or dry powder inhaler

These are handheld devices that allow children to self-administer medications on an intermittent basis. **(15.1)**

INDICATIONS

Respiratory conditions that necessitate bronchodilators or corticosteroids

CONSIDERATIONS

Provide instructions to the child and parents for use of an MDI

- Remove the cap from the inhaler.
- Shake the inhaler five to six times.
- Attach the spacer. (Encourage a spacer for children to facilitate proper inhalation of the medication.)
- Hold the inhaler with the mouthpiece at the bottom.
- Hold the inhaler with the thumb near the mouthpiece, and the index and middle fingers at the top.
- Instruct the child on an MDI placement technique.
  - **Open-mouth method:** Hold the inhaler approximately 3 to 4 cm (1.2 to 1.6 in) away from the front of the mouth.
  - **Closed-mouth method:** Place the inhaler between the lips and instruct the child to form a seal around the MDI.
- Take a deep breath and then exhale.
- Tilt the head back slightly, and press the inhaler. While pressing the inhaler, begin a slow, deep breath that lasts for 3 to 5 seconds to facilitate delivery to the air passages.
- Hold the breath for approximately 5 to 10 seconds to allow the medication to deposit in the airways.
- If an additional puff is needed, wait 1 min between puffs.
- Take the inhaler out of the mouth and slowly exhale through the nose.
- Resume normal breathing.

Provide instructions to the child and parents for the use of a DPI

- Do not shake the device.
- Take the cover off the mouthpiece.
- Follow the directions of the manufacturer for preparing the medication (turning the wheel of the inhaler).
- Exhale completely.
- Place the mouthpiece between the lips and take a deep breath through the mouth.
- Hold breath for 5 to 10 seconds.
- Take the inhaler out of the mouth and slowly exhale through pursed lips.
- Resume normal breathing.
- If more than one puff is prescribed, wait the length of time directed before administering the second puff.
- Remove the canister and rinse the inhaler, cap, and spacer once a day with warm running water. Dry the inhaler before reuse.

COMPLICATIONS

Improper medication dosage related to improper use

- Inhalation is too rapid.
- Inability to coordinate inhalation with spray.
- Not holding breath for adequate period.

NURSING ACTIONS: Ensure the child uses the inhaler with proper technique.

CLIENT EDUCATION: Reinforce proper technique with client and family.

Fungal infections

Fungal infections of the oral cavity can occur with corticosteroid use.

NURSING ACTIONS

- Check mouth for manifestations of infections.
- Assist the child with rinsing their mouth after administration.

CLIENT EDUCATION: Reinforce with the child and guardians to clean the MDI and spacer after each use and to have the child rinse out the mouth and expectorate. ○Pcc

Chest physiotherapy

Chest physiotherapy is a set of techniques that includes manual or mechanical percussion, vibration, cough, forceful expiration (or huffing), and breathing exercises, which are generally performed by a respiratory therapist. Gravity and positioning loosen respiratory secretions and move them into the central airways, where they can be eliminated by coughing or suctioning to rid excessive secretions from specific areas of the lungs.

INDICATIONS

CLIENT PRESENTATION: Thick secretions with an inability to clear the airway

CONTRAINDICATION: Decreased cardiac reserves, pulmonary embolism, or increased intracranial pressure

CONSIDERATIONS

PREPROCEDURE NURSING ACTIONS

- Schedule treatments before meals or at least 1 hr after meals and at bedtime to decrease the likelihood of vomiting or aspirating.
- Administer a bronchodilator medication or nebulizer treatment prior to postural drainage if prescribed.

INTRAPROCEDURE NURSING ACTIONS

- Perform hand hygiene, provide privacy, and explain the procedure to the child and parents.
- Ensure proper positioning to promote drainage of specific areas of the lungs.
  - **Apical sections of the upper lobes:** Fowler's position
  - **Posterior sections of the upper lobes:** Sitting position with child leaning forward curled over pillows
  - **Anterior segments of both upper lobes:** Supine and rotated slightly away from side being drained
  - **Superior segments of both lower lobes:** Prone with hips elevated on pillows.
- Apply manual percussion by using cupped hand or a special device to clap rhythmically on the chest wall to break up secretions.
- Electronic percussion is applied by a vest device worn by the child.
- Have the child remain in each postural drainage position for 20 to 30 min to allow time for percussion, vibration, and postural drainage. Older children can tolerate longer periods.
- Individualize the position used and the duration and frequency of treatment.
- Discontinue the procedure if the child reports faintness or dizziness.

POSTPROCEDURE NURSING ACTIONS

- Perform lung auscultation and check the amount, color, and character of the expectorated secretions.
- Document interventions and repeat the procedure as prescribed (typically three or four times per day).

Oxygen therapy

- Oxygen therapy increases the oxygen concentration of the air that is being breathed.
- Oxygen can be delivered via nasal cannula, face mask, face tent, CPAP, BiPAP, tent, hood, or mechanical ventilator. (15.2)
- Humidification of oxygen moistens the airways, which promotes loosening and mobilization of pulmonary secretions and prevents drying and injury of respiratory structures.
- While the client is receiving oxygen, continue to monitor vital signs, including SaO_2 for changes, and intervene as needed.

INDICATIONS

Hypoxemia

Hypoxemia develops when there is an inadequate level of oxygen in the blood. Hypovolemia, hypoventilation, and interruption of arterial flow can lead to hypoxemia.

EARLY MANIFESTATIONS
- Tachypnea
- Tachycardia
- Restlessness
- Pallor of the skin and mucous membranes
- Evidence of respiratory distress (use of accessory muscles, nasal flaring, tracheal tugging, adventitious lung sounds)

LATE MANIFESTATIONS
- Confusion and stupor
- Cyanosis of skin and mucous membranes
- Bradypnea
- Bradycardia
- Hypotension or hypertension

CONSIDERATIONS

PREPARATION OF THE CLIENT
- Warm oxygen to prevent hypothermia.
- Use a calm, nonthreatening approach.
- Reinforce all procedures to the child and parents.
- Place the client in semi-Fowler's or Fowler's position to facilitate breathing and to promote chest expansion.
- Ensure that equipment is working properly.

ONGOING CARE
- Provide oxygen therapy at the lowest liter flow that corrects hypoxemia.
- Check/monitor lung sounds and respiratory rate, rhythm, and effort to determine the need for supplemental oxygen.
- Do not allow oxygen to blow directly onto infants' faces.
- Change linens and clothing frequently.
- Monitor the child's temperature closely in an oxygen tent for hypothermia.
- Check/monitor oxygenation status with pulse oximetry and ABGs.

- Apply the oxygen delivery device prescribed.
- Provide oral hygiene as needed.
- Promote turning, coughing, deep breathing, and use of incentive spirometry and suctioning.
- Promote rest and decrease environmental stimuli.
- Provide emotional support for children who appear anxious.
- Collect data about nutritional status and provide supplements as prescribed.
- Check/monitor skin integrity closely for pressure injuries. Move devices and inspect the skin several times daily. Provide moisture and pressure-relief devices as indicated.
- Check/monitor and document response to oxygen therapy.
- Monitor oxygen saturations to maintain the prescribed oxygen saturation.
- Discontinue oxygen gradually.

COMPLICATIONS

Combustion

Oxygen is combustible. Qs

NURSING ACTIONS
- Place "No Smoking" or "Oxygen in Use" signs to alert others of the combustion hazard.
- Know where the closest fire extinguisher is located.
- Have the child wear a cotton gown, because synthetics or wools can create sparks of static electricity.
- Ensure that all electric machinery (monitors, suction machines) are grounded.
- Avoid toys that can induce a spark.
- Do not use volatile, flammable materials (alcohol, acetone) near children who are receiving oxygen.
- Educate the child and others about the fire hazards of smoking with oxygen use. Qpcc

---

15.2 Oxygen therapy delivery systems

DELIVERY SYSTEM	NURSING ACTIONS
Oxygen hood Small plastic hood that fits over the infant's head	• Ensure that neck, chin, or shoulders do not rub against the hood. • Secure a pulse oximeter for continuous SaO₂ monitoring.
Nasal cannula Disposable plastic tube with two prongs for insertion into the nostrils that delivers an oxygen concentrations of 24% to 40% FiO₂ at a flow rate of 1 to 6 L/min	• Nasal cannulas are safe, easy to apply, and well tolerated. • The child is able to eat, talk, and ambulate while wearing a cannula. • Cannulas can be used by infants and older children who are cooperative. • Check the patency of the nares. • Ensure that the prongs fit in the nares properly. • A nasal cannula can cause skin breakdown and dry mucous membranes. • Supply the child with a water-soluble gel if the nares are dry. • Provide humidification for flow rates greater than 4 L/min. • Prongs can become dislodged easily. Monitor the child frequently.
Pediatric face mask Pediatric-size mask that covers the nose and mouth	• Used for short-term therapy. • Used at a flow rate of 5 to 10 L/min to minimize carbon dioxide rebreathing. • Face masks require a snug fit and might not be tolerated. • Used for supplying high oxygen flow rate or for children who are mouth breathers.

Oxygen toxicity

- Oxygen toxicity can result from high concentrations of oxygen, long duration of oxygen therapy, and the child's degree of lung disease.
- Hypoventilation and increased $PaCO_2$ levels allow for rapid progression into unconscious state.

MANIFESTATIONS: Nonproductive cough, substernal pain, nasal stuffiness, nausea, vomiting, fatigue, headache, sore throat, and hypoventilation

NURSING ACTIONS

- Use the lowest level of oxygen necessary to maintain an adequate SaO_2.
- Monitor ABGs and notify the provider if $PaCO_2$ levels rise outside of the expected reference range.
- Decrease the oxygen flow rate gradually.

Suctioning

Suctioning can be accomplished orally, nasally, endotracheally, or through a tracheostomy tube.

INDICATIONS

To remove mucus plugs and excessive secretions

CLIENT PRESENTATION: Early manifestations of hypoxemia (restlessness, tachypnea, tachycardia, decreased SaO_2 levels, adventitious breath sounds, visualization of secretions, cyanosis, absence of spontaneous cough)

CONSIDERATIONS

Nasal suctioning

- Use clean technique.
- Use a mushroom tip catheter.

Oral suctioning

- Use clean technique.
- Use a hard catheter tip.
- Insert in sides of mouth.

Endotracheal and tracheal suctioning

PREPROCEDURE NURSING ACTIONS

- Perform hand hygiene, provide privacy, and explain the procedure to the child.
- Don the required personal protective equipment. Assist the child to a high-Fowler's or Fowler's position for suctioning if possible.
- Perform through a tracheostomy or an endotracheal tube. Select a catheter with a diameter one half the diameter of the tracheostomy tube.
- Ask for assistance if necessary.
- Hyperoxygenate and hyperventilate the child using a bag-valve-mask resuscitator or specialized ventilator function with an FiO_2 of 100%.
- Monitor breath sounds and vital signs, including oxygen saturation (SaO_2) by pulse oximeter. Oxygen saturation should be monitored continually during the procedure.

INTRAPROCEDURE NURSING ACTIONS

- Use correct surgical aseptic technique as identified in appropriate resources.
- Maintain ongoing collection of data of oxygen status while performing the procedure.
- Limit suction time to less than 5 seconds for infants and less than 10 seconds for children.
- Allow the child to rest 30 to 60 seconds after each aspiration for oxygen saturation to return to normal.

POSTPROCEDURE NURSING ACTIONS: Document the child's response.

COMPLICATIONS

Hypoxia

NURSING ACTIONS

- Stop the procedure.
- Hyperoxygenate the child.

Artificial airways

- A tracheotomy is a sterile surgical incision into the trachea through the skin and muscles for the purpose of establishing an airway.
- A tracheotomy can be performed as an emergency procedure for epiglottitis, croup, or foreign-body aspiration, or as a scheduled surgical procedure.
- A tracheostomy is the stoma/opening that results from a tracheotomy to provide and secure a patent airway. A tracheostomy can be permanent or temporary.
- Artificial airways can be placed orotracheally, nasotracheally, or through a tracheostomy to assist with respiration.
- Pediatric tracheostomy tubes made of plastic and/or with a cuff to prevent dislodgement.

INDICATIONS

CLIENT PRESENTATION: Obstruction of the upper airway requiring the use of artificial ventilation

CONSIDERATIONS

- Check/monitor:
  - Oxygenation, ventilation (respiratory rate, effort, SaO_2), and vital signs hourly.
  - Thickness, quantity, odor, and color of mucous secretions.
  - The stoma and skin surrounding the stoma for manifestations of inflammation or infection (redness, swelling, or drainage).
- Provide adequate humidification and hydration to thin secretions and decrease the risk of mucus plugging.
- Suction only as often as necessary to maintain patency of the tube. Do not suction routinely. This can cause mucosal damage, bleeding, and bronchospasm.
- Check/monitor the need for suctioning. Suction as necessary when checking for findings that indicate the need to do so (audible/noisy secretions, crackles, restlessness, tachypnea, tachycardia, and mucus in the airway).

- Maintain surgical aseptic technique when suctioning to prevent infection.
- Provide emotional support to the child and guardians.
- Provide oral hygiene every 2 hr.
- Provide tracheostomy care as indicated by the provider.
- Check ties frequently and change if soiled.
- Keep an emergency tracheostomy tube (one size smaller) at the bedside.

CLIENT EDUCATION

- Provide reinforcement of discharge teaching regarding the following.
  - Tracheostomy care
  - Monitor skin at the tracheostomy site for drainage or breakdown. This area should be cleaned with soap and water.
  - Findings that the family should immediately report to the provider (manifestations of infection or copious secretions)
  - Ways to promote improved nutrition
- Provide written material for parents to reinforce instructions. Qᴘᴄᴄ

COMPLICATIONS

Accidental decannulation

Accidental decannulation or dislodgement in the first 72 hr after surgery is an emergency because the tracheostomy tract has not matured and replacement can be difficult.

NURSING ACTIONS: Keep a new tube and obturator at the bedside.

CLIENT EDUCATION: Ensure that tracheostomy is tied or secured properly.

Occlusion

Occlusion is a situation in which the tube is clogged with secretions and prevents adequate air exchange.

NURSING ACTIONS: Maintain a patent airway with suctioning.

CLIENT EDUCATION: Suction to prevent occlusion.

Active Learning Scenario

A nurse is reinforcing teaching with a child how to use a metered-dose inhaler. What information should be included? Use the ATI Active Learning Template: Nursing Skill to complete this item.

DESCRIPTION OF SKILL: Outline the steps for using a metered-dose inhaler.

Application Exercises

1. A nurse is reinforcing teaching with an adolescent to self-administer a corticosteroid medication using a metered-dose inhaler (MDI). Which of the following instructions should the nurse include? (Select all that apply.)
   A. Shake the device prior to use.
   B. Rinse and expectorate after administration.
   C. Inhale slowly with medication administration.
   D. Exhale quickly after medication administration.
   E. Wait 30 seconds between puffs.

2. A nurse caring for a child who is receiving oxygen therapy and is on a continuous oxygen saturation monitor that is reading 89%. Which of the following actions should the nurse take first?
   A. Increase the oxygen flow rate.
   B. Encourage the child to take deep breaths.
   C. Ensure proper placement of the sensor probe.
   D. Place the child in the Fowler's position.

3. A nurse is collecting data from an infant who has a respiratory infection. Which of the following findings is an early indication of acute hypoxemia?
   A. Nonproductive cough
   B. Hypoventilation
   C. Tachypnea
   D. Nasal stuffiness

4. A nurse is caring for a child who is receiving oxygen. Which of the following findings indicates oxygen toxicity?
   A. Increased blood pressure
   B. Hyperventilation
   C. Decreased $PaCO_2$
   D. Unconsciousness

5. A nurse is caring for a child who is receiving a bronchodilator medication by nebulized aerosol therapy. Which of the following actions should the nurse take? (Select all that apply.)
   A. Instruct the child that the treatment will last 30 min.
   B. Obtain vital signs prior to the procedure.
   C. Tell the child to take slow deep breaths.
   D. Determine if the child should use a mask.
   E. Attach the device to an air source.

Application Exercises Key

1. A. **CORRECT:** MDIs require shaking for 3 to 4 seconds prior to use to aerosolize the medication.
   B. **CORRECT:** Corticosteroids can cause an oral fungal infection. The client should rinse and expectorate following medication administration.
   C. **CORRECT:** The client should breathe in slowly (about 3 to 5 seconds) to administer the medication into the lungs.
   D. After inhalation of the medication, the client should hold their breath for 5 to 10 seconds.
   E. The client should wait 1 min between puffs.

Ⓝ *NCLEX® Connection: Pharmacological Therapies, Medication Administration*

2. A. Increasing the oxygen flow rate for a child who has an oxygen saturation of 89% is important, but is not the priority.
   B. Encouraging the child to take deep breaths to increase oxygenation is important, but is not the priority.
   C. **CORRECT:** The first action to take using the nursing process approach is to collect data. Ensuring the sensor probe is properly placed is the nurse's priority action.
   D. Placing the child in Fowler's position to increase oxygenation is important, but is not the priority.

Ⓝ *NCLEX® Connection: Physiological Adaptation, Alterations in Body Systems*

3. A. Nonproductive cough is a manifestation of a respiratory infection.
   B. Hypoventilation is a manifestation of oxygen toxicity.
   C. **CORRECT:** Tachypnea is an early indication of hypoxemia in an infant.
   D. Nasal stuffiness is a manifestation of a respiratory infection.

Ⓝ *NCLEX® Connection: Physiological Adaptation, Basic Pathophysiology*

4. A. Increased blood pressure is not a manifestation of oxygen toxicity.
   B. Hypoventilation is a manifestation of oxygen toxicity.
   C. An increased $PaCO_2$ is a manifestation of oxygen toxicity.
   D. **CORRECT:** Children who exhibit oxygen toxicity progress into an unconscious state rapidly.

Ⓝ *NCLEX® Connection: Physiological Adaptation, Unexpected Response to Therapies*

5. A. Nebulized medications take approximately 10 to 15 min to deliver.
   B. **CORRECT:** Baseline vital signs should be obtain prior to a nebulized medication for purposes of comparison with how the client tolerates the medication.
   C. **CORRECT:** The client should take slow, deep breaths to inhale the medication deeply into the respiratory tract.
   D. **CORRECT:** Nebulized medications can be delivered by mask, mouthpiece, or blow-by. Determine the best method of delivery.
   E. **CORRECT:** Nebulized medications need to have an air source to break the medication into small particles for inhalation.

Ⓝ *NCLEX® Connection: Pharmacological Therapies, Medication Administration*

Active Learning Scenario Key

Using the ATI Active Learning Template: Nursing Skill

DESCRIPTION OF SKILL

- Remove the cap from the inhaler
- Shake the inhaler five to six times.
- Attach the spacer. (A spacer should be encouraged for children to facilitate proper inhalation of the medication.)
- Hold the inhaler with the mouthpiece at the bottom.
- Hold the inhaler with the thumb near the mouthpiece and the index and middle fingers at the top.
  - Open-mouth technique: Hold the inhaler approximately 3 to 4 cm (1.2 to 1.6 in) away from the front of the mouth.
  - Closed-mouth method: Place the inhaler between the lips and instruct the child to form a seal around the inhaler.
- Take a deep breath and then exhale.
- Tilt the head back slightly, and press the inhaler. While pressing the inhaler, begin a slow, deep breath that lasts for 3 to 5 seconds to facilitate delivery to the air passages.
- Hold the breath for approximately 5 to 10 seconds to allow the medication to deposit in the airways.
- If an additional puff is needed, wait 1 min between puffs.
- Take the inhaler out of the mouth and slowly exhale through the nose.
- Resume normal breathing.

Ⓝ *NCLEX® Connection: Pharmacological Therapies, Medication Administration*

UNIT 2 **SYSTEM DISORDERS**
SECTION: RESPIRATORY DISORDERS

CHAPTER 16 *Acute and Infectious Respiratory Illnesses*

Acute and infectious respiratory illnesses prevalent in children include tonsillitis, nasopharyngitis, pharyngitis, croup syndromes, bacterial tracheitis, bronchitis, bronchiolitis, allergic rhinitis, and pneumonia.

Tonsillitis and tonsillectomy

Tonsils are masses of lymph-type tissue found in the pharyngeal area. They filter pathogenic organisms (viral and bacterial), which helps to protect the respiratory and gastrointestinal tracts. In addition, they contribute to antibody formation.

Tonsils are highly vascular, which helps them to protect against infection because foreign materials (viral or bacterial organisms), enter the body through the mouth.

Palatine tonsils are located on both sides of the oropharynx. These are the tonsils removed during a tonsillectomy.

Pharyngeal tonsils, also known as the adenoids, are removed during an adenoidectomy.

Enlarged tonsils
- In some instances, enlarged tonsils can block the nose and throat. This can interfere with breathing, nasal and sinus drainage, sleeping, swallowing, and speaking.
- Enlarged tonsils also can disrupt the function of the Eustachian tube, which can cause otitis media or impede hearing.

Acute tonsillitis occurs when the tonsils become inflamed and reddened. Acute tonsillitis can become chronic.

DATA COLLECTION

RISK FACTORS
- Exposure to a viral or bacterial agent
- Immature immune systems (younger children)

EXPECTED FINDINGS
- Report of sore throat with difficulty swallowing
- History of otitis media and hearing difficulties

PHYSICAL FINDINGS
- Mouth odor
- Mouth breathing
- Snoring
- Nasal qualities in the voice
- Fever
- Tonsil inflammation with redness and edema
- Difficulty swallowing or eating

LABORATORY TESTS

Throat culture for group A beta-hemolytic streptococci (GABHS)

PATIENT-CENTERED CARE

NURSING CARE

Tonsillitis
- Provide treatment for manifestations of viral tonsillitis (rest, warm fluids, warm salt-water gargles).
- Administer antibiotic therapy as prescribed for bacterial tonsillitis.

MEDICATIONS

Antipyretics/analgesics: acetaminophen

Hydrocodone is indicated for the child having difficulty drinking fluids.

Antipyretics

Decrease fever and manage pain

NURSING ACTIONS: Be aware of allergies.

CLIENT EDUCATION: Reinforce the appropriate dosing for acetaminophen and ibuprofen.

Antibiotics

For treatment of GABHS infection

NURSING ACTIONS: Be aware of allergies.

CLIENT EDUCATION: Reinforce with the guardians to administer antibiotics for the full course of treatment.

THERAPEUTIC PROCEDURES

Tonsillectomy and/or adenoidectomy

PREOPERATIVE NURSING ACTIONS: Maintain NPO status.

POSTOPERATIVE NURSING ACTIONS
- Positioning
  - Place in position to facilitate drainage.
  - Elevate head of bed when child is fully awake.
- Data collection
  - Check for evidence of bleeding, which includes frequent swallowing, clearing the throat, restlessness, bright red emesis, tachycardia, and/or pallor.
  - Check the airway and vital signs.
  - Monitor for difficulty breathing related to oral secretions, edema, and/or bleeding.
- Comfort measures
  - Administer liquid analgesics or tetracaine lollipops as prescribed.
  - Provide an ice collar.
  - Avoid administering codeine postoperatively.
  - Offer ice chips or sips of water to keep throat moist.
  - Administer pain medication on a regular schedule.

- Diet
  - Encourage clear liquids and fluids after a return of the gag reflex, avoiding red-colored liquids, citrus juice, and milk-based foods initially.
  - Advance the diet with soft, bland foods.
- Instruction
  - Discourage coughing, throat clearing, and nose blowing in order to protect the surgical site.
  - Avoid straws, as they can damage the surgical site.
  - Alert guardians that there can be clots or blood-tinged mucus in vomitus.

CLIENT EDUCATION

- Notify the provider if bright red bleeding occurs.
- Get plenty of rest.

CLIENT EDUCATION

- Contact the provider if the child experiences difficulty breathing, lack of oral intake, increase in pain, and/or indications of infection.
- Ensure that the child does not put objects in the mouth.
- Administer pain medications for discomfort.
- Intake plenty of fluids, advance to a soft diet, and avoid foods that are irritating or highly seasoned.
- Limit activity to decrease the potential for bleeding.
- Full recovery usually occurs in approximately 14 days.
- Observe for manifestations of hemorrhage, dehydration, and infection, and notify the provider if necessary.

COMPLICATIONS

Hemorrhage

NURSING ACTIONS
- Use a good light source and possibly a tongue depressor to directly observe the throat.
- Check for findings of bleeding (tachycardia, repeated swallowing and clearing of throat, hemoptysis). Hypotension is a late manifestation of shock.
- Contact the provider immediately if there is any indication of bleeding.

CLIENT EDUCATION: Instruct family to report indications of bleeding (frequent swallowing, clearing the throat, restlessness, bright red emesis, tachycardia, pallor).

Dehydration

NURSING ACTIONS
- Encourage oral fluids.
- Monitor I&O.

CLIENT EDUCATION
- Increase intake of oral fluids.
- Observe for manifestations of dehydration.

Chronic infection

Chronically infected tonsils with GABHS can pose a potential threat to other parts of the body. Some children who frequently have tonsillitis can develop other diseases (rheumatic fever and kidney infection).

CLIENT EDUCATION: Seek medical attention when the child presents with manifestations of tonsillitis.

Common respiratory illnesses

Disorders can affect both the upper (oronasopharynx, pharynx, larynx, and upper part of the trachea) and lower (bronchi, bronchioles, and alveoli) respiratory tracts. Infections of the respiratory tract can affect more than one area.

The information in this section is applicable to a range of common respiratory illnesses.

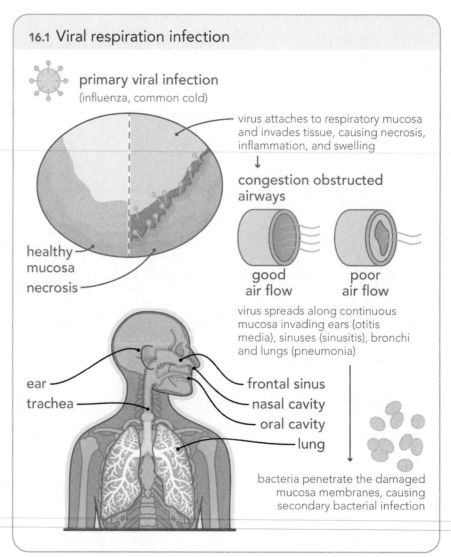

16.1 Viral respiration infection

primary viral infection
(influenza, common cold)

virus attaches to respiratory mucosa and invades tissue, causing necrosis, inflammation, and swelling

congestion obstructed airways

good air flow   poor air flow

healthy mucosa
necrosis

virus spreads along continuous mucosa invading ears (otitis media), sinuses (sinusitis), bronchi and lungs (pneumonia)

ear
trachea

frontal sinus
nasal cavity
oral cavity
lung

bacteria penetrate the damaged mucosa membranes, causing secondary bacterial infection

DATA COLLECTION

RISK FACTORS

Age
- Infants between 3 and 6 months of age are at increased risk due to the decrease of maternal antibodies acquired at birth and the lack of antibody protection.
- Viral infections are more common in toddlers and preschoolers. The incidence of these infections decreases by age 5.
- Certain viral agents can cause serious illness during infancy, but only cause a mild illness in older children.

Anatomy
- A short, narrow airway can become easily obstructed with mucus or edema.
- A short respiratory tract allows infections to travel quickly to the lower airways.
- Infectious agents have easy access to the middle ear through the short and open Eustachian tubes of infants and young children.

Decreased resistance
- Compromised immune system
- Anemia
- Nutritional deficiencies
- Allergies
- Chronic medical conditions (asthma, cystic fibrosis, chronic lung disease, cardiac anomalies)
- Exposure to second-hand smoke

Seasonal variables
- Children who have asthma have a greater incidence of respiratory infections during cold weather.
- Respiratory syncytial virus (RSV) and other common respiratory infections are more common during the winter and spring.
- Infections caused by *Mycoplasma pneumoniae* are more frequent during autumn and early winter.

EXPECTED FINDINGS

- Nursing history that includes recent infections, medications taken, immunization status, and family coping
- Reports of sore throat, decreased activity level, chest pain, fatigue, difficulty breathing, shortness of breath, cough, and decreased appetite

LABORATORY TESTS

Throat culture or rapid antigen testing to rule out GABHS infection

PATIENT-CENTERED CARE

NURSING CARE

- Closely monitor progression of illness and ensuing respiratory distress. Observe for increased heart and respiratory rate, retractions, nasal flaring, and restlessness.
- Make emergency equipment for intubation readily accessible.
- Position the child to have optimal ventilation without increasing distress that would contribute to increasing respiratory distress.
- Implement isolation precautions as indicated.

CLIENT EDUCATION

- Use a cool-air vaporizer to provide humidity.
- Rest during febrile illness.
- Maintain adequate fluid intake. Infants can be given commercially prepared oral rehydration solutions, and older children can be given sports drinks.
- Administer medications using accurate dosages and appropriate time intervals.
- Develop strategies to decrease the spread of infection. Strategies include performing good hand hygiene; covering the nose and mouth with tissues when sneezing and coughing; properly disposing of tissues; not sharing cups, eating utensils, and towels; and keeping infected children from contact with children who are well.
- Seek further medical attention for the child if manifestations worsen or respiratory distress occurs.

Nasopharyngitis

Also known as the common cold: Self-limiting virus that persists for 10 to 14 days.

DATA COLLECTION

EXPECTED FINDINGS

- Nasal inflammation, dryness and irritation of nasal passages and the pharynx
- Fever, decreased appetite, and restlessness

PATIENT-CENTERED CARE

NURSING CARE

Instruct guardians about home management.
- Give antipyretic for fever.
- Encourage rest.
- Provide vaporized air (cool mist).
- Give decongestants for children older than 6 years.
- Give cough suppressants with caution (avoid over sedation).
- Antihistamines are not recommended.
- Antibiotics are not indicated.

Acute streptococcal pharyngitis

GABHS: Infection of the upper airway (strep throat)

DATA COLLECTION

EXPECTED FINDINGS

- Onset is abrupt and characterized by pharyngitis, headache, fever, and abdominal pain.
- Tonsils and pharynx can be inflamed and covered with exudate, usually appears by second day of illness.

LABORATORY TESTS

Throat culture or rapid antigen testing to determine GABHS infection

PATIENT-CENTERED CARE

NURSING CARE

- Administer antibiotics as prescribed.
  - Oral penicillin in a dose sufficient to control the acute local manifestations and is administered for at least 10 days.
  - Amoxicillin once a day for 10 days is also effective
  - IM penicillin G benzathine is also appropriate.
  - Oral erythromycin for children allergic to penicillin.
- Administer antipyretics for fever.
- Clarithromycin, azithromycin, clindamycin, oral cephalosporins, and amoxicillin with clavulanic acid are also effective to treat GABHS.

Bronchitis (tracheobronchitis)

- Associated with an upper respiratory infection and inflammation of large airways
- Self-limiting

DATA COLLECTION

EXPECTED FINDINGS

- Persistent dry, hacking cough as a result of inflammation
- Resolves in 5 to 10 days

LABORATORY TESTS

Test nasopharyngeal secretions

PATIENT-CENTERED CARE

NURSING CARE

Instruct guardians about home management.
- Give antipyretics for fever.
- Give a cough suppressant.
- Provide increased humidity (cool mist vaporizer).

Bronchiolitis

- Mostly caused by Respiratory Syncytial Virus (RSV)
- Primarily affects the bronchi and bronchioles
- Occurs at the bronchiolar level

DATA COLLECTION

EXPECTED FINDINGS

INITIALLY: Rhinorrhea, intermittent fever, pharyngitis, coughing, sneezing, wheezing, possible ear or eye infection

WITH ILLNESS PROGRESSION: Increased coughing and wheezing, fever, tachypnea and retractions, refusal to nurse or bottle feed, copious secretions

SEVERE ILLNESS: Tachypnea (greater than 70/min), listlessness, apneic spells, poor air exchange, poor breath sounds, cyanosis

LABORATORY TESTS

Test nasopharyngeal secretions using either rapid immunofluorescent antibody-direct fluorescent antibody staining or enzyme-linked immunosorbent assay techniques for RSV antigen detection.

PATIENT-CENTERED CARE

NURSING CARE

- Supplemental oxygen to maintain oxygen saturation equal to or greater than 90%.
- Encourage fluid intake if able to tolerate oral fluids. Otherwise IV fluids until acute phase has passed.
- Maintain airway.
- Medications as prescribed. Corticosteroid use is controversial. Bronchodilators are not recommended.
- Antibiotics if a coexisting bacterial infection is present.
- CPT is not recommended.
- Nasopharyngeal or nasal suctioning as needed.
- Encourage breastfeeding.

Allergic rhinitis

Caused by seasonal reaction to allergens most often in the autumn or spring

DATA COLLECTION

EXPECTED FINDINGS

Watery rhinorrhea; nasal obstruction; itchiness of the nose, eyes, pharynx and conjunctiva; snoring; fatigue; malaise; headache; and poor performance in school

LABORATORY TESTS

Nasal smear to determine amount of eosinophils in nasal secretions, blood exam for total IgE and elevated eosinophils, skin tests and various challenge tests.

PATIENT-CENTERED CARE

NURSING CARE

Instruct guardians about home management.
- Avoid allergens.
- Give nasal corticosteroids (first-line medications used).
- Give antihistamines, beta adrenergic decongestants, mast cell stabilizers, leukotriene modifiers, and ipratropium.

Bacterial pneumonia

- Bacterial pneumonia often caused by *Streptococcus pneumoniae*, Group A streptococci, *Staphylococcus aureus*, *Mycoplasma catarrhalis*, *Mycoplasma pneumoniae*.
- Viral pneumonia are more common among children of all ages and usually precedes an viral upper respiratory infection.

DATA COLLECTION

EXPECTED FINDINGS

Bacterial

- High fever
- Cough that can be unproductive or productive of white sputum
- Tachypnea
- Retractions and nasal flaring
- Chest pain
- Dullness with percussion
- Adventitious breath sounds (rhonchi, fine crackles)
- Pale color that can progress to cyanosis
- Irritability, restless, lethargic
- Abdominal pain, diarrhea, lack of appetite, and vomiting

Viral

- Fever (mild/severe)
- Cough (productive or non-productive)
- Fatigue

LABORATORY TESTS

- Radiographic examination to detect presence of infiltrates
- Gram stain and culture of sputum in older children
- Nasopharyngeal specimens
- Blood cultures
- Occasionally lung aspiration and biopsy
- Elevated antistreptolysin titer if streptococcal infection present

PATIENT-CENTERED CARE

NURSING CARE

Viral

- Administer oxygen.
- Monitor continuous oximetry.
- Administer antipyretics for fever.
- Monitor I&O.
- CPT and postural drainage.

Bacterial

- Encourage rest.
- Administer IV antibiotics.
- Promote increased oral intake.
- Monitor I&O.
- Administer antipyretics for fever.
- CPT and postural drainage can be helpful.
- Administer IV fluids.
- Administer oxygen.
- Monitor continuous oximetry.

CLIENT EDUCATION: The pneumococcal conjugate vaccine is encouraged for the prevention of pneumonia.

COMPLICATIONS

Pneumothorax

Accumulation of air in the pleural space

MANIFESTATIONS: Dyspnea, chest pain, back pain, labored respirations, decreased oxygen saturations, and tachycardia

NURSING INTERVENTIONS
- Prepare the client for an emergent needle aspiration to remove air in pleural space, with insertion of chest tube to closed drainage.
- Provide for chest tube management.
- Check respiratory status.
- Administer oxygen.

Pleural effusion

Accumulation of fluid in the pleural space

MANIFESTATIONS: Decreased breath sounds, vomiting, tachypnea, fatigue, irritability, and hypoxia

NURSING INTERVENTIONS
- Prepare the client for an emergent needle aspiration to remove fluid in the pleural space, with insertion of chest tube to closed drainage.
- Provide for chest tube management.
- Check respiratory status.
- Administer oxygen as prescribed.

Croup syndromes: Bacterial epiglottitis (acute supraglottitis)

- Medical emergency
- Usually caused by *Haemophilus influenza*

DATA COLLECTION

EXPECTED FINDINGS

- Predictive indicators: Absence of cough, drooling, and agitation
- Sitting upright with chin pointing out, mouth opened, and tongue protruding (tripod position)
- Dysphonia (thick, muffled voice and froglike croaking sound)
- Dysphagia (difficulty swallowing)
- Inspiratory stridor (noisy inspirations)
- Suprasternal and substernal retractions
- Sore throat, high fever, and restlessness

DIAGNOSTIC PROCEDURES

Lateral neck radiograph of the soft tissues

PATIENT-CENTERED CARE

NURSING CARE

- Protect airway.
- Avoid throat culture or using a tongue blade.
- Assist with preparations for intubation.
- Provide humidified oxygen.
- Monitor continuous oximetry.
- Administer corticosteroids, and collaborate with the RN to ensure that the child receives IV fluids as prescribed.
- Begin initial antibiotic therapy IV, then transition to oral to complete a 10-day course, as prescribed.
- Droplet isolation precautions for first 24 hr after IV antibiotics initiated.

Croup syndromes: Acute laryngotracheobronchitis and acute spasmodic laryngitis

Acute laryngotracheobronchitis: Causative agents include RSV, influenza A and B, and *Mycoplasma pneumonia*, parainfluenza types 1, 2, and 3.

Acute spasmodic laryngitis
- Self-limiting illness that can result from allergens
- Characterized by paroxysmal attacks of laryngeal obstruction that occur mainly at night

DATA COLLECTION

EXPECTED FINDINGS

Acute laryngotracheobronchitis
- Low-grade fever, restlessness, hoarseness, barky cough, dyspnea, inspiratory stridor, and retractions
- INFANTS AND TODDLERS: nasal flaring, intercostal retractions, tachypnea, and continuous stridor

Acute spasmodic laryngitis: Croupy barky cough, restlessness, difficulty breathing, hoarseness, and nighttime episodes of laryngeal obstruction

PATIENT-CENTERED CARE

NURSING CARE

- Provide humidity with cool mist.
- Administer oxygen if needed.
- Monitor continuous oximetry.
- Administer nebulized racemic epinephrine as prescribed.
- Administer corticosteroids: oral or IM (dexamethasone), or nebulized (budesonide).
- Encourage oral intake if tolerated.
- Administer IV fluids as prescribed.

Home management: Spasmodic croup

- Reinforce to guardians to provide cool mist for the child's room.
- Advise guardians to run hot shower and sit with their child in the steamy environment.

Influenza A and B

Mild, moderate, or severe

DATA COLLECTION

EXPECTED FINDINGS

- Sudden onset of fever and chills
- Dry throat and nasal mucosa
- Dry cough
- Flushed face
- Photophobia
- Myalgia
- Fatigue

LABORATORY TESTS

- Analyze nasopharyngeal secretions for viral culture or rapid detection testing.
- Influenza A and B detected by fluorescent antibody and indirect immunofluorescent antibody staining.

PATIENT-CENTERED CARE

NURSING CARE

Reinforce with guardians about home management.
- Promote increased fluid intake.
- Rest.
- Acetaminophen or ibuprofen for fever.
- Give medications, as prescribed.

MEDICATIONS

Amantadine (type A)

- Shortens the length of the illness.
- Administer within 24 to 48 hr of onset of manifestations.

Zanamivir (type A and B)

- Treatment of influenza for children 7 and older or for prophylaxis for children 5 and older.
- Start within 48 hr of manifestations.
- Inhaled two times per day for 5 days.

Oseltamivir (type A and B)

- Decreases manifestations.
- Give orally for 5 days.
- Start within 48 hr of manifestations.

Influenza vaccine (prevention)

- Inactivated influenza vaccine recommended for children 6 months and older.
- Live vaccination should not be used in children who have heart or lung disease, diabetes or kidney failure, are immunocompromised, have respiratory conditions, are pregnant, or have a history of Guillain-Barré syndrome.
- Clients who have experienced a severe allergic reaction to eggs should receive the influenza vaccine in a medical setting that is able to manage severe allergic reactions should they occur.

Active Learning Scenario

A nurse is reinforcing teaching with the guardian of a child who has an infectious respiratory illness. What should the nurse include in the teaching? Use the ATI Active Learning Template: Basic Concept to complete this item.

RELATED CONTENT: Identify at least three strategies to decrease the spread of infection.

Application Exercises

1. A nurse is caring for a child who has bronchiolitis. Which of the following actions should the nurse take? (Select all that apply.)
   - A. Administer oral prednisone.
   - B. Initiate chest percussion and postural drainage.
   - C. Administer humidified oxygen.
   - D. Suction the nasopharynx as needed.
   - E. Administer oral penicillin.

2. A nurse is reinforcing teachings with a group of guardians about influenza. Which of the following information should the nurse include?
   - A. "Amantadine will prevent the illness."
   - B. "The influenza vaccine is recommend for children 4 months and older."
   - C. "Zanamivir can be given to children 1 year and older."
   - D. "Oseltamivir should be given within 48 hours of onset of manifestations."

3. A nurse is collecting data from a child who is postoperative following a tonsillectomy. Which of the following is a clinical finding of postoperative bleeding?
   - A. Hgb 11.6 and Hct 37%
   - B. Inflamed and reddened throat
   - C. Frequent swallowing and clearing of the throat
   - D. Blood-tinged mucus

4. A nurse is assisting with the care of a child in the postoperative period following a tonsillectomy. Which of the actions should the nurse take?
   - A. Encourage the child to blow their nose gently.
   - B. Administer analgesics on a schedule.
   - C. Offer orange juice.
   - D. Position the child supine.

5. A nurse is collecting data from a child who has epiglottitis. Which of the following findings should the nurse expect? (Select all that apply.)
   - A. Hoarseness
   - B. Difficulty swallowing
   - C. Low-grade fever
   - D. Drooling
   - E. Dry, barking cough
   - F. Stridor

Application Exercises Key

1. A. Corticosteroids are not indicated for a client who has bronchiolitis.
   B. Chest percussion and postural drainage are not indicated for a client who has bronchiolitis.
   C. **CORRECT:** Humidified oxygen provides moisture to the airway and is an action to take.
   D. **CORRECT:** Suctioning the nasopharynx will assist the client to clear secretions and is an appropriate action to take.
   E. Antibiotics are not indicated for a client who has bronchiolitis.

   Ⓝ NCLEX® Connection: Physiological Adaptation, Alterations in Body Systems

2. A. Amantadine can shorten the length of the illness.
   B. The influenza vaccine is recommended yearly for children 6 months and older.
   C. Zanamivir is approved for children over the age of 5 years.
   D. **CORRECT:** Oseltamivir decrease flu manifestations in clients who have findings for less than 48 hr.

   Ⓝ NCLEX® Connection: Physiological Adaptation, Alterations in Body Systems

3. A. Hgb 11.6 and Hct 37% are within the expected reference range.
   B. Inflamed and reddened throat is an expected finding following a tonsillectomy.
   C. **CORRECT:** Frequent swallowing and clearing of the throat indicates that there is an increased amount of fluid in the back of the throat, which is a clinical finding in the client who is experiencing postoperative bleeding.
   D. Blood-tinged mucus is an expected finding following a tonsillectomy.

   Ⓝ NCLEX® Connection: Physiological Adaptation, Unexpected Response to Therapies

4. A. Blowing the nose causes pressure and could increase the risk of bleeding.
   B. **CORRECT:** Analgesics should be administered on a scheduled basis to provide pain relief.
   C. Citrus juices (orange juice) can cause discomfort and should be avoided postoperatively.
   D. The client should be positioned on the abdomen or side-lying following a tonsillectomy.

   Ⓝ NCLEX® Connection: Reduction of Risk Potential, Potential for Complications from Surgical Procedures and Health Alterations

5. A. Hoarseness and difficulty speaking is a manifestation of laryngotracheobronchitis.
   B. **CORRECT:** Difficulty swallowing is a manifestation of epiglottitis.
   C. A high fever is a manifestation of epiglottitis.
   D. **CORRECT:** Drooling is a manifestation of epiglottitis.
   E. Dry, barking cough is a manifestation of croup.
   F. **CORRECT:** Stridor is a manifestation of epiglottitis.

   Ⓝ NCLEX® Connection: Physiological Adaptation, Basic Pathophysiology

Active Learning Scenario Key

Using the ATI Active Learning Template: Basic Concept
RELATED CONTENT
- Perform appropriate hand hygiene.
- Cover the nose and mouth with tissues when sneezing and coughing.
- Dispose of tissues properly.
- Do not share cups, eating utensils, or towels.
- Keep infected children from contact with children who are well.

Ⓝ NCLEX® Connection: Safety and Infection Control, Standard Precautions/Transmission–Based Precautions/Surgical Asepsis

UNIT 2   **SYSTEM DISORDERS**
SECTION: RESPIRATORY DISORDERS

CHAPTER 17 *Asthma*

Asthma is a chronic childhood inflammatory disorder of the airways that results in intermittent and reversible airflow obstruction of the bronchioles. It causes school absences and is considered one of the leading causes of hospitalizations among children. The obstruction occurs because the mast cells release histamines and leukotrienes which causes inflammation or airway hyper-responsiveness. Asthma diagnoses are classified into one of four categories based on effects on the child: intermittent, mild persistent, moderate persistent, and severe persistent. (17.1) Q EBP

DATA COLLECTION

RISK FACTORS

- Family history of asthma or allergies
- Sex (boys affected more than girls until adolescence, then the incidence is greater among girls)
- Exposure to tobacco smoke
- Low birth weight
- Being overweight

TRIGGERS TO ASTHMA

- Allergens
  - Indoor: mold, cockroach antigen, dust, dust mites
  - Outdoor: grasses, pollen, trees, shrubs, molds, spores, air pollution, weeds
  - Irritants: Tobacco smoke, wood smoke, odors, sprays
- Exercise
- Cold air or changes in weather or temperature

- Environmental change (new home or school)
- Infections/viruses (colds)
- Animal hair or dander
- Medications: Aspirin, nonsteroidal anti-inflammatory drugs, antibiotics, beta blockers
- Strong emotions: Fear, anger, laughing, crying
- Conditions: Gastroesophageal reflux, tracheoesophageal fistula
- Food allergies or additives (sulfites)
- Endocrine factors: Menses, pregnancy, thyroid disease

EXPECTED FINDINGS

- Chest tightness
- History regarding current and previous asthma exacerbations
  - Onset and duration
  - Precipitating factors
  - Changes in medication regimen
  - Medications that relieve manifestations
  - Other medications
  - Self-care methods used to relieve manifestations
  - Home/school environment
  - Heating/cooling source in the home

PHYSICAL FINDINGS

- Dyspnea
- Cough
- Audible wheezing
- Coarse lung sounds, wheezing throughout possible crackles
- Mucus production
- Restlessness, irritability
- Anxiety
- Sweating
- Use of accessory muscles
- Decreased oxygen saturation (low SaO_2)
- Tripod positioning
- Sitting retractions
- Inaudible breath sounds or crackles (severe obstruction)

LABORATORY TESTS

CBC (increased WBC, eosinophils)

17.1 Effects of asthma on the child

		Intermittent	Mild persistent	Moderate persistent	Severe persistent
Frequency of findings		0 to 2 times/week	More than twice/week, but not daily	Daily	Continually
Nighttime findings	0- to 4-year-old	None	1 to 2 times/month	3 to 4 times/month	Frequent
	5- to 11-year-old	Two times a month or less	3 to 4 times/month	More than once/week, but not daily	
Activity limitations		None	Minor	Some	Extreme
Use of a short-acting beta agonist		Less than twice/week	More than 2 days/week, but not daily	Daily	Several times/day

DIAGNOSTIC PROCEDURES

Pulmonary function tests
- The most accurate tests for diagnosing asthma and its severity Q EBP
- Baseline test at time of diagnosis
- Repeat testing after treatment is initiated and child is stabilized
- Test every 1 to 2 years

Peak expiratory flow rates (PEFR)
- Uses a flow meter to measure the amount of air that can be forcefully exhaled in 1 second
- Each child needs to establish personal best

Bronchoprovocation testing
- Exposure to methacholine, cold air, or histamine
- Exercise challenge

Skin prick testing: Identify allergens that trigger asthma

Chest x-ray: Showing hyperexpansion and infiltrates

PATIENT-CENTERED CARE

NURSING CARE
- Avoid allergens whenever possible.
- Monitor airway patency, respiratory rate, symmetry, effort, and use of accessory muscles.
- Auscultate breath sounds in all lung fields.
- Monitor for shortness of breath, dyspnea, and audible wheezing. An absence of wheezing can indicate severe constriction of the alveoli.
- Monitor vital signs and oxygen saturation.
- Check CBC and chest x-ray results, possible ABGs.
- Position the child to maximize ventilation.
- Administer oxygen therapy as prescribed. Keep endotracheal intubation equipment nearby. Qs
- Assist with initiating and maintaining IV access as prescribed.
- Maintain a calm and reassuring demeanor.
- Encourage appropriate vaccinations and prompt medical attention for infections.
- Administer medications. The provider can prescribe antibiotics if a bacterial infection is confirmed.
- Reinforce with the family and the child about when to use each of the prescribed medications (rescue medications vs. maintenance medications).

MEDICATIONS

A stepwise approach is used for treatment based upon the severity.

Bronchodilators (inhalers)

Short-acting beta$_2$ agonists (SABA) (albuterol, levalbuterol, terbutaline)
- Used for acute exacerbations
- Prevention of exercised-induced asthma

Long-acting beta$_2$ agonists (LABA) (formoterol, salmeterol)
- Used to prevent exacerbations and reduce use of SABA.
- Must be used along with anti-inflammatory therapy.
- Cannot be used to treat acute exacerbations.

Cholinergic antagonists (anticholinergic medications; atropine, ipratropium) block the parasympathetic nervous system, providing relief of acute bronchospasms.

NURSING ACTIONS
- Reinforce with the child and family about the proper use of metered-dose inhaler or nebulizer.
- Monitor the child for dizziness, nasal dryness, sore throat, vision changes, cardiac and CNS stimulation when taking ipratropium.

CLIENT EDUCATION
- Older children who are taking ipratropium can suck on hard candies to help with dry mouth.
- Administer prior to exercise or activity.
- Rinse mouth after using inhaler.
- Watch the child for irritability, tremors, insomnia, and nervousness while taking albuterol.

Anti-inflammatory agents

Decrease airway inflammation.

Corticosteroids can be given parenterally (methylprednisolone), orally (prednisone), or by inhalation (fluticasone).
- Oral systemic steroids can be given for short periods (3 or 10 days).
- Inhaled corticosteroids are administered daily as a preventive measure.
- Monitor child's growth.

Leukotriene modifiers (zafirlukast, montelukast)
- Decrease in airway resistance

Mast cell stabilizers (cromolyn)
- Long-term control

Monoclonal antibodies (omalizumab) are used to treat moderate to severe persistent allergic asthma uncontrolled by inhaled corticosteroids in children 12 years old and older.

Combination medications contain an inhaled corticosteroid and a LABA (fluticasone/salmeterol)

NURSING ACTIONS
- Observe the oral mucosa for infection secondary to use of inhaled medication.
- Monitor weight, blood pressure, electrolytes, glucose, and growth with oral corticosteroid use.

CLIENT EDUCATION
- Drink plenty of fluids to promote hydration.
- Take oral corticosteroids with food.
- Rinse the mouth after the use of a corticosteroid inhaler.
- Watch for redness, sores, or white patches in the mouth, and report them to the provider.
- Follow prescription for medication administration (dosage, tapering off medication, length of time to take).

Theophylline: Used when the child is not responding to maximum therapy. Frequent monitoring of theophylline blood levels is recommended because of the risk for toxicity.

INTERPROFESSIONAL CARE

- Assist with obtaining a consult for respiratory services for inhalers and breathing treatments.
- Contact nutritional services for weight loss or gain related to medications or diagnosis.
- Assist with obtaining a consult for rehabilitation if the child has prolonged weakness and needs assistance with increasing level of activity.

CLIENT EDUCATION

- Identify personal triggering agents.
- Avoid triggering agents.
- Provide the family and child with an asthma action plan.
- Properly self-administer medications (nebulizers, inhalers, and spacer).
- Use a peak flow meter. (Use at the same time each day.)
  - Ensure the marker is zeroed.
  - Have the child stand up straight.
  - Remove gum or food from mouth.
  - Close lips tightly around the mouthpiece (ensure the tongue is not occluding).
  - Blow out as hard and as quickly as possible.
  - Read the number on the meter.
  - Repeat these steps two more times for a total of three attempts (wait at least 30 seconds between attempts.)
  - Record highest number.
- Keep a record of PEFR results. Readings over time show the child's "best" efforts, and provide a warning of increased airway impairment.
- Learn how to interpret PEFR results and what measures to take for their zone. **(17.2)**
- Learn how to recognize an asthma exacerbation (decreased PEFR, increased use of SABA, difficulty speaking or eating). Qs
- Perform infection prevention techniques.
  - Promote good nutrition.
  - Reinforce importance of good hand hygiene.
  - Reduce allergens in the child's environment
- Perform prompt medical attention for infections.
- Keep immunizations, including seasonal influenza and pneumonia vaccines, up to date.
- Perform regular exercise as part of asthma therapy.
  - Promotes ventilation and perfusion
  - Maintains cardiac health
  - Enhances skeletal muscle strength
- Children can require medication before exercise to prevent induced spasms of the bronchus.

COMPLICATIONS

Status asthmaticus

A life-threatening episode of airway obstruction that is often unresponsive to common treatment. It is considered a prolonged severe asthma attack.

MANIFESTATIONS include wheezing, labored breathing, nasal flaring, lack of air movement in lungs with an inability to speak, use of accessory muscles, distended neck veins, tachycardia, tachypnea, hypoxia, diaphoresis, and risk for cardiac and respiratory arrest.

NURSING ACTIONS
- Monitor oxygen saturations continuously.
- Place on continuous cardiorespiratory monitoring.
- Position the child sitting upright, standing, or leaning slightly forward.
- Administer humidified oxygen.
- Administer three nebulizer treatments of a beta$_2$ agonist, 20 to 30 min apart or continuously. Ipratropium bromide can be added to the nebulizer to increase bronchodilation.
- Assist with obtaining IV access.
- Monitor ABGs and blood electrolytes.
- Administer corticosteroid and anticholinergics.
- Ensure that emergency intubation supplies are readily available.
- Magnesium sulfate IV decreases inflammation and improves pulmonary function and peak flow rate among children who have moderate to severe asthma when treated in the emergency department or pediatric ICU.
- Heliox (a mixture of helium and oxygen) can be administered via a non-rebreathing mask to decrease airway resistance and work of breathing.
- Ketamine (smooth muscle relaxant) can be administered to decrease airway resistance.

Respiratory failure

Persistent hypoxemia related to asthma can lead to respiratory failure.

NURSING ACTIONS
- Monitor oxygenation levels and acid-base balance.
- Assist with preparations for intubation and mechanical ventilation as indicated.

17.2 Analysis of peak flow rates according to colored zones

	% OF PERSONAL BEST	ANALYSIS
Green	80% to 100%	Good control. Follow routine plan.
Yellow	50% to 79%	Caution. This zone warns of an acute attack. Use maintenance medications. Notify provider if the peak flow rate stays in this zone.
Red	Less than 50%	Emergent action needed. Use a short-acting bronchodilator. Notify provider if the peak flow rate does not improve.

Application Exercises

1. A nurse is collecting data from a child who has asthma. Which of the following are indications of deterioration in the child's respiratory status? (Select all that apply.)

   A. Oxygen saturation 95%

   B. Wheezing

   C. Retraction of sternal muscles

   D. Warm extremities

   E. Nasal flaring

2. A nurse is reinforcing teaching to an adolescent about the appropriate use of their asthma medications. Which of the following medications should the nurse instruct the client to use as needed before exercise?

   A. Fluticasone/salmeterol

   B. Montelukast

   C. Prednisone

   D. Albuterol

3. A nurse is contributing to the plan of care for a child who has asthma. Which of the following interventions should the nurse include in the plan of care? (Select all that apply.)

   A. Perform chest percussion.

   B. Place the child in an upright position.

   C. Monitor oxygen saturation.

   D. Administer bronchodilators.

   E. Administer dornase alfa daily.

4. A nurse is reinforcing teaching with a child who has asthma about how to use a peak flow meter. Which of the following information should the nurse include in the teaching? (Select all that apply.)

   A. Zero the meter before each use.

   B. Record the average of the attempts.

   C. Perform three attempts.

   D. Deliver a long, slow breath into the meter.

   E. Sit in a chair with feet on the floor.

5. A nurse is preparing to assist the charge nurse with discussing risk factors for asthma with a group of newly licensed nurses. Which of the following conditions should the nurse include in the teaching? (Select all that apply.)

   A. Family history of asthma

   B. Family history of allergies

   C. Exposure to smoke

   D. Low birth weight

   E. Being underweight

Active Learning Scenario

A nurse is reinforcing teaching with a child about asthma triggers. What information should the nurse include in the teaching? Use the ATI Active Learning Template: System Disorder to complete this item.

CLIENT EDUCATION: List at least eight possible asthma triggers.

Application Exercises Key

1. A. Expect a child experiencing respiratory difficulty to have an oxygen saturation below the expected reference range.
   B. **CORRECT:** Bronchoconstriction causes wheezing, which is an indicator of deterioration in a child's respiratory status.
   C. **CORRECT:** Increased work of breathing causes retraction of the sternal muscles, which is an indicator of deterioration in a child's respiratory status.
   D. Expect a child experiencing respiratory difficulty to exhibit restlessness and irritability.
   E. **CORRECT:** Increased work of breathing causes nasal flaring, which is an indicator of deterioration in a child's respiratory status.

   Ⓝ *NCLEX® Connection: Physiological Adaptation, Unexpected Response to Therapies*

2. A. Reinforce to the adolescent that fluticasone/salmeterol is a combination of LABA and corticosteroid medications, and to use it for maintenance control of asthma.
   B. Reinforce to the adolescent that montelukast affects the immune response to prevent medication, and to use it for maintenance control of asthma.
   C. Reinforce to the adolescent that prednisone is an anti-inflammatory medication used short-term for exacerbations of asthma.
   D. **CORRECT:** Albuterol is a beta$_2$ agonist used for bronchodilation. Reinforce to the adolescent the medicine is quick-acting, should be administered prior to exercise, and is used to provide immediate relief of bronchoconstriction.

   Ⓝ *NCLEX® Connection: Pharmacological Therapies, Expected Actions/Outcomes*

3. A. Use chest percussion to promote movement of mucus plugs for a child who has cystic fibrosis.
   B. **CORRECT:** Children who are experiencing an asthma exacerbation have decreased oxygenation. Place the child an upright position to promote ventilation.
   C. **CORRECT:** Children who are experiencing an asthma exacerbation have decreased oxygenation. Monitor oxygen saturation to detect changes in the child's condition.
   D. **CORRECT:** Children who are experiencing an asthma exacerbation experience bronchoconstriction. Administer bronchodilators to promote ventilation.
   E. Administer dornase alfa to a child who has cystic fibrosis to help with removal of respiratory secretions.

   Ⓝ *NCLEX® Connection: Coordinated Care, Collaboration with Interdisciplinary Team*

4. A. **CORRECT:** Reinforce to the child to zero the monitor before each use to achieve accurate results.
   B. Reinforce to the child to record the highest number reading.
   C. **CORRECT:** The child should perform three attempts to achieve accurate results.
   D. Reinforce to the child to breathe hard and fast when using the peak flow meter to measure airflow.
   E. Reinforce to the child to stand upright when using a peak flow meter.

   Ⓝ *NCLEX® Connection: Reduction of Risk Potential, Diagnostic Tests*

5. A. **CORRECT:** A familial history of asthma is a risk factor for the development asthma.
   B. **CORRECT:** A familial history of allergies is a risk factor for the development of asthma.
   C. **CORRECT:** Exposure to smoke is a risk factor for the development of asthma.
   D. **CORRECT:** Low birth weight is a risk factor for the development of asthma.
   E. Being overweight is a risk factor for the development of asthma.

   Ⓝ *NCLEX® Connection: Health Promotion and Maintenance, Health Promotion/Disease Prevention*

Active Learning Scenario Key

Using the ATI Active Learning Template: System Disorder

CLIENT EDUCATION
- Allergens
  - Indoor: mold, cockroach antigen, dust mites
  - Outdoor: grasses, pollen, trees, shrubs, molds, spores, air pollution
- Exercise/activity
- Cold air or changes in weather or temperature
- Tobacco smoke
- Infections/colds
- Animal hair or dander
- Medications
- Strong odors
- Emotions
- Food allergies or additives

Ⓝ *NCLEX® Connection: Physiological Adaptation, Alterations in Body Systems*

CHAPTER 18 *Cystic Fibrosis*

Cystic fibrosis is a respiratory disorder that results from inheriting a mutated gene. It is characterized by mucus glands that secrete an increase in the quantity of thick, tenacious mucus, which leads to mechanical obstruction of organs (pancreas, lungs, liver, small intestine, and reproductive system); an increase in organic and enzymatic constituents in the saliva; an increase in the sodium and chloride content of sweat; and autonomic nervous system abnormalities.

DATA COLLECTION

RISK FACTORS

- Both biological parents carry the recessive trait for cystic fibrosis.
- Caucasian ethnicity

EXPECTED FINDINGS

- Family history of cystic fibrosis
- Medical history of respiratory infections, growth failure
- Meconium ileus at birth manifested as distention of the abdomen, vomiting, and inability to pass stool. Meconium ileus is the earliest indication of cystic fibrosis in the newborn.

RESPIRATORY FINDINGS

- Stasis of mucus increases the risk for respiratory infections.
- Early manifestations
  ○ Wheezing, rhonchi
  ○ Dry, nonproductive cough
- Increased involvement
  ○ Dyspnea
  ○ Paroxysmal cough
  ○ Obstructive emphysema and atelectasis on chest x-ray
- Advanced involvement
  ○ Cyanosis
  ○ Barrel-shaped chest
  ○ Clubbing of fingers and toes
  ○ Multiple episodes of bronchitis or bronchopneumonia

GASTROINTESTINAL FINDINGS

- Large, frothy, bulky, greasy, foul-smelling stools (steatorrhea)
- Voracious appetite (early), loss of appetite (late)
- Failure to gain weight or weight loss
- Delayed growth patterns
- Distended abdomen (infant)
- Thin arms and legs (infant)
- Deficiency of fat-soluble vitamins
- Anemia
- Reflux
- Prolapse rectum (infant, child)
- Constipation

INTEGUMENTARY FINDINGS

Sweat, tears, and saliva have an excessively high content of sodium and chloride.

ENDOCRINE AND REPRODUCTIVE SYSTEM FINDINGS

- Viscous cervical mucus
- Decreased or absent sperm
- Decreased insulin production

LABORATORY TESTS

Blood specimen: Nutritional panel to detect a deficiency of fat-soluble vitamins (A, D, E, and K)

Sputum culture for detection of infection: *Pseudomonas aeruginosa, Haemophilus influenzae, Burkholderia cepacia, Staphlococcus aureus, Escherichia coli,* or *Klebsiella pneumoniae*

DIAGNOSTIC PROCEDURES

DNA testing: To isolate the mutation

Pulmonary function tests (PFTs): evaluate the small airways

Chest x-ray: Can indicate diffuse atelectasis and obstructive emphysema

Abdominal x-ray: Detect meconium ileus

Stool analysis: For presence of fat and enzymes

Duodenal analysis: Analyze pancreatic trypsin levels (NG tube)

Sweat chloride test
- The child must be well hydrated to ensure accurate test results.
- A device that uses an electrical current stimulates sweat production. Ⓠᴇʙᴘ
- Collection of sweat from two different sites for adequate sample.
- Expected reference range is chloride content less than 40 mEq/L and sodium content less than 70 mEq/L.

> Diagnostic confirmation of cystic fibrosis: Chloride greater than 40 mEq/L for infants less than 3 months of age and greater than 60 mEq/L for all others; sodium greater than 90 mEq/L

PATIENT-CENTERED CARE

NURSING CARE

- Check lung sounds and respiratory status.
- Vital signs with oxygen saturation.
- Assist with obtaining IV access. Use of a peripherally inserted central catheter or IV port allows for home IV antibiotic therapy.
- Obtain sputum for culture and sensitivity.
- Provide support to the child and family.

Pulmonary management

- Assist in providing airway clearance therapy (ACT) to promote expectoration of pulmonary secretions. Usually prescribed twice a day in the morning and evening. Avoid ACT immediately before or after meals. Several methods of ACT are available.
  - Chest physiotherapy (CPT) with postural drainage as prescribed (manual or mechanical percussion).
  - Positive expiratory therapy (PEP) uses a device (a flutter mucus clearance device) to encourage the client to breathe with forceful exhalations.
  - Active-cycle-of-breathing techniques ("huffing" or forced expiration) are encouraged.
  - Autogenic drainage uses an electronic chest vibrator or handheld percussor along with breathing techniques.
  - High-frequency chest compression uses a mechanical chest device combined with nebulization therapy.
- Administer aerosol therapy as prescribed (bronchodilator, human deoxyribonuclease). Often recommended prior to ACT.
- Administer IV or aerosolized antibiotics.
- Encourage physical aerobic exercise.
- Provide oxygen as prescribed (monitor for carbon dioxide retention).
- Monitor for hemoptysis or pneumothorax.

Gastrointestinal management

- Provide a well-balanced diet high in protein and calories.
- Give three meals a day with snacks.
- Encourage oral fluid intake.
- Administer pancreatic enzymes within 30 min of eating a meal or snack.
- Administer vitamin supplements: multivitamin; vitamins A, D, E, and K.
- Administer laxatives or stool softeners for constipation. Polyethylene-glycol electrolyte solution is administered orally or via nasogastric tube.
- Administer histamine-receptor antagonist and motility medications for GERD.
- Administer possible formula supplements in addition to breastfeedings or via gastric tube.
- Encourage to add salt to food during hot weather (dehydration).
- Assist with a referral to a dietitian. Child should receive regular nutritional evaluations.

Endocrine management

- Cystic fibrosis related diabetes (CFRD) necessitates monitoring of blood glucose levels and quarterly glycosylated hemoglobin (A1C) levels.
- Administer insulin. Oral glycemic medications are not effective for CFRD.

MEDICATIONS

Respiratory medications

Short-acting beta$_2$ agonists (albuterol)

Cholinergic antagonists (anticholinergics [ipratropium bromide])

Fluticasone propionate/salmeterol
NURSING ACTIONS
- Monitor for tremors and tachycardia when the child is taking albuterol.
- Observe for dry mouth when the child is taking ipratropium.
- Reinforce how to properly use an MDI, PEP, or nebulizer.
CLIENT EDUCATION: Rinse mouth after fluticasone propionate/salmeterol.

Dornase alfa (aerosol)
Decreases the viscosity of mucus and improves lung function
NURSING ACTIONS
- Monitor sputum thickness and ability of client to expectorate.
- Monitor the child for improvement in PFTs.
- Reinforce how to use a nebulizer.
CLIENT EDUCATION
- Administer once or twice a day.
- This medication can cause laryngitis.

Antibiotics

- Administer through IV or aerosol.
- Specific to treat pulmonary infection. Common medications include tobramycin, ticarcillin, or piperacillin-tazobactam. ◯ EBP

NURSING ACTIONS
- Check for allergies.
- High doses may be prescribed. Collect blood specimens before and after some IV antibiotics to maintain therapeutic levels.

Pancreatic enzymes

Pancrelipase treats pancreatic insufficiency associated with cystic fibrosis.

NURSING ACTIONS
- Monitor stools for adequate dosing (1 to 2 stools/day).
- Monitor weight.
- Administer capsules with all meals and snacks.
- Child can swallow or sprinkle capsule's content on food. Do not sprinkle on hot foods or add to bottles or formula.
- Increase dosage of enzymes when eating high-fat foods.
- Capsule contents can be added to a small amount of formula or breast milk for an infant.

Vitamins

Daily multivitamin and fat-soluble vitamins A, E, D, and K

INTERPROFESSIONAL CARE

- Respiratory and physical therapy, social services, pulmonologist, pharmacist, pediatrician, infectious disease specialists, and dietitians may be involved in the care of the child who has cystic fibrosis.
- Adolescents who have advanced disease can be considered for lung transplants.

CLIENT EDUCATION

- Ensure that the family has information regarding access to medical equipment and medications.
- Reinforce teaching about equipment and medications prior to discharge.
- Instruct the family about ways to provide CPT and breathing exercises.
- Visit the provider regularly.
- Stay up-to-date on immunizations, including a yearly influenza vaccine and pneumococcal vaccine.
- Practice regular dental hygiene
- Reinforce the importance of diet and ways to increase calorie intake.
- Identify indications of infection and notify the provider if necessary.
- Know methods to manage chronic illness in children.
- Change diapers frequently.
- Monitor for impairments of skin integrity.
- Encourage regular physical activity and frequent position changes. Encourage the child to rest prior to meals and before physiotherapy.
- Encourage the family to participate in a support group and use community resources.
- Identify specific needs based on the client's developmental level. For example, older adolescents are at a higher risk for depression due to the emotional and physical effects of cystic fibrosis.
- Provide home palliative care for the child or adolescent in the terminal stages of CF.

COMPLICATIONS

RESPIRATORY: Respiratory infections, respiratory colonizations, bronchial cysts, emphysema, pneumothorax, nasal polyps

GASTROINTESTINAL: Meconium ileus, prolapse of the rectum, intestinal obstruction, GERD

ENDOCRINE: Diabetes mellitus

Application Exercises

1. A nurse is reviewing the diagnostic findings for a preschool age child who is suspected of having cystic fibrosis. Which of the following findings should the nurse identify as an indication of cystic fibrosis?
   A. Sweat chloride content 85 mEq/L
   B. Increased blood levels of fat-soluble vitamins
   C. 72 hr stool analysis sample indicating hard, packed stools
   D. Chest x-ray negative for atelectasis

2. A nurse is assisting with the admission of a child who has cystic fibrosis. Which of the following medications should the nurse expect the provider to prescribe? (Select all that apply.)
   A. Tobramycin
   B. Loperamide
   C. Fat-soluble vitamins
   D. Albuterol
   E. Dornase alfa

3. A nurse is collecting data from a child who has cystic fibrosis. Which of the following findings should the nurse expect? (Select all that apply.)
   A. Wheezing
   B. Clubbing of fingers and toes
   C. Barrel-shaped chest
   D. Thin, watery mucus
   E. Rapid growth spurts

4. A nurse is reinforcing discharge teaching for a child who has cystic fibrosis. Which of the following instructions should the nurse include?
   A. Provide a low-calorie, low-protein diet.
   B. Administer pancreatic enzymes with meals and snacks.
   C. Implement a fluid restriction during times of infection.
   D. Restrict physical activity.

Active Learning Scenario

A nurse is caring for a child who has cystic fibrosis. What nursing interventions should the nurse anticipate providing? Use the ATI Active Learning Template: System Disorder to complete this item.

NURSING CARE

- Describe at least three general nursing actions.
- Describe three nursing actions related to the management of pulmonary function.
- Describe two nursing actions related to gastrointestinal system management.
- Describe two nursing actions related to endocrine system management.

Application Exercises Key

1. A. **CORRECT:** Children who have cystic fibrosis excrete an excessive amount of sodium and chloride in their sweat. A sweat chloride content of 85 mEq/L is above the expected reference range and is an indication of cystic fibrosis.
   B. Children who have cystic fibrosis are expected to have decreased blood levels of fat-soluble vitamins.
   C. Children who have cystic fibrosis are expected to have large, bulky, frothy, greasy, foul-smelling stools (steatorrhea).
   D. Children who have cystic fibrosis are expected to have obstructive emphysema and atelectasis on chest x-ray.

   Ⓝ *NCLEX® Connection: Reduction of Risk Potential, Laboratory Values*

2. A. **CORRECT:** Children who have cystic fibrosis have pulmonary infections. Administering antibiotics is an expected part of the plan of care.
   B. Children who have cystic fibrosis have constipation and are expected to have a laxative or stool softener as part of the plan of care. Loperamide is an antidiarrheal medication.
   C. **CORRECT:** Children who have cystic fibrosis have difficulty absorbing fat. Supplementation of the fat-soluble vitamins is an expected part of the plan of care.
   D. **CORRECT:** Children who have cystic fibrosis have mucus plugs. Administering a bronchodilator is an expected part of the plan of care.
   E. **CORRECT:** Children who have cystic fibrosis have mucus plugs. Administering dornase alfa, which decreases the viscosity of the mucus, is an expected part of the plan of care.

   Ⓝ *NCLEX® Connection: Pharmacological Therapies, Expected Actions/Outcomes*

3. A. **CORRECT:** Wheezing is an expected finding of cystic fibrosis.
   B. **CORRECT:** Clubbing is an expected finding of cystic fibrosis.
   C. **CORRECT:** A barrel-shaped chest is an expected finding of cystic fibrosis.
   D. Thick, viscous mucus is an expected finding of cystic fibrosis.
   E. Delayed growth is an expected finding of cystic fibrosis.

   Ⓝ *NCLEX® Connection: Physiological Adaptation, Basic Pathophysiology*

4. A. Children who have cystic fibrosis should eat a high-calorie, high-protein diet to allow for proper growth.
   B. **CORRECT:** Children who have cystic fibrosis have pancreatic insufficiency. Provide instruction about administering pancreatic enzymes within 30 min of a meal or snack.
   C. Children who have cystic fibrosis should increase fluids to assist in thinning thick mucus.
   D. Children who have cystic fibrosis should engage in daily aerobic activity to assist with lung expansion and to stimulate mucus expectoration.

   Ⓝ *NCLEX® Connection: Physiological Adaptation, Alterations in Body Systems*

Active Learning Scenario Key

Using the ATI Active Learning Template: System Disorder

NURSING CARE

General Nursing Actions
- Check lung sounds and respiratory status.
- Check vital signs with oxygen saturation.
- Assist with obtaining IV access (peripherally inserted central catheter).
- Obtain sputum for culture and sensitivity.
- Provide support to the child and family.

Pulmonary Management
- Assist with performing ACT as prescribed. Avoid immediately before and after meals.
- Administer aerosol therapy (bronchodilator, human deoxyribonuclease).
- Administer IV antibiotics (tobramycin, ticarcillin, or gentamicin).
- Encourage physical aerobic exercise.
- Provide oxygen as prescribed. (Monitor for carbon dioxide retention.)

Gastrointestinal Management
- Consume a well-balanced diet high in protein and calories.
- Eat three meals a day with snacks.
- Encourage oral fluid intake.
- Administer pancreatic enzymes within 30 min of eating.
- Take vitamin supplements: multivitamin, vitamins A, D, E, and K.
- Administer laxatives or stool softeners for constipation.
- Administer histamine-receptor antagonist and motility medications for GERD.
- Administer possible formula supplements in addition to breastfeeding or via a gastric tube.
- Assist with obtaining a referral for a dietitian

Endocrine Management
- Monitor blood glucose levels.
- Administer insulin as prescribed.

Ⓝ *NCLEX® Connection: Physiological Adaptation, Basic Pathophysiology*

When reviewing the following chapters, keep in mind the relevant topics and tasks of the NCLEX outline, in particular:

Pharmacological Therapies

EXPECTED ACTIONS/OUTCOMES: Reinforce education to client regarding medications.

MEDICATION ADMINISTRATION

Administer a subcutaneous, intradermal, or intramuscular medication.

Collect required data prior to medication administration.

Reduction of Risk Potential

DIAGNOSTIC TESTS: Perform diagnostic testing.

POTENTIAL FOR COMPLICATIONS OF DIAGNOSTIC TESTS/ TREATMENTS/PROCEDURES: Use precautions to prevent injury and/or complications associated with a procedure or diagnosis.

Physiological Adaptation

ALTERATIONS IN BODY SYSTEMS

Provide care to correct client alteration in body system.

Reinforce education to the client regarding care and condition.

BASIC PATHOPHYSIOLOGY

Identify signs and symptoms related to an acute or chronic illness.

Consider general principles of client disease process when providing care.

UNIT 2   SYSTEM DISORDERS
SECTION: CARDIOVASCULAR AND HEMATOLOGIC DISORDERS

CHAPTER 19 *Cardiovascular Disorders*

Heart disease in children can be congenital or acquired.

Anatomic abnormalities present at birth can lead to congenital heart disease (CHD) most commonly, heart failure, and hypoxemia.

Heart failure occurs when the heart is unable to meet the metabolic and physical demands of the body due to inadequate blood flow.

Hyperlipidemia has increased due to changing lifestyles and a decrease in socioeconomic status. This results in obesity in childhood, which leads to heart disease in adulthood.

Congenital heart disease

Anatomic defects of the heart prevent normal blood flow to the pulmonary and/or systemic system. Defects are categorized by blood flow patterns in the heart.
- Increased pulmonary blood flow: ASD, VSD, PDA
- Decreased pulmonary blood flow: Tetralogy of Fallot, tricuspid atresia
- Obstruction to blood flow: Coarctation of the aorta, pulmonary stenosis, aortic stenosis
- Mixed blood flow: Transposition of the great arteries, truncus arteriosus, hypoplastic left heart syndrome

DATA COLLECTION

RISK FACTORS

MATERNAL FACTORS
- Infection
- Alcohol or other substance use disorder during pregnancy
- Diabetes mellitus

GENETIC FACTORS
- History of congenital heart disease in other family members
- Syndromes (Trisomy 21 [Down syndrome])
- Presence of other congenital anomalies or chromosomal abnormalities

EXPECTED FINDINGS

Defects that increase pulmonary blood flow

Defects with increased pulmonary blood flow allow blood to shift from the high pressure left side of the heart to the right, lower pressure side of the heart.
- Increased pulmonary blood volume on the right side of the heart increases pulmonary blood flow.
- These defects include manifestations and findings of heart failure.

Ventricular septal defect (VSD) (19.1)
A hole in the septum between the right and left ventricle that results in increased pulmonary blood flow (left-to-right shunt)
- Loud, harsh murmur auscultated at the left sternal border
- Heart failure
- Many VSDs close spontaneously early in life

Atrial septal defect (ASD)
A hole in the septum between the right and left atria that results in increased pulmonary blood flow (left-to-right shunt)
- Loud, harsh murmur with a fixed split second heart sound
- Heart failure
- Asymptomatic (possibly)

Patent ductus arteriosus (PDA)
A condition in which the normal fetal circulation conduit between the pulmonary artery and the aorta fails to close and results in increased pulmonary blood flow (left-to-right shunt)
- Systolic murmur (machine hum)
- Wide pulse pressure
- Bounding pulses
- Asymptomatic (possibly)
- Heart failure
- Rales

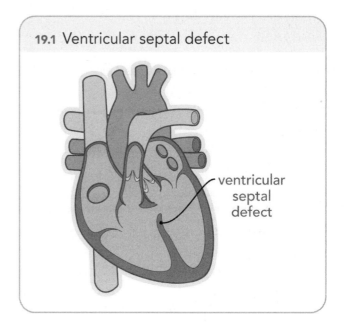

19.1 Ventricular septal defect

ventricular septal defect

Obstructive defects

Obstructive defects include those where blood flow exiting the heart meets an area of narrowing (stenosis), which causes obstruction of blood flow.
- The pressure that occurs before the defect is increased (ventricle) and the pressure that occurs after the defect is decreased. This results in a decrease in cardiac output.
- These children can present with manifestations of heart failure.

Pulmonary stenosis (19.2)
A narrowing of the pulmonary valve or pulmonary artery that results in obstruction of blood flow from the ventricles
- Systolic ejection murmur
- Asymptomatic (possibly)
- Cyanosis varies with defect, worse with severe narrowing
- Cardiomegaly
- Heart failure

Aortic stenosis
A narrowing of the aortic valve
- INFANTS: Faint pulses, hypotension, tachycardia, poor feeding tolerance
- CHILDREN: Intolerance to exercise, dizziness, chest pain, possible ejection murmur

Coarctation of the aorta (19.3)
A narrowing of the lumen of the aorta, usually at or near the ductus arteriosus, that results in obstruction of blood flow from the ventricle
- Elevated blood pressure in the arms
- Bounding pulses in the upper extremities
- Decreased blood pressure in the lower extremities
- Cool skin of lower extremities
- Weak or absent femoral pulses
- Heart failure in infants
- Dizziness, headaches, fainting, or nosebleeds in older children

Defects that decrease pulmonary blood flow

- Defects that decrease pulmonary blood flow have an obstruction of pulmonary blood flow and an anatomic defect (ASD or VSD) between the right and left sides of the heart.
- In these defects, there is a right to left shift allowing deoxygenated blood to enter the systemic circulation.
- Hypercyanotic spells (blue, or "Tet," spells) manifest as acute cyanosis and hyperpnea.

Tricuspid atresia
A complete closure of the tricuspid valve that results in mixed blood flow. An atrial septal opening needs to be present to allow blood to enter the left atrium.
- Infants: Cyanosis, dyspnea, tachycardia
- Older children: Hypoxemia, clubbing of fingers

Tetralogy of Fallot (19.4)
Four defects that result in mixed blood flow: Pulmonary stenosis, ventricular septal defect, overriding aorta, right ventricular hypertrophy
- Cyanosis at birth: progressive cyanosis over the first year of life
- Systolic murmur
- Episodes of acute cyanosis and hypoxia (blue or "Tet" spells)

Mixed defects

Transposition of the great arteries
A condition in which the aorta is connected to the right ventricle instead of the left, and the pulmonary artery is connected to the left ventricle instead of the right. A septal defect or a PDA must exist in order to oxygenate the blood.
- Murmur depending on presence of associated defects
- Severe to less cyanosis depending on the size of the associated defect
- Cardiomegaly
- Heart failure

Truncus arteriosus
Failure of septum formation, resulting in a single vessel that comes off of the ventricles
- Heart failure
- Murmur
- Variable cyanosis
- Delayed growth
- Lethargy
- Fatigue
- Poor feeding habits

Hypoplastic left heart syndrome
Left side of the heart is underdeveloped. An ASD or patent foramen ovale allows for oxygenation of the blood.
- Mild cyanosis
- Heart failure
- Lethargy
- Cold hands and feet
- Once PDA closes, progression of cyanosis and decreased cardiac output result in eventual cardiac collapse

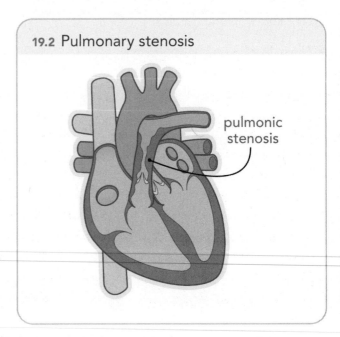

19.2 Pulmonary stenosis

pulmonic stenosis

PATIENT-CENTERED CARE

THERAPEUTIC PROCEDURES

Ventricular septal defect

NONSURGICAL PROCEDURE/THERAPIES
- Closure during cardiac catheterization
- Careful observations for spontaneous closure
- Diuretics

SURGICAL PROCEDURES
- Pulmonary artery banding
- Complete repair with patch (increased risk for heart block)

Atrial septal defect

NONSURGICAL PROCEDURES/THERAPIES
- Closure during cardiac catheterization
- Diuretics
- Low dose aspirin 6 months after procedure

SURGICAL PROCEDURE:
- Patch closure
- Cardiopulmonary bypass

Patent ductus arteriosus

NONSURGICAL PROCEDURES/THERAPIES
- Administration of indomethacin (to allow for closure)
- Insertion of coils to occlude PDA during cardiac catheterization
- Administration of diuretics (furosemide)
- Provide extra calories for infants

SURGICAL PROCEDURE: Thoracoscopic repair (ligate vessels)

Pulmonary stenosis

NONSURGICAL PROCEDURES/THERAPIES: Balloon angioplasty with cardiac catheterization

SURGICAL PROCEDURES
- INFANTS: Brock procedure
- CHILDREN: pulmonary valvotomy

Aortic stenosis

NONSURGICAL PROCEDURES/THERAPIES
- Balloon dilation with cardiac catheterization
- Administer beta blockers, calcium channel blockers

SURGICAL PROCEDURES
- Norwood procedure
- Aortic valvotomy

Coarctation of the aorta

NONSURGICAL PROCEDURES/THERAPIES
- Infants and children: Balloon angioplasty
- Adolescents: Placement of stents

SURGICAL PROCEDURE: Repair of defect recommended for infants less than 6 months of age

Tricuspid atresia

SURGICAL PROCEDURES: Surgery in 3 stages: shunt placement, Glenn procedure, modified Fontan procedure

Tetralogy of Fallot

SURGICAL PROCEDURES
- Shunt placement until able to undergo primary repair
- Complete repair within the first year of life

Transposition of the great arteries

SURGICAL PROCEDURE/THERAPIES
- Surgery to switch the arteries within the first 2 weeks of life.
- IV prostaglandin E (keep ducts open)

Truncus arteriosus

SURGICAL PROCEDURE: Surgical repair within the first month of life

Hypoplastic left heart syndrome

SURGICAL PROCEDURES: Surgery in three stages starting shortly after birth: Norwood procedure, Glenn shunt, and Fontan procedure

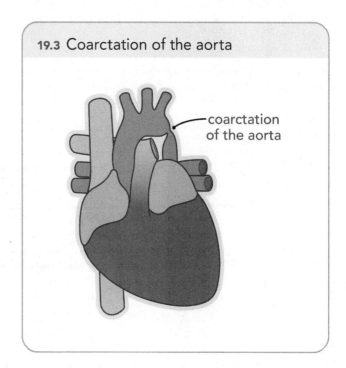

19.3 Coarctation of the aorta

coarctation of the aorta

Pulmonary artery hypertension

Pulmonary artery hypertension (PAH) is high blood pressure in the arteries of the lungs that is a progressive and eventually fatal disease. There is no cure for pulmonary hypertension.

DATA COLLECTION

RISK FACTORS

Although anyone can develop PAH, there can be a genetic link in children who have family who have PAH.

EXPECTED FINDINGS

- Dyspnea with exercise
- Chest pain
- Syncope

DIAGNOSTIC PROCEDURES

- Radiography (chest x-ray)
- Electrocardiogram
- Echocardiography
- Cardiac catheterization

PATIENT-CENTERED CARE

NURSING CARE

- Support the child and family regarding diagnosis and decisions of treatment options.
- Assist with preparing the child and family for possible lung transplantation.

CLIENT EDUCATION
- Avoid high altitude areas because of hypoxia.
- Consider supplemental oxygen therapy.
- It is important to adhere to the medication schedule.
- The prostacyclin infusion cannot be interrupted for any reason.

Infective (bacterial) endocarditis

- Infective endocarditis is an infection of the inner lining of the heart and the valves that can enter the bloodstream.
- Causative organisms include *Streptococcus viridans*, *Candida albicans*, and *Staphylococcus aureus*.

DATA COLLECTION

RISK FACTORS

- Congenital or acquired heart disease
- Indwelling catheters

EXPECTED FINDINGS

- Fever, malaise, new murmur, myalgias, arthralgias, diaphoresis, weight loss, splinter hemorrhages under fingernails
- Neonates: Feeding problems, respiratory distress, tachycardia, heart failure, septicemia

LABORATORY TESTS

- CBC
- Erythrocyte sedimentation rate (ESR): elevated
- Urinalysis
- Blood cultures (positive for diagnosis)

DIAGNOSTIC PROCEDURES

- Electrocardiogram (ECG; vegetations present)
- Echocardiogram

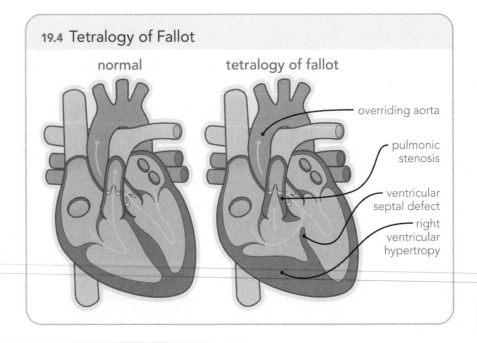

19.4 Tetralogy of Fallot

normal   tetralogy of fallot

overriding aorta

pulmonic stenosis

ventricular septal defect

right ventricular hypertropy

PATIENT-CENTERED CARE

NURSING CARE

- Ensure administration of antibiotics parenterally for an extended length of time (2 to 8 weeks) usually via a peripherally inserted central catheter.
- Maintain a high level of oral care.
- Advise the family's regular dentist of existing cardiac problems in high-risk children to ensure preventative treatment.

MEDICATIONS

High-dose anti-infectives are given for 2 to 8 weeks IV.

CLIENT EDUCATION ○PCC

- High risk children require prophylactic antibiotics prior to dental and surgical procedures
- Observe for manifestations and findings of infection.
- Schedule follow-up appointments.
- Follow the American Heart Association's recommendations for infective endocarditis prophylaxis. Only high-risk children should receive prophylactic antibiotic therapy.
- High-risk children should receive prophylactic antibiotic therapy prior to dental procedures, surgical procedures that involve the respiratory tract, and procedures on infected skin or musculoskeletal tissue.
- The high-risk group requiring prophylaxis treatment includes children who have artificial heart valves; previous diagnosis of infective endocarditis; unrepaired cyanotic congenital heart disease; repaired congenital heart disease using prosthetic material or device during the first 6 months of the procedure; and residual defects after congenital heart disease repair.
- Observe for manifestations of endocarditis (low-grade fever, malaise, decreased appetite with weight loss).
- Children can require long-term antibiotics at home.

19.5 Clubbed fingers

COMPLICATIONS

- Heart failure
- Myocardial infarction
- Embolism

Cardiomyopathy

Cardiomyopathy refers to abnormalities of the myocardium which interfere with its ability to contract effectively. Can lead to heart failure.

CLASSIFICATIONS

Dilated (DCM): Most common

Hypertrophic (HCM): Autosomal genetic increase in heart muscle mass leads to abnormal diastolic function

Restrictive: Rare; prevents filling of the ventricles and causes a decrease in diastolic volume

DATA COLLECTION

RISK FACTORS

Genetic factors, infection, deficiency states, metabolic conditions, collagen diseases, drug toxicity, dysrhythmias

EXPECTED FINDINGS

- Tachycardia and dysrhythmias
- Dyspnea
- Hepatosplenomegaly
- Fatigue and poor growth
- DCM: Palpations, syncope, infant poor feeding-respiratory distress
- HCM: Chest pain, syncope, dyspnea

PATIENT-CENTERED CARE

THERAPEUTIC MEASURES

- Beta blockers, calcium channel blockers, ACE inhibitors, anticoagulants
- Heart transplant

DIAGNOSTIC PROCEDURES

- Radiography (chest x-ray)
- ECG
- Echocardiogram
- Cardiac catheterization

COMPLICATIONS

- Infection
- Embolic complications (restrictive)

Shock

Cardiogenic shock results from impaired cardiac function that leads to a decrease in cardiac output.

Anaphylactic shock results from a hypersensitivity to a foreign substance that leads to massive vasodilation and capillary leak and can occur in response to an allergy to latex or drugs, insect stings, or blood transfusions.

DATA COLLECTION

RISK FACTORS

- Cardiogenic shock can be seen in children following cardiac surgery and with acute dysrhythmias, congestive heart failure, trauma, or cardiomyopathy.
- Anaphylaxis can be seen in children who have allergies, asthma, or a family history of anaphylaxis.

EXPECTED FINDINGS

- Dyspnea
- Breath sounds with crackles
- Grunting
- Hypotension
- Tachycardia
- Weak peripheral pulses

MANIFESTATIONS OF HEART FAILURE
- **Impaired myocardial function:** Sweating, tachycardia, fatigue, pallor, cool extremities with weak pulses, hypotension, gallop rhythm, cardiomegaly
- **Pulmonary congestion:** Tachypnea, dyspnea, retractions, nasal flaring, grunting, wheezing, cyanosis, cough, orthopnea, exercise intolerance
- **Systemic venous congestion:** Hepatomegaly, peripheral edema, ascites, neck vein distention, periorbital edema, weight gain

MANIFESTATIONS OF HYPOXEMIA: Cyanosis, poor weight gain, tachypnea, dyspnea, clubbing, polycythemia (19.5)

MANIFESTATIONS OF ANAPHYLAXIS: Urticaria, periorbital or perioral angioedema, stridor, bronchospasm

LABORATORY TESTS

- ABGs including pH
- Hemoglobin, hematocrit, and blood electrolytes

DIAGNOSTIC PROCEDURES

ECG monitoring

To identify cardiac dysrhythmias

NURSING ACTIONS
- Assist with the application of electrodes.
- Assist with maintaining the child in a quiet position.

CLIENT EDUCATION: Tell the child that the test will not be painful.

Radiography (chest x-ray)

To determine heart size and blood flow

NURSING ACTIONS: Assist with positioning the child.

Echocardiography

To determine cardiac defects and heart function by use of ultrasound

NURSING ACTIONS: Assist with positioning the child.

Cardiac catheterization

An invasive test used for diagnosing, repairing some defects, and evaluating dysrhythmias. A radiopaque catheter is peripherally inserted and threaded into the heart with the use of fluoroscopy. A contrast medium (can be iodine-based) is injected, and images of the blood vessels and heart are taken as the medium is diluted and circulated throughout the body.

PREPROCEDURE NURSING ACTIONS
- Collect data related to nursing history and physical exam. Evidence of infection (a severe diaper rash) can necessitate canceling the procedure if femoral access is required.
- Check for allergies to iodine and shellfish.
- Assist with providing age-appropriate instruction.
- Reinforce how long the procedure will take, how the child will feel, and what care will be required after the procedure.
- Provide for NPO status 4 to 6 hr prior to the procedure. (If the procedure is performed as outpatient, be sure the child and family are given instructions in advance.)
- Assist with obtaining baseline vital signs, including oxygen saturation.
- Locate and mark the dorsalis pedis and posterior tibial pulses on both extremities. Document the quality of the pulses.
- Ensure the administration of pre-sedation as prescribed based on the child's age, height, weight, condition, and type of procedure being performed.

POSTPROCEDURE NURSING ACTIONS
- Provide for continuous cardiac monitoring and oxygen saturation to observe for bradycardia, dysrhythmias, hypotension, and hypoxemia.
- Monitor heart and respiratory rate for 1 full minute.
- Palpate pulses for equality and symmetry.
- Monitor temperature and color of affected extremity. A cool extremity with skin that blanches can indicate arterial obstruction.
- Monitor insertion site (femoral or antecubital area) for bleeding or hematoma.
- Maintain clean dressing.
- Prevent bleeding by maintaining the affected extremity in a straight position for 4 to 8 hr.
- Monitor I&O for adequate urine output, hypovolemia, or dehydration.
- Monitor for hypoglycemia. IV fluids with dextrose can be necessary.
- Encourage oral intake, starting with clear liquids.
- Encourage the child to void to promote excretion of the contrast medium.

CLIENT EDUCATION

- Fluid intake can help with the removal of the dye from the body.
- Monitor the site for infection.
- Use mild analgesics for pain.
- Keep dressing clean and dry.
- No strenuous exercise.

PATIENT-CENTERED CARE

NURSING CARE

- Remain calm when providing care.
- Keep the child well-hydrated.
- Conserve the child's energy by providing frequent rest periods; clustering care; providing small, frequent meals; bathing PRN; and keeping crying to a minimum in cyanotic children.
- Perform daily weight and I&O to monitor fluid status and nutritional status.
- Monitor heart rate, blood pressure, blood electrolytes, and kidney function to monitor for complications.
- Provide support and resources for guardians to promote developmental growth in the child.
- Monitor family coping and provide support.
- Administer prescribed medications.
- Maintain fluid and electrolyte balance.
  - Administer potassium supplements if prescribed. These might not be indicated if the child is concurrently taking an ACE inhibitor.
  - Maintain sodium and fluid restrictions if prescribed.
- Decrease workload of the heart.
  - Maintain bed rest.
  - Position the infant in a car seat or hold at a 45° angle. Keep safety restraints low and loose on the abdomen.
  - Allow the child to sleep with several pillows and encourage a semi-Fowler's or Fowler's position while awake.
- Provide adequate nutrition.
  - Plan to feed the infant using a feeding schedule of every 3 hr. The infant should be rested, which occurs soon after awakening.
  - Use a soft preemie nipple or a regular nipple with a slit to provide an enlarged opening.
  - Hold the infant in a semi-upright position.
  - Allow the infant to rest during feedings, taking approximately 30 min to complete the feeding.
  - Gavage feed the infant if he is unable to consume enough formula or breast milk.
  - Increase caloric density of formula gradually from 20 kcal/oz to 30 kcal/oz.
  - Encourage clients who are breastfeeding to alternate feedings with high-density formula or fortified breast milk.
- Increase tissue oxygenation.
  - Provide cool, humidified oxygen via an oxygen hood (or tent), mask, or nasal cannula.
  - Suction the airway as indicated.
  - Monitor oxygen saturation every 2 to 4 hr.

MEDICATIONS

Digoxin

Improves myocardial contractility

NURSING ACTIONS

- Monitor pulse and withhold the medication as prescribed. Generally, if an infant's pulse is less than 90/min, the medication should be withheld. In children, the medication should be withheld if the pulse is less than 70/min.
- Monitor for toxicity as evidenced by bradycardia, dysrhythmias, nausea, vomiting, or anorexia.
- Anticipate the administration of digoxin immune fab as an antidote for toxicity.
- Therapeutic blood levels can vary between conditions and children. Consider manifestations and digoxin level when toxicity is suspected.

Captopril or enalapril

Angiotensin-converting enzyme (ACE) inhibitors reduce afterload by causing vasodilation, resulting in decreased pulmonary and systemic vascular resistance.

NURSING ACTIONS

- Monitor blood pressure before and after the medication is administered.
- Monitor for evidence of hyperkalemia.

CLIENT EDUCATION: Monitor blood pressure frequently.

Metoprolol or carvedilol

Beta blockers decrease heart rate and blood pressure, and promote vasodilation.

NURSING ACTIONS

- Monitor blood pressure and pulse prior to administration.
- Monitor for adverse effects (dizziness, hypotension, and headache).

Furosemide or chlorothiazide

Potassium-wasting diuretics rid the body of excess fluid and sodium.

NURSING ACTIONS

- Encourage a diet high in potassium.
- Monitor I&O.
- Monitor for adverse effects (hypokalemia, nausea, vomiting, and dizziness).
- Monitor weight daily.

INTERPROFESSIONAL CARE

Dietitians should be consulted to assist the family with appropriate food choices.

CLIENT EDUCATION Q_{PCC}

Cardiac catheterization

- Monitor for possible complications (bleeding, infection, thrombosis).
- Limit activity for 24 hr.
- Encourage fluids.

Digoxin administration

- Take pulse prior to medication administration. Notify provider if pulse is lower than specified rate.
- Administer digoxin every 12 hr.
- Direct oral elixir toward the side and back of mouth when administering. Q_S
- Give water following administration to prevent tooth decay if the child has teeth.
- If a dose is missed, do not give an extra dose or increase the next dose.
- If the child vomits, do not re-administer the dose.
- Observe for manifestations of digoxin toxicity (decreased heart rate, decreased appetite, nausea, vomiting). Notify the provider if these occur.
- Keep the medication in a locked cabinet.

Diuretic administration

- Offer small amounts of fluids in small cups or containers
- Observe for adverse effects of diuretics, which can include nausea, vomiting, and diarrhea.
- Observe for manifestations of blood potassium level imbalances (muscle weakness, irritability, excessive drowsiness, and increased or decreased heart rate).
- Encourage the child to eat foods high in potassium (bran cereals, bananas, legumes, leafy vegetables, oranges, and orange juice.)

CLIENT EDUCATION
- Monitor weight daily.
- Report evidence of worsening heart failure (increased sweating and decreased urinary output [fewer wet diapers or less frequent toileting]).

COMPLICATIONS

Cardiac catheterization (potential)

- Nausea, vomiting
- Low-grade fever
- Loss of pulse in the catheterized extremity
- Transient dysrhythmias
- Acute hemorrhage from entry site
- Hypoglycemia: Monitor blood glucose levels

NURSING ACTIONS
- Apply direct continuous pressure at 2.5 cm (1 in) above the catheter entry site to localize pressure over the location of the vessel puncture.
- Position the child flat to reduce the gravitational effect on the rate of bleeding.
- Notify the provider immediately.
- Prepare for the possible administration of replacement fluids and/or medication to control emesis.

CLIENT EDUCATION
- Monitor for infection.
- Monitor for bleeding.

Hypoxemia

A hypercyanotic spell can result in severe hypoxemia, which leads to cerebral hypoxia, and should be treated as an emergency.

NURSING ACTIONS: Immediately place the child in the knee-chest position, attempt to calm the child, and call for help.

Heart failure requiring transplant

Cardiomyopathy and congenital heart disease are causes of heart failure.

NURSING ACTIONS
- Maintain pharmacological support as ordered (oxygen, diuretics, digoxin, afterload reducers [ACE inhibitors]).
- Provide family and child support.

CLIENT EDUCATION
- Adhere to the medication regimen.
- Be aware of infection control precautions.

Rheumatic fever

Rheumatic fever is an inflammatory disease that occurs as a reaction to Group A beta-hemolytic streptococcus (GABHS) infection of the throat.

DATA COLLECTION

RISK FACTORS

Rheumatic fever usually occurs within 2 to 6 weeks following an untreated or partially treated upper respiratory infection (strep throat) with GABHS.

EXPECTED FINDINGS

- History of recent upper respiratory infection
- Fever
- Tachycardia, cardiomegaly, new or changed heart murmur, muffled heart sounds, pericardial friction rub, and report of chest pain, which can indicate carditis
- Nontender, subcutaneous nodules over bony prominence
- Large joints (knees, elbows, ankles, wrists, shoulders) with painful swelling, indicating polyarthritis Q_{PCC}
  - Findings can be present for a few days and then disappear without treatment, frequently returning in another joint.
- Pink, nonpruritic macular rash on the trunk and inner surfaces of extremities that appears and disappears rapidly, indicating erythema marginatum
- CNS involvement (chorea) including involuntary, purposeless muscle movements; muscle weakness; involuntary facial movements; difficulty performing fine motor activities; labile emotions; and random, uncoordinated movements of the extremities
- Irritability, poor concentration, and behavioral problems

LABORATORY TESTS

Throat culture for GABHS: currently recommend screen all school-aged children who have sore throats

Blood antistreptolysin O titer: Elevated or rising titer, most reliable diagnostic test

C-reactive protein (CRP): Elevated in response to an inflammatory reaction

Erythrocyte sedimentation rate: Elevated in response to an inflammatory reaction

DIAGNOSTIC PROCEDURES

Radiography (chest x-ray)

To determine if the child has cardiomegaly

Cardiac function

- ECG to reveal the presence of conduction disturbances and to evaluate the function of the heart and valves
- Echocardiography to document pericardial effusions

NURSING ACTIONS: Position the child correctly for the procedure.

CLIENT EDUCATION: Explain the need for decreased movement during the procedure.

Jones criteria

The diagnosis of rheumatic fever is made on the basis of modified Jones criteria. The child should demonstrate the presence of two major criteria or the presence of one major and two minor criteria following an acute infection with GABHS infection.

MAJOR CRITERIA
- Carditis
- Subcutaneous nodules
- Polyarthritis
- Rash (erythema marginatum)
- Chorea

MINOR CRITERIA
- Fever
- Arthralgia

PATIENT-CENTERED CARE

NURSING CARE

- Encourage bed rest during the acute illness.
- Administer antibiotic as prescribed.
- Encourage nutritionally balanced meals.
- Monitor for chorea (nervousness, behavioral changes, decreased attention span).

MEDICATIONS

Antibiotic prophylaxis

Follow the prescribed prophylactic treatment regimen, which can include one of the following.
- Two daily oral doses of penicillin V
- Monthly IM injection of penicillin G
- Daily oral dose of sulfadiazine

The length of treatment varies according to residual heart disease, ranging from 5 years to indefinitely.

NURSING ACTIONS
- Monitor for an allergic response (anaphylaxis, hives, rashes).
- Monitor for nausea, vomiting, or diarrhea.

CLIENT EDUCATION: Encourage compliance with medication regimen.

CLIENT EDUCATION ⵇPCC

- Promote rest during the acute phase.
- Provide information and reassurance related to the development of chorea and its self-limiting nature.
- Consume a diet of well-balanced meals.
- Seek medical care if infection recurrence is suspected.
- Child may need valve repair or replacement surgery.
- Follow up with cardiologist regularly.

COMPLICATIONS

Carditis and heart disease, atrial fibrillation, embolism

Dyslipidemia

Dyslipidemia refers to disorders of lipid metabolism that can result in abnormalities in the lipid profile. Cholesterol is part of the lipoprotein complex in blood.

Triglycerides come from two sources: Naturally made in the body from carbohydrates, and the end product of fat ingestion

Total cholesterol: The sum of all forms of cholesterol

High density lipoprotein (HDL) cholesterol: "Good" cholesterol, having low level of cholesterol and triglycerides and high level of protein

Low density lipoprotein (LDL) cholesterol: "Bad" cholesterol, having a high level of cholesterol, low level of triglycerides, and moderate levels of protein

DATA COLLECTION

RISK FACTORS

- Family history
- Genetic
- Obesity
- Lack of exercise
- History of health condition: diabetes, hypertension
- Congenital heart disease and transplant recipients
- Cancer survivors
- History of Kawasaki disease with coronary artery aneurysms
- Chronic inflammatory diseases
- Medications: birth control pills, diuretics, beta-blockers

LABORATORY TESTS

Lipid profile: fasting for 12 hr prior to test

Fasting blood glucose

PATIENT-CENTERED CARE

NURSING CARE

- Assist in screening children who are at risk. Recommend two screenings between 2 to 8 years and the results of both tests are averaged.
- Determine if the child had a febrile illness 3 weeks prior to screening. (Illness will alter results.)

CLIENT EDUCATION Qpcc

- Keep a diet history for review by the dietitian.
- Diet to lower cholesterol: low fat, whole grains, fruit and vegetables.
- Use olive oil and canola oil.
- Maintain an exercise program (60 min/day of aerobic exercise for 5 days/week).

MEDICATION

Cholestyramine and colestipol

- Used in children who do not respond to conventional treatment
- Used in children 10 years and older who have LDL 190 mg/dL or higher, or 160 mg/dL in those who have risk factors

NURSING ACTIONS

- Powdered medication mixed in 4 to 6 oz water or juice, then administered immediately.
- Monitor for adverse effects: Constipation, abdominal pain, flatulence, nausea and abdominal bloating.
- Monitor laboratory findings: Liver function tests, CBC, creatinine kinase, and fasting lipid profile at 4- and 8-week intervals and with any dosage change.

CLIENT EDUCATION

- Understand how to administer medications.
- Observe for adverse effects of medications.
- Discontinue medication if experiencing dark urine or muscle aches, and notify the provider.
- Take multivitamin supplements while taking this medication.

HMG-CoA reductase inhibitors (statins)

NURSING ACTIONS

- Monitor for liver function and creatine kinase (CK) prior to start of therapy and during therapy.
- Can cause rhabdomyolysis (dark urine and muscle aches).
- Most effective in older children and adolescents.

CLIENT EDUCATION: Take in the evening.

INTERPROFESSIONAL CARE

Dietary counseling

COMPLICATIONS

Atherosclerosis and coronary heart disease

NURSING ACTIONS: Identify children who are at risk and promote early screening.

CLIENT EDUCATION: Practice healthy eating habits.

Kawasaki disease

Acute systemic vasculitis, resolves in less than 8 weeks. Also known as "mucocutaneous lymph node syndrome."

DATA COLLECTION

RISK FACTORS

Etiology unknown

EXPECTED FINDINGS

Acute phase

Onset of high fever, lasting 5 days to 2 weeks, that is unresponsive to antipyretics
- Irritability
- Red eyes without drainage
- Bright red, chapped lips
- Strawberry tongue with white coating or red bumps on the posterior aspect
- Red oral mucous membranes with inflammation including the pharynx
- Swelling of hand and feet with red palms and soles
- Nonblistering rash
- Bilateral joint pain

- Enlarged lymph nodes
- Desquamation of the perineum
- Cervical lymphadenopathy.
- Cardiac manifestations: Myocarditis, decreased left ventricular function, pericardial effusion, and mitral regurgitation

Subacute phase

Resolution of fever and gradual subsiding of other manifestations
- Irritability
- Peeling skin around the nails, on the palms and soles
- Temporary arthritis

Convalescent

No manifestations seen except altered laboratory findings. Resolution in about 6 to 8 weeks from onset.

LABORATORY TESTS

CBC, CRP, ESR, blood albumin, elevated liver enzymes, lumbar puncture to determine if the child has aseptic meningitis and inflammation

DIAGNOSTIC PROCEDURES

Radiography (chest x-ray)

Echocardiogram to evaluate heart size and the functioning of the ventricles and valves. A follow-up study is recommended 4 to 6 weeks after treatment.

PATIENT-CENTERED CARE

NURSING CARE

- Monitor vital signs and cardiac status. Maintain cardiac monitoring.
- Monitor for manifestations of heart failure (decreased urine output, gallop heart rhythm, tachycardia, respiratory distress).
- Monitor I&O.
- Obtain daily weight.
- Ensure IV fluids are administered to prevent dehydration.
- Offer clear liquids and soft, non-acidic foods.
- Ensure IV gamma globulin is administered according to facility policy.
- Administer aspirin as prescribed.
- Provide care to promote comfort due to findings.
  - Perform oral hygiene. Apply lip balm as needed.
  - Apply cool cloths to skin.
  - Apply skin lotions to maintain hydration.
  - Provide for a calm, quiet environment.
  - Promote rest by clustering care.

MEDICATION

Gamma globulin

NURSING ACTIONS
- Ensure the administration via IV infusion.
- High dosage: 2 g/kg over 8 to 12 hr.
- Ideally, administer within the first 10 days of illness.
- Repeat for children who remain febrile.
- Monitor vital signs.
- Monitor for manifestations of an allergic reaction.

Aspirin

HIGH DOSE: 80 to 100 mg/kg/day divided every 6 hr

ONCE AFEBRILE: 3 to 5 mg/kg/day to continue until platelet count returns to expected range which can be approximately 6 to 8 weeks

> If coronary abnormalities develop, continue aspirin therapy indefinitely.

CLIENT EDUCATION

- Understand disease progression.
- Maintain follow-up appointments.
- The irritability can last 2 months.
- Arthritic manifestations can last several weeks.
- Skin manifestations are painless, but the skin could be tender.
- Perform passive ROM exercises in the bathtub.
- Avoid live immunizations for 11 months.
- Notify the provider of any fever.

CARE AFTER DISCHARGE
- Avoid smoking.
- Maintain a heart healthy diet.
- Screen for heart disease as child ages.
  - Blood cholesterol testing
  - Blood pressure monitoring
  - Periodic imaging of the heart

COMPLICATIONS

Coronary artery dilation or aneurysm formation

- Most common in the subacute phase
- Echocardiogram to monitor for changes
- Administer anticoagulation medications as prescribed (enoxaparin)

Application Exercises

1. A nurse is collecting data from an infant who has coarctation of the aorta. Which of the following findings should the nurse expect? (Select all that apply.)
   A. Weak femoral pulses
   B. Cool skin of lower extremities
   C. Severe cyanosis
   D. Clubbing of the fingers
   E. Low blood pressure

2. A nurse is collecting data from an infant who has heart failure. Which of the following findings should the nurse expect? (Select all that apply.)
   A. Bradycardia
   B. Cool extremities
   C. Peripheral edema
   D. Increased urinary output
   E. Nasal flaring

3. A nurse is reinforcing teaching with the caregiver of an infant who has a prescription for digoxin. Which of the following statements should the nurse make?
   A. "Do not offer your baby fluids after giving the medication."
   B. "Digoxin increases your baby's heart rate."
   C. "Give the correct dose of medication at regularly scheduled times."
   D. "If your baby vomits a dose, you should repeat the dose to ensure that the correct amount is received."

4. A nurse is assisting with the care of a 2-year-old child who has a heart defect and is scheduled for cardiac catheterization. Which of the following actions should the nurse take?
   A. Place on NPO status for 12 hr prior to the procedure.
   B. Check for iodine or shellfish allergies prior to the procedure.
   C. Elevate the affected extremity following the procedure.
   D. Limit fluid intake following the procedure.

5. A nurse is collecting data from a child who has rheumatic fever. Which of the following findings should the nurse expect? (Select all that apply.)
   A. Erythema marginatum (rash)
   B. Continuous joint pain of the digits
   C. Tender, subcutaneous nodules
   D. Decreased erythrocyte sedimentation rate
   E. Elevated C-reactive protein

Active Learning Scenario

A nurse is reinforcing teaching with the adoptive parent of a child who has Kawasaki disease. What should the nurse include? Use the ATI Active Learning Template: System Disorder to complete this item.

EXPECTED FINDINGS: Identify for the acute, subacute, and convalescent phase.

NURSING CARE: List seven nursing actions for this child.

Application Exercises Key

1. A. **CORRECT:** Narrowing of the lumen of the aorta results in obstruction of blood flow from the ventricle, resulting in weak or absent femoral pulses.
   B. **CORRECT:** Narrowing of the lumen of the aorta results in obstruction of blood flow from the ventricle, resulting in cool skin of the lower extremities.
   C. A client who has coarctation of the aorta exhibits adequate oxygenation of blood. Severe cyanosis is not present.
   D. Clubbing of the fingers is a manifestation of chronic hypoxemia and will not be observed in an infant who has coarctation of the aorta.
   E. **CORRECT:** Hypotension occurs when the heart is unable to meet the body's demands and is a manifestation of coarctation of the aorta.

   Ⓝ NCLEX® Connection: Physiological Adaptation, Basic Pathophysiology

2. A. A client who has heart failure will exhibit tachycardia as the heart attempts to meet the body's demands.
   B. **CORRECT:** A client who has heart failure will exhibit cool extremities as the heart is unable to adequately circulate oxygenated blood.
   C. **CORRECT:** A client who has heart failure will exhibit peripheral edema as the heart is unable to adequately circulate blood through the body and back to the heart.
   D. With heart failure, the heart is unable to keep up with the body's demands. A decrease in urinary output is a manifestation of heart failure.
   E. **CORRECT:** A client who has heart failure will exhibit nasal flaring due to inadequate oxygenation of blood.

   Ⓝ NCLEX® Connection: Physiological Adaptation, Basic Pathophysiology

3. A. Digoxin can be given without regard to food or fluids.
   B. Digoxin slows the heart rate by increasing contractility of the heart.
   C. **CORRECT:** The correct amount of digoxin should be administered at regularly scheduled times to maintain therapeutic blood levels.
   D. It is not recommended to repeat digoxin following an emesis because it is impossible to determine how much medication was lost.

   Ⓝ NCLEX® Connection: Pharmacological Therapies, Medication Administration

4. A. The child should remain NPO 4 to 6 hr prior to the procedure.
   B. **CORRECT:** Iodine-based dyes can be used in this procedure, so the child is monitored for allergies to iodine or shellfish which could lead to anaphylaxis.
   C. The affected extremity should be maintained in a straight position following the procedure.
   D. Fluids should be encouraged after the procedure to maintain adequate urine output and promote excretion of the dye.

   Ⓝ NCLEX® Connection: Reduction of Risk Potential, Potential for Complications from Surgical Procedures and Health Alterations

5. A. **CORRECT:** Rheumatic fever is caused by Group A beta-hemolytic streptococcus. An erythema marginatum (rash) is a manifestation.
   B. A client who has rheumatic fever exhibits migratory joint pain of the large joints.
   C. A client who has rheumatic fever exhibits nontender subcutaneous nodules of bony prominences.
   D. Rheumatic fever is caused by Group A beta-hemolytic streptococcus, which results in an elevated erythrocyte sedimentation rate.
   E. **CORRECT:** Rheumatic fever is caused by Group A beta-hemolytic streptococcus. An increase in C-reactive protein is a manifestation.

   Ⓝ NCLEX® Connection: Physiological Adaptation, Pathophysiology

Active Learning Scenario Key

Using the ATI Active Learning Template: System Disorder
EXPECTED FINDINGS

Acute phase: onset of high fever that is unresponsive to antipyretics, with development of other manifestations
- Fever greater than 38.9° C (102° F) lasting 5 days to 2 weeks and unresponsive to antipyretics
- Irritability
- Red eyes without drainage
- Bright red, chapped lips
- Strawberry tongue with white coating or red bumps on the posterior aspect
- Red oral mucous membranes
- Swelling of hands and feet with red palms and soles
- Non-blistering rash
- Bilateral joint pain
- Enlarged lymph nodes
- Subacute phase: resolution of the fever and gradual subsiding of other manifestations
- Irritability
- Peeling skin around the nails, on the palms and soles

Convalescent phase: no manifestations seen except altered laboratory findings. Resolution in about 6 to 8 weeks from onset.

NURSING CARE
- Monitor vital signs, ECG, and cardiac status.
- Monitor for indications of heart failure (decreased urine output, gallop heart rhythm, tachycardia, respiratory distress).
- Monitor I&O. Obtain daily weight.
- Monitor IV fluids. Offer clear liquids and soft foods.
- Monitor IV gamma globulin according to facility policy.
- Administer aspirin as prescribed.
- Provide care to include oral hygiene, cool cloths to extremities, application of skin lotion; providing for a quiet environment to promote rest; cluster nursing care.

   Ⓝ NCLEX® Connection: Physiological Adaptation, Unexpected Response to Therapies

CHAPTER 20 *Hematologic Disorders*

Blood disorders that can affect children include epistaxis, iron deficiency anemia, sickle cell anemia, and hemophilia.

Epistaxis

- Short, isolated occurrences of epistaxis (nosebleeds) are common in childhood.
- Although epistaxis is rarely an emergency, it causes anxiety for the child and the child's caregivers.

DATA COLLECTION

RISK FACTORS

- Trauma (picking or rubbing the nose) can cause mucous membranes in the nose, which are vascular and fragile, to tear and bleed.
- Low humidity, allergic rhinitis, upper respiratory infection, blunt injury, or a foreign body in the nose can precipitate a nosebleed.
- Medications that affect clotting factors can increase bleeding.
- Epistaxis can be the result of underlying diseases (von Willebrand disease, hemophilia, idiopathic thrombocytopenia purpura, leukemia).

PHYSICAL FINDINGS
- Active bleeding from nose
- Restlessness and agitation

PATIENT-CENTERED CARE

NURSING CARE

- Maintain a calm demeanor with the child and family.
- Have the child sit up with the head tilted slightly forward to prevent aspiration of blood. Qs
- Apply pressure to the lower nose with the thumb and forefinger for at least 10 min.
- Do not pack cotton or tissue into the nostril or ask the child to blow their nose because this could displace the clot.
- Encourage the child to breathe through their mouth while pressure is being applied to their nose to control the bleeding.
- Apply ice or a cold cloth across the bridge of the nose if bleeding continues.

CLIENT EDUCATION
- For recurrences, sit up and slightly forward so blood does not flow down the throat and cause coughing.
- Bleeding usually stops within 10 min.

Iron deficiency anemia

- Iron deficiency anemia is the most prevalent anemia worldwide.
- Adolescents are at risk due to poor diet, rapid growth, menses, strenuous activities, and obesity.
- The production of hemoglobin (Hgb) requires iron. Iron deficiency will result in decreased Hgb levels.
- Iron deficiency anemia usually results from an inadequate dietary supply of iron, and is the most preventable mineral disturbance.

DATA COLLECTION

RISK FACTORS

- Premature birth resulting in decreased iron stores
- Excessive intake of cows' milk in toddlers
  - Milk is not a good source of iron.
  - Milk takes the place of iron-rich solid foods.
- Malabsorption disorders
- Poor dietary intake of iron
- Increased iron requirements (blood loss)

Infants: GERD, pyloric stenosis

Older Child: GI polyps, colitis

Adolescents: Menorrhagia

EXPECTED FINDINGS

- Tachycardia
- Pallor
- Brittle, spoon-shaped fingernails
- Fatigue, irritability, and muscle weakness
- Systolic heart murmur
- Cravings for non-nutritive substances (ice, dirt, paper)

LABORATORY TESTS

CBC: Decreased RBC count, Hgb, and Hct

Hgb levels: Vary with age

RBC indices: Decreased, indicating microcytic/hypochromic RBCs
- **Mean corpuscular volume:** Average size of RBC
- **Mean corpuscular Hgb:** Average weight of RBC
- **Mean corpuscular hemoglobin concentration:** Amount of Hgb relative to size of cell

Reticulocyte count: Can be decreased (indicates bone marrow production of RBCs)

Total iron binding capacity: Elevated

Transferrin: 10% indicative of anemia

Stool analysis: Guaiac test

PATIENT-CENTERED CARE

NURSING CARE

- Provide iron supplements for preterm and low-birth-weight infants by the age of 2 months. Q̃EBP
- Provide iron supplements to full term infants by the age of 4 to 6 months.
- Recommend iron-fortified formula for infants when solids are introduced
- Modify the infant's diet to include high iron and vitamin C.
- Monitor formula intake in infants.
  - Limit formula intake to 32 oz (960 mL) per day.
  - Encourage intake of iron-rich foods.
  - Provide iron-fortified cereal when solid foods are introduced.
  - Allow frequent rest periods.
- If packed RBCs are required, follow protocols for administration.

MEDICATIONS

Iron supplements

NURSING ACTIONS
- Give 1 hr before or 2 hr after milk, tea, or antacid to prevent decreased absorption.
- Gastrointestinal (GI) upset (diarrhea, constipation, nausea) is common at the start of therapy. These will decrease over time.
- If tolerated, administer iron supplements on an empty stomach. Give with meals and start with reduced dose and gradually increase if GI distress occurs.
- Give with vitamin C (ascorbic acid) to increase absorption.
- Use a straw with liquid preparation to prevent staining of teeth.
- Use a Z-track into deep muscle for parenteral injections. Do not massage after injection.

CLIENT EDUCATION
- Expect stools to turn a tarry green color if dose is adequate.
- Brush teeth after oral dose to minimize or prevent staining.

SEVERE ANEMIA THERAPY

Monitoring during IV administration ferrous sulfate

- Very painful infusion
- Requires close monitoring of the child during administration

Blood transfusion

PRBC preferred

Supplemental oxygen

Used for severe hypoxia

CLIENT EDUCATION

- Diarrhea, constipation, or nausea can occur at the start of therapy, but these adverse effects are usually self-limiting.
- Understand appropriate iron administration.
- Increase fiber and fluids if constipation develops.
- To prevent toxicity, store no more than 1 month's supply in a child-proof bottle out of reach of children.
- Allow adequate time for the child to rest.
- The length of treatment will be determined by the child's response to the treatment. If Hgb levels are not increased after 1 month of therapy, further evaluation is warranted.
- Return for follow-up laboratory tests to determine the effectiveness of treatment.
- Schedule universal anemia screens at 12 months of age.

Dietary sources of iron
- **INFANTS:** Iron-fortified cereals and formula or exclusive breastfeeding
- **OLDER CHILDREN:** Dried beans and lentils; peanut butter; green, leafy vegetables; iron-fortified breads and flour; poultry; and red meat

COMPLICATIONS

Developmental delay

NURSING ACTIONS
- Monitor level of functioning.
- Improve nutritional intake.
- Refer to appropriate developmental services.

CLIENT EDUCATION: Provide support to the family.

Sickle cell anemia

Sickle cell disease (SCD) is a group of diseases in which abnormal sickle hemoglobin S (HbS) replaces normal adult hemoglobin (Hgb A).

Sickle cell anemia (SCA) is the homozygous and most common form of SCD.
- Manifestations and complications of SCA are the result of RBC sickling, which leads to increased blood viscosity, obstruction of blood flow, and tissue hypoxia. Manifestations of SCA are not usually apparent until later in infancy due to the presence of fetal Hgb.
- Tissue hypoxia causes tissue ischemia, which results in pain.
- Increased destruction of RBCs occurs.

Sickle cell trait: Child has the genes but is asymptomatic.

Sickle cell crisis is the acute exacerbation of SCA.

DATA COLLECTION

RISK FACTORS

- SCD is an autosomal recessive genetic disorder.
- SCA primarily affects African-Americans. Other forms of SCD can affect individuals of Mediterranean, Indian, or Middle Eastern descent.
- Children who have the sickle cell trait do not manifest the disease but can pass the trait to their offspring.

EXPECTED FINDINGS

- Family history of sickle cell anemia or sickle cell trait
- Reports of pain
- Shortness of breath, fatigue
- Pallor, pale mucous membranes
- Jaundice
- Hands and feet cool to touch
- Dizziness
- Headache

Vaso-occlusive crisis (painful episode)

Acute (related to dehydration and decreased oxygen)
- Severe pain, usually in bones, joints, and abdomen
- Swollen joints, hands, and feet
- Abdominal pain
- Hematuria
- Obstructive jaundice
- Visual disturbances

Chronic
- Increased risk of respiratory infections and osteomyelitis
- Retinal detachment and blindness
- Systolic murmurs
- Renal failure and enuresis
- Liver cirrhosis; hepatomegaly
- Seizures
- Skeletal deformities; shoulder or hip avascular necrosis

Sequestration

- Excessive pooling of blood primarily in the spleen (splenomegaly), and sometimes in the liver (hepatomegaly)
- Reduced circulating blood volume results in hypovolemia and can progress to shock
- Hypovolemic shock: irritability, tachycardia, pallor, decreased urinary output, tachypnea, cool extremities, thready pulse, hypotension

Aplastic crisis

- Extreme anemia as a result of a temporary decreased RBC production
- Typically triggered by an infection with a virus

Hyperhemolytic crisis

Increased rate of RBC destruction leading to anemia, jaundice, and/or reticulocytosis

LABORATORY TESTS

Screening for SCA in newborns is mandatory in all 50 US states and territories.

CBC to detect anemia.

Sickle-turbidity screening tool detects the presence of HbS but will not differentiate the trait from the disease.

Hemoglobin electrophoresis separates the various forms of Hgb and is the definitive diagnosis of sickle cell anemia or sickle cell trait.

Sickle-cell crisis

Hgb: decreased

WBC count: elevated

Bilirubin and reticulocyte levels: elevated

Peripheral blood smear reveals sickled cells

DIAGNOSTIC PROCEDURES

Transcranial Doppler (TCD) test
- Used to monitor intracranial vascular flow and detect the risk for cerebrovascular accident (CVA). Qs
- A TCD is performed annually on children ages 2 to 16 years who have SCD.

PATIENT-CENTERED CARE

NURSING CARE

- Promote rest to decrease oxygen consumption.
- Administer oxygen as prescribed if hypoxia is present.
- Provide intense hydration therapy while maintaining fluid and electrolyte balance.
  - Monitor I&O.
  - Give oral fluids.
  - Ensure administration of IV fluids with electrolyte replacement.
  - Caution with potassium replacement.
- Ensure administration of blood products, usually packed RBCs, and exchange transfusions per facility protocol. Monitor for manifestations of hypervolemia and transfusion reaction.
- Treat and prevent infection.
  - Administer antibiotics.
  - Perform frequent hand hygiene.
  - Give oral prophylactic penicillin. QEBP
  - Administer pneumococcal conjugate vaccine, meningococcal vaccine, and *Haemophilus influenzae* type B vaccine.
- Monitor and report laboratory results

Pain management

- Use an interprofessional approach.
- Treat mild to moderate pain with acetaminophen or ibuprofen. Manage severe pain with opioid analgesics.
- Apply comfort measures (warm packs to painful joints).
- Schedule administration of analgesics to prevent pain.

MEDICATIONS

Opioids

Codeine, morphine sulfate, oxycodone, hydromorphone, and methadone provide analgesia for pain management.

NURSING ACTIONS
- Administer orally (immediate- or sustained-release) or IV (for severe pain).
- Administer on a regular schedule to maintain control, or prevent pain if possible.
- Use patient-controlled analgesia if appropriate.

CLIENT EDUCATION
- Avoid activities that require mental alertness. Qs
- Analgesics can be necessary in high doses, and addiction is rare.

ANTINEOPLASTICS

Hydroxyurea not FDA approved for SCA but used widely to increase oxygenation to the cells.

NURSING ACTIONS
- Administer PO.
- Monitor nutrition intake.

CLIENT EDUCATION: Antineoplastics can cause anorexia.

THERAPEUTIC PROCEDURES

Exchange transfusions: Replaces the sickled blood cells with normal blood cells.

Hematopoietic stem cell transplant: Permanent solution for SCD. High risk of neurologic complications.

CLIENT EDUCATION

- Provide emotional support, and refer to social services if appropriate.
- Observe for manifestations of crisis and infection and notify the provider promptly.
- Promote rest and provide adequate nutrition for the child.
- Practice good hand hygiene and avoid individuals who have colds/infections/viruses.
- Adhere to fluid intake requirements (i.e., how many bottles or glasses of fluid should be consumed daily) to prevent dehydration.
- Consider genetic counseling.
- Maintain up-to-date immunizations.
- Wear a medical identification wristband or medical identification tags.
- Attend school regularly and avoid contact sports.

COMPLICATIONS

Stroke

Sickled cells can occlude blood vessels.

NURSING ACTIONS
Monitor and report manifestations.
- Seizures
- Abnormal behavior
- Weakness of, or inability to move, an extremity
- Slurred speech
- Visual changes
- Vomiting
- Severe headache

CLIENT EDUCATION: Blood transfusions are usually performed monthly to prevent a repeat stroke.

Acute chest syndrome

- Can be life-threatening
- Common in adolescents
- Increased risk for pneumonia due to decreased oxygen to lung tissue

NURSING ACTIONS
Monitor and report manifestations.
- Chest, back, or abdominal pain
- Fever of 38.5° C (101.3° F) or higher
- Cough
- Tachypnea
- Dyspnea, wheezing
- Retractions
- Decreased oxygen saturations

CLIENT EDUCATION
- May need blood transfusion
- Take antibiotics as prescribed

Infections
- Risk for infections (streptococcus pneumoniae, *H. influenzae*)
- Spleen decrease in size
- Increased risk for septicemia

Other complications

- Kidney scarring
- Visual acuity decreased
- Priapism (males)

Hemophilia

Hemophilia is a group of bleeding disorders characterized by difficulty controlling bleeding. Deficiencies in the clotting factors.

- Bleeding time is extended due to lack of a factor required for blood to clot. Bleeding is internal or external.
- Bleeding tendencies are sometimes recognized during infancy following circumcision, but might not become apparent until the infant becomes more active and prone to injuries during the toddler years.
- Hemophilia varies in severity based on the percentage of clotting factor a child's body contains. For example, a child who has mild hemophilia can have up to 40% of the normal factor VIII in their body, while a child who has severe hemophilia has very little factor VIII.
- Both hemophilia A and B are X-linked recessive disorders.

Hemophilia A

- Deficiency of factor VIII
- Referred to as classic hemophilia
- Accounts for 80% of cases

Hemophilia B

- Deficiency of factor IX
- Referred to as Christmas disease

Von Willebrand

Inherited lack of the von Willebrand factor protein characterized by the inability of the platelets to aggregate

DATA COLLECTION

EXPECTED FINDINGS

Episodes of bleeding, excessive bleeding, reports of joint pain and stiffness, impaired mobility, easy bruising, and activity intolerance

PHYSICAL FINDINGS

- Active bleeding, which includes bleeding gums, epistaxis, hematuria, and/or tarry stools
- Hematomas and/or bruising, even with minor injuries
- Hemarthrosis as evidenced by joint pain, stiffness, warmth, swelling, redness, loss of range of motion, and deformities
- Headache, slurred speech, and a decreased level of consciousness

LABORATORY TESTS

- Prolonged partial thromboplastin time (aPTT)
- Factor-specific assays to determine deficiency
- Platelets and prothrombin time are within expected reference ranges
- Whole blood clotting time is within expected range or prolonged

DIAGNOSTIC PROCEDURES

DNA testing: Detects classic hemophilia trait in females

PATIENT-CENTERED CARE

NURSING CARE

Management of bleeding in the hospital

- Administer injections via the subcutaneous route instead of the intramuscular route whenever possible.
- Avoid unnecessary skin punctures and use surgical aseptic technique.
- Venipunctures are preferred over finger or heel sticks for blood sampling.
- Monitor urine, stool, and nasogastric fluid for occult blood.
- Do not administer aspirin or any products that contain aspirin.
- Acetaminophen is an acceptable substitute for aspirin.
- Control localized bleeding.
  - Administer factor replacement.
  - Observe for adverse effects, which include headache, flushing, low sodium, and alterations in heart rate and blood pressure.
  - Encourage the child to rest and immobilize the affected joints.
  - Elevate and apply ice to the affected joints.

MEDICATIONS

1-deamino-8-d-arginine vasopressin (DDAVP)

DDAVP is a synthetic form of vasopressin that increases plasma factor VIII (antihemophilic factor).

- Effective for mild, but not severe, hemophilia
- Not effective for hemophilia B, which involves a factor IX deficiency

NURSING ACTIONS: Can be given prior to dental or surgical procedures

Factor VIII, products that contain factor VIII, pooled plasma, and recombinant products

Used to prevent and treat hemorrhage

NURSING ACTIONS: Administer by IV infusion.

CLIENT EDUCATION
- Treatment can require numerous doses.
- Periodic administration has proven effective for preventing bleeding complications.

Corticosteroids

Used to treat hematuria, acute episodes of hemarthrosis, and chronic synovitis

NURSING ACTIONS: Monitor for infection and bleeding.

CLIENT EDUCATION: Maintain good hand hygiene and avoid individuals with colds/infection/viruses.

E-aminocaproic acid (EACA)

Inhibits clot destruction

Nonsteroidal anti-inflammatory agents

Used with caution to treat chronic synovitis

NURSING ACTIONS: Monitor for infection.

CLIENT EDUCATION
- Administer cautiously due to potential inhibition of platelet function.
- Take the medication with food.

INTERPROFESSIONAL CARE

An interprofessional approach includes the pediatrician, hematologist, orthopedist, nurse, nurse practitioner, physical therapist, school nurse, and social worker.

CLIENT EDUCATION

- Prevent bleeding at home. Qs
  - Environment should be made as safe as possible to prevent injury.
  - Provide a safe home and a play environment.
  - Set activity restrictions to avoid injury. Acceptable activities include low-contact sports (bowling, fishing, swimming, golf). While participating in these activities, children should wear protective equipment.
  - Use soft-bristled toothbrushes.
- Perform regular exercise and physical therapy after active bleeding is controlled.
- Maintain up-to-date immunizations.
- Wear medical identification.
- Observe for manifestations of internal bleeding and hemarthrosis.
- Control bleeding episodes using the RICE (rest, ice, compression, elevation) method.
- Participate in a support group.
- Administer factor replacement.
- Adhere to active ROM; passive ROM contraindicated with acute episodes due to risk of damage to the capsule of the joints.

COMPLICATIONS

Uncontrolled bleeding

Intracranial hemorrhage, airway obstruction from bleeding in mouth, neck, or chest

NURSING ACTIONS
- Monitor vital signs for evidence of impending shock.
- Take measures to control bleeding.
- Administer appropriate factor replacement during bleeding episodes to treat excessive bleeding or hemarthrosis.
- Ensure administration of a blood transfusion as prescribed.
- Identify neurological manifestations that can indicate presence of an intracranial bleed.
- Provide prophylaxis treatment. Regimens include infusion of factor VIII concentrate:
  - Prior to joint bleed
  - Three times a week or every other day after the first joint bleed.

CLIENT EDUCATION: Report manifestations of bleeding.

Joint deformity

- Most often elbows, knees, and ankles.
- Repeated episodes of hemarthrosis (bleeding into joint spaces) lead to impaired range of motion, pain, tenderness, and swelling, which can develop into joint deformities.

NURSING ACTIONS
- Take appropriate measures to rest, immobilize, elevate, and apply ice to the affected joints during active bleeding.
- Encourage active range of motion after active bleeding is controlled.
- Encourage maintenance of ideal weight to minimize stress on joints.
- Encourage maintenance of regular exercise and physical therapy.

Application Exercises

1. A nurse is reinforcing teaching about the management of epistaxis to an adolescent. Which of the following positions should the nurse instruct the adolescent to take when experiencing a nosebleed?

   A. Sit up and lean forward.

   B. Sit up and tilt the head up.

   C. Lie in a supine position.

   D. Lie in a prone position.

2. A nurse is providing reinforcement teaching about epistaxis to the parent of a school-age child. Which of the following should the nurse include as an action to take when managing an episode of epistaxis? (Select all that apply.)

   A. Press the nares together for at least 10 min.

   B. Breathe through the nose until bleeding stops.

   C. Pack cotton or tissue into the naris that is bleeding.

   D. Apply a cold cloth across the bridge of the nose.

   E. Insert petroleum into the naris after the bleeding stops.

3. A nurse is reinforcing teaching to the parent of a child who has a new prescription for liquid oral iron supplements. Which of the following statements by the parent indicates an understanding?

   A. "I should take my child to the emergency department if his stools become dark."

   B. "My child should avoid eating citrus fruits while taking the supplements."

   C. "I should give the iron with milk to help prevent an upset stomach."

   D. "My child should take the supplement through a straw."

4. A nurse is preparing to administer iron dextran IM to a school-age child who has iron deficiency anemia. Which of the following actions by the nurse is appropriate?

   A. Administer the dose in the deltoid muscle.

   B. Use the Z-track method when administering the dose.

   C. Avoid injecting more than 2 mL with each dose.

   D. Massage the injection site for 1 min after administering the dose.

5. A nurse is caring for an infant whose screening test reveals a potential diagnosis of sickle cell disease. Which of the following tests should be performed to distinguish if the infant has the trait or the disease?

   A. Sickle solubility test

   B. Hemoglobin electrophoresis

   C. Complete blood count

   D. Transcranial Doppler

Active Learning Scenario

A nurse is caring for a child who has a new diagnosis of hemophilia A. Use the ATI Active Learning Template: System Disorder to complete this item.

EXPECTED FINDINGS: List two physical findings associated with hemophilia.

CLIENT EDUCATION: List three concepts to reinforce in the teaching with the family and child.

Application Exercises Key

1. A. **CORRECT:** Instruct the adolescent to sit up and lean to prevent aspiration when experiencing a nosebleed.
   B. Sitting up and tilting the head up could cause aspiration of blood and is not the correct position when experiencing a nosebleed.
   C. Lying in a supine position could cause aspiration of blood and is not the correct position when experiencing a nosebleed.
   D. Lying in a prone position could cause aspiration of blood and is not the correct position when experiencing a nosebleed.

   Ⓝ *NCLEX® Connection: Reduction of Risk Potential, Potential for Alterations in Body Systems*

2. A. **CORRECT:** Pressing the nares together for at least 10 min is an appropriate action to take when managing an episode of epistaxis.
   B. The child should breathe through the mouth until the bleeding stops.
   C. Packing cotton or tissue into the naris that is bleeding is not an appropriate action when managing an episode of epistaxis because this could displace a clot.
   D. **CORRECT:** Applying an ice pack across the bridge of the nose is an appropriate action when managing an episode of epistaxis.
   E. Inserting petroleum into the naris after the bleeding stops is not an appropriate action when managing an episode of epistaxis.

   Ⓝ *NCLEX® Connection: Reduction of Risk Potential, Potential for Complications from Surgical Procedures and Health Alterations*

3. A. The child's stools will become a tarry-green color if the iron supplement dose is adequate.
   B. Vitamin C increases absorption of the iron and should be encouraged while taking the supplement.
   C. Milk prevents absorption of the iron. The supplement should be given 1 hr before or 2 hr after consuming milk.
   D. **CORRECT:** The child should take the supplement through a straw to prevent or minimize staining of the teeth.

   Ⓝ *NCLEX® Connection: Pharmacological Therapies, Medication Administration*

4. A. Administer the dose in to a large muscle mass.
   B. **CORRECT:** Use the Z-track method when administering the dose.
   C. Avoid injecting more than 1 mL with each dose.
   D. To reduce irritation and skin staining, do not massage the injection site after administering the dose.

   Ⓝ *NCLEX® Connection: Pharmacological Therapies, Medication Administration*

5. A. The sickle solubility test is a screening tool that detects the presence of abnormal hemoglobin, but does not distinguish between the trait and the disease.
   B. **CORRECT:** The hemoglobin electrophoresis test should be performed to distinguish if the infant has the trait or the disease.
   C. A complete blood count tests for anemia. It indicates the average size of the red blood cells, and the amount of hemoglobin in the red blood cells. It will not distinguish between sickle cell disease and sickle cell trait.
   D. The transcranial Doppler is performed to monitor intracranial vascular flow and detect the risk for cerebrovascular accident. It will not distinguish between sickle cell disease and sickle cell trait.

   Ⓝ *NCLEX® Connection: Reduction of Risk Potential, Diagnostic Tests*

Active Learning Scenario Key

Using the ATI Active Learning Template: System Disorder

EXPECTED FINDINGS
- Active bleeding (possibly from the gums, epistaxis, hematuria, and/or GI tract)
- Hematomas and bruising occur easily even with minor injuries
- Joint pain and stiffness, warmth, swelling, redness, loss of range of motion of the joints
- Cerebral bleeding can cause headaches, slurred speech, and decreased level of consciousness

CLIENT EDUCATION
- Prevent bleeding at home.
- Provide a safe home and a play environment that is free of clutter.
- Place padding on corners of furniture.
- Set activity restrictions to avoid injury. Stress importance of wearing protective equipment during activities.
- Caution with contact sports.
- Recommend the use of soft-bristled toothbrushes or oral water irrigations.
- Encourage regular exercise and physical therapy when not actively bleeding.
- Encourage recommended immunizations remain up-to-date.
- Reinforce the importance of wearing a medical identification.
- Reinforce manifestations of internal bleeding and hemarthrosis
- Inform of the RICE (rest, ice, compression, elevation) method to control active bleeding.

Ⓝ *NCLEX® Connection: Physiological Adaptation, Alterations in Body Systems*

N NCLEX® Connections

When reviewing the following chapters, keep in mind the
relevant topics and tasks of the NCLEX outline, in particular:

Reduction of Risk Potential

DIAGNOSTIC TESTS: Perform diagnostic testing.

**POTENTIAL FOR COMPLICATIONS OF DIAGNOSTIC
TESTS/TREATMENTS/PROCEDURES:** Identify client
response to diagnostic tests/treatments/procedures.

THERAPEUTIC PROCEDURES: Reinforce client
teaching on treatments and procedures.

Physiological Adaptation

ALTERATIONS IN BODY SYSTEMS
Reinforce education to the client regarding care and condition.

Identify signs and symptoms of an infection.

BASIC PATHOPHYSIOLOGY
Identify signs and symptoms related to an acute or chronic illness.

Consider general principles of client disease process when providing care.

FLUID AND ELECTROLYTE IMBALANCES
Identify signs and symptoms of client fluid and/or electrolyte imbalances.

Provide care for a client with a fluid and electrolyte balance.

CHAPTER 21 *Acute Infectious Gastrointestinal Disorders*

Diarrhea can be mild to severe, and acute or chronic. It can result in mild to severe dehydration.

Acute diarrhea is a sudden increase in frequency and change in consistency of stool. It is usually secondary to an infectious agent in the GI tract, upper respiratory infection, urinary tract infection, antibiotic use, or laxative use. Self-resolution occurs in less than 14 days if dehydration does not occur. Acute infectious diarrhea is caused by a variety of viral, bacterial, or parasitic pathogens.

Chronic diarrhea is an increase in frequency and change of consistency of stools for more than 14 days. It is caused by chronic conditions (malabsorption syndrome, food allergies, or inflammatory bowel disease). Chronic nonspecific diarrhea has no identified cause.

Dehydration is a body fluid disturbance when the output exceeds intake. It results from causes (fluid losses through the skin, or respiratory, urinary, or GI tract).

DATA COLLECTION

RISK FACTORS

Lack of normal elimination pattern, lack of clean water, poor hygiene, crowded living environments, poor sanitation, and nutritional deficiency

EXPECTED FINDINGS

- Reports of fatigue, malaise, change in behavior, change in stool pattern, poor appetite, weight loss, and pain.
- Monitor for manifestations of dehydration.

Rotavirus

Viral infection

MANIFESTATIONS
- Most common cause of diarrhea in children younger than 5 years
- Affects children of all ages
- Fever
- Onset of watery stools
- Diarrhea for 5 to 7 days
- Vomiting for approximately 2 days

TRANSMISSION: Fecal-oral

INCUBATION PERIOD: 48 hr

Yersinia enterocolitis

Bacterial infection

MANIFESTATIONS
- Mucoid, possibly bloody diarrhea
- Abdominal pain, fever, and vomiting

TRANSMISSION: Pets and food

INCUBATION PERIOD: 1 to 3 weeks

Escherichia coli

Bacterial infection

MANIFESTATIONS
- Watery diarrhea for 1 to 2 days, followed by abdominal cramping and bloody diarrhea
- Could lead to hemolytic uremic syndrome

TRANSMISSION: Depends on strain of *E. coli*

INCUBATION PERIOD: 3 to 4 days

Salmonella nontyphoidal groups

Bacterial infection

MANIFESTATIONS
- Mild to severe nausea, vomiting, abdominal cramping, bloody diarrhea, and fever (can be afebrile in infants)
- Diarrhea can last 2 to 3 weeks
- Possible headache, confusion, drowsiness, and seizures
- Can lead to meningitis or septicemia

TRANSMISSION: Person to person, undercooked meats and poultry

INCUBATION PERIOD: 6 to 72 hr

Clostridium difficile

Bacterial infection

Infection can occur from overgrowth of *C. difficile* following antibiotic therapy.

MANIFESTATIONS
- Mild, watery diarrhea for a few days
- Possible less severe manifestations in children than adults
- Possible leukocytosis, hypoalbuminemia, and high fever in certain children
- Possible pseudomembranous colitis

TRANSMISSION: Contact with colonized spores.

INCUBATION PERIOD: Nonspecified

Clostridium botulinum

Bacterial infection

MANIFESTATIONS
- Manifestations depend on strain
- Abdominal pain, cramping, and diarrhea
- Possible respiratory or CNS problems

TRANSMISSION: Contaminated food products

INCUBATION PERIOD: 12 to 26 hr

Shigella groups: Shigellosis

Bacterial infection

MANIFESTATIONS
- Sick appearance
- Fever, fatigue, and anorexia
- Cramping abdomen followed by watery or bloody diarrhea lasting 5 to 10 days

TRANSMISSION: Contaminated food or water

INCUBATION PERIOD: 1 to 7 days

Norovirus; norwalk

Viral infection

MANIFESTATIONS
- Abdominal cramps, nausea and vomiting, malaise, watery diarrhea
- Lasts 2 to 3 days

TRANSMISSION: Contaminated water

INCUBATION PERIOD: 12 to 48 hr

Staphylococcus

Bacterial infection

MANIFESTATIONS: Diarrhea, nausea, and vomiting

TRANSMISSION: Inadequately cooked or refrigerated food

INCUBATION PERIOD: 1 to 8 hr

Enterobius vermicularis (pinworm)

Helminthic infection

MANIFESTATIONS: Perianal itching, enuresis, sleeplessness, restlessness, and irritability due to itching

TRANSMISSION: Fecal-oral

Ingested or inhaled eggs hatch in the upper intestine, and mature. After mating, worms migrate out of the intestine and lay eggs. Eggs can survive for 2 to 3 weeks on surfaces.

Giardia lamblia: parasitic pathogen

MANIFESTATIONS
- Children 5 years of age or younger
  - Diarrhea
  - Vomiting
  - Anorexia
- Older children
  - Abdominal cramps
  - Intermittent loose, malodorous, pale, greasy stools

TRANSMISSION: Person to person, food, animals

The nonmotile stage of protozoa can survive in the environment for months.

LABORATORY TESTS

- CBC with differential to determine anemia and/or infection.
- Hct, Hgb, BUN, creatinine, and urine-specific gravity levels are usually elevated with dehydration.
- Stool specimen analysis:
  - Occult blood
  - Cultures
- Urinalysis if dehydration is suspected.

DIAGNOSTIC PROCEDURES

Tape test

Performed to check for *Enterobius vermicularis*.

CLIENT EDUCATION
- Guardians should place transparent tape over the child's anus at bedtime, preferably after the child is asleep. The caregiver should remove the tape just prior to the child awaking, if possible, prior to the child toileting or bathing.
- The specimen should be brought to the laboratory for microscopic evaluation for the presence of pinworm ova.
- Guardians should use good hand hygiene during this procedure.

Infectious gastroenteritis

Rotavirus: Enzyme immunoassay (ELISA) (stool sample)

E. coli: Sorbitol-MacConkey agar (stool sample)

Salmonella: Gram-stain, stool culture

C. difficile: Stool culture

C. botulinum: Blood and stool culture

Staphylococcus: Identification of organism in stool, blood, food, or aspirate

G. lamblia: Enzyme immunoassay (stool sample)

Shigellosis: Stool culture

Norovirus: Polymerase chain reaction assays (PCR), stool sample

Yersinia enterocolitis: Identification of organism in stool culture, ELISA

PATIENT-CENTERED CARE

NURSING CARE

- Obtain baseline height and weight.
- Obtain the child's weight at the same time each day.
- Avoid taking a rectal temperature.
- Check and monitor I&O (urine and stool).
- Assist with initiating IV fluids as ordered.
- Administer antibiotic as prescribed (*Shigella, C. difficile, and G. lamblia*).
- Avoid antibiotics (*E. coli, Salmonella*).
- Avoid antimotility agents (*E. coli, Salmonella, Shigella*).

Oral rehydration therapy

- Start replacement with an oral replacement solution (ORS) of 75 to 90 mEq of sodium/L at 40 to 50 mL/kg over 4 hr. **QEBP**
- Determine the need for further rehydration after initial replacement.
- Monitor the administration of maintenance therapy with ORS of 40 to 60 mEq of sodium/L and limit to 150 mL/kg/day.
  - Give ORS alternately with intake of other liquids (breast milk, formula, milk).
  - Give infants water, breast milk, or lactose-free formula if supplementary fluid is needed.
  - Older children can resume their regular diets for additional intake.
- Replace each diarrheal stool with 10 mL/kg of ORS for ongoing diarrhea.

MEDICATIONS

Metronidazole and tinidazole

Indicated for *C. difficile* and *G. lamblia*

NURSING ACTIONS
- Monitor for allergies.
- Monitor for GI upset.

CLIENT EDUCATION: Take the medication as prescribed and report any GI disturbances.

Mebendazole, albendazole, and pyrantel pamoate

Indicated for *Enterobius vermicularis*

NURSING ACTIONS
- Administer in a single dose that can need to be repeated in 2 weeks.
- Administer mebendazole for children older than 2 years of age.

CLIENT EDUCATION: Entire family should be treated at the same time.

CLIENT EDUCATION

- Guardians should inform the child's school or day care of the infection/infestation. The child should stay home during the incubation period.
- Reinforce with the family to use commercially prepared ORS when the child experiences diarrhea. Foods and fluids to avoid include
  - Fruit juices, carbonated sodas, and gelatin, which all have high carbohydrate content, low electrolyte content, and a high osmolality
  - Caffeine, due to its mild diuretic effect
  - Chicken or beef broth, which has too much sodium and not enough carbohydrates
- Perform prevention measures, including immunization for rotavirus.
- Provide frequent skin care to prevent skin breakdown.
- Reinforce with the family how to prevent the spread of infectious diseases.
  - Change bed linens and underwear daily for several days. Avoid shaking linens to prevent the spread of disease.
  - Keep the child's toys away from other children. Cleanse toys and child care areas thoroughly to prevent further spread or reinfestation.
  - Shower frequently.
  - Avoid undercooked or under-refrigerated food.
  - Perform proper hand hygiene after toileting and after changing diapers.
  - Do not share dishes and utensils. Wash them in hot, soapy water or in the dishwasher.
  - Clip nails and discourage nail biting and thumb sucking.
  - Clean toilet areas.

COMPLICATIONS

Dehydration

TYPES OF DEHYDRATION

- **Isotonic**
  - Water and sodium are lost in nearly equal amounts.
  - Major loss of fluid from extracellular fluid leads to a reduced volume of circulating fluid.
  - Hypovolemic shock can result.
  - Blood sodium is within normal limits (130 to 150 mEq/L).
- **Hypotonic**
  - Electrolyte loss is greater than water loss.
  - Water changes from extracellular fluid to intracellular fluid.
  - Physical manifestations are more severe with smaller fluid loss.
  - Shock is likely.
  - Blood sodium is less than 130 mEq/L.
- **Hypertonic**
  - Water loss is greater than electrolyte loss.
  - Fluid shifts from intracellular to extracellular.
  - Shock is less likely.
  - Neurologic changes (change in level of consciousness, irritability, hyperreflexia) can occur.
  - Blood sodium concentration is greater than 150 mEq/L.

LEVELS OF DEHYDRATION

- **Mild**
  - WEIGHT LOSS
    - 3% to 5% in infants
    - 3% to 4% in children
  - MANIFESTATIONS
    - Behavior, mucous membranes, anterior fontanel, pulse, and blood pressure within expected findings
    - Capillary refill greater than 2 seconds
    - Possible slight thirst
- **Moderate**
  - WEIGHT LOSS
    - 6% to 9% in infants
    - 6% to 8% in children
  - MANIFESTATIONS
    - Capillary refill between 2 and 4 seconds
    - Possible thirst and irritability
    - Pulse slightly increased with normal to orthostatic blood pressure
    - Dry mucous membranes and decreased tears and skin turgor
    - Slight tachypnea
    - Normal to sunken anterior fontanel on infants

- **Severe**
  - WEIGHT LOSS
    - Greater than 10% in infants
    - 10% in children
  - MANIFESTATIONS
    - Capillary refill greater than 4 seconds
    - Tachycardia present, and orthostatic blood pressure can progress to shock
    - Extreme thirst
    - Very dry mucous membranes and tented skin
    - Hyperpnea
    - No tearing with sunken eyeballs
    - Sunken anterior fontanel
    - Oliguria or anuria

NURSING ACTIONS

- Oral rehydration is attempted first for mild and moderate cases of dehydration.
  - **Mild:** 50 mL/kg rehydration fluid within 4 hr
  - **Moderate:** 100 mL/kg rehydration fluid within 4 hr
  - **Replacement of diarrhea losses** with 10 mL/kg each stool
- Administer parenteral fluid therapy as prescribed.
  - Initiate when a child is unable to drink enough oral fluids to correct fluid losses, and those with severe dehydration or continued vomiting.
  - Isotonic solution at 20 mL/kg IV bolus with possible repeat for isotonic and hypotonic dehydration.
  - Hypertonic dehydration: rapid fluid replacement is contraindicated because of the risk of cerebral edema.
  - Administer maintenance IV fluids as prescribed.
  - Avoid potassium replacement until kidney function is verified.
- Check capillary refill.
- Check vital signs.
- Monitor weight.
- Maintain accurate I&O.

CLIENT EDUCATION

- Increase oral fluids.
- Resume normal diet as soon as possible.
- Monitor how many times the child voids.

Application Exercises

1. A nurse is caring for a child who has had watery diarrhea for the past 3 days. Which of the following is an action for the nurse to take?

   A. Offer chicken broth.

   B. Assist with initiating oral rehydration therapy.

   C. Assist with starting an infusion of a hypertonic IV solution.

   D. Keep NPO until the diarrhea subsides.

2. A nurse is caring for a child who is suspected to have *Enterobius vermicularis*. Which of the following actions should the nurse take?

   A. Perform a tape test.

   B. Collect stool specimen for culture.

   C. Test the stool for occult blood.

   D. Assist with initiating an infusion of IV fluids.

3. A nurse is collecting data from a child who has a rotavirus infection. Which of the following are expected findings? (Select all that apply.)

   A. Fever

   B. Vomiting

   C. Watery stools

   D. Bloody stools

   E. Confusion

4. A nurse is reinforcing teaching with a group of parents about *Salmonella*. Which of the following information should the nurse include? (Select all that apply.)

   A. Incubation period is nonspecific.

   B. It is a bacterial infection.

   C. Bloody diarrhea is common.

   D. Transmission can be from house pets.

   E. Antibiotics are used for treatment.

5. A nurse is reinforcing teaching a group of caregivers about *E. coli*. Which of the following information should the nurse include? (Select all that apply.)

   A. Severe abdominal cramping occurs.

   B. Watery diarrhea is present for more than 5 days.

   C. It can lead to hemolytic uremic syndrome.

   D. It is a foodborne pathogen.

   E. Antibiotics are given for treatment.

Active Learning Scenario

A nurse is reinforcing teaching with the guardian of a child who has an acute gastrointestinal infection. What information should the nurse include? Use the ATI Active Learning Template: System Disorder to complete this item.

CLIENT EDUCATION: Describe at least 10 points to review regarding care after discharge.

Application Exercises Key

1. A. Chicken broth is avoided for children who
      have diarrhea because of its increased sodium
      and inadequate carbohydrates.
   B. **CORRECT:** Oral rehydration therapy is recommended to
      replace lost electrolytes for children who have diarrhea.
   C. Isotonic IV solutions are recommended for children
      who experience severe dehydration.
   D. Children who experience diarrhea are at risk for
      dehydration. Keeping them NPO is contraindicated.

   Ⓝ *NCLEX® Connection: Physiological Adaptation,*
   Fluid and Electrolyte Imbalances

2. A. **CORRECT:** A tape test is used when diagnosing
      Enterobius vermicularis infection.
   B. Stool cultures are obtained to diagnose
      Salmonella or *C. difficile* infection.
   C. A manifestation of *E. coli* is bloody stools.
   D. IV fluids are initiated for children who are dehydrated.

   Ⓝ *NCLEX® Connection: Reduction of Risk Potential,*
   Diagnostic Tests

3. A. **CORRECT:** Fever is a manifestation of rotavirus infection.
   B. **CORRECT:** Vomiting for approximately 2 days
      is a manifestation of rotavirus infection.
   C. **CORRECT:** Foul-smelling, watery stools is a
      manifestation of rotavirus infection.
   D. Bloody stools are a manifestation of *E. coli.*
   E. Confusion is a manifestation of *Salmonella.*

   Ⓝ *NCLEX® Connection: Physiological Adaptation,*
   Alterations in Body Systems

4. A. The incubation period of *Salmonella* is 6 to 72 hr.
   B. **CORRECT:** *Salmonella* is classified as a bacterial infection.
   C. **CORRECT:** *Salmonella* manifestations include bloody
      diarrhea, nausea, vomiting, and abdominal cramping.
   D. **CORRECT:** *Salmonella* can be transmitted to children from
      household pets (cats, dogs, hamsters, and turtles).
   E. *Salmonella* is a bacterial infection. Antibiotics
      are not recommended for treatment.

   Ⓝ *NCLEX® Connection: Health Promotion and Maintenance, Health*
   Promotion and Disease Prevention

5. A. **CORRECT:** Severe abdominal cramping
      is a manifestation of *E. coli.*
   B. Watery diarrhea lasts 1 to 2 days, then
      advances to bloody diarrhea.
   C. **CORRECT:** *E. coli* can lead to hemolytic uremic syndrome.
   D. **CORRECT:** *E. coli* is a foodborne pathogen.
   E. Antibiotics can worsen an *E. coli* infection.
      They are not recommended.

   Ⓝ *NCLEX® Connection: Health Promotion and Maintenance, Health*
   Promotion and Disease Prevention

Active Learning Scenario Key

Using the ATI Active Learning Template: System Disorder

CLIENT EDUCATION

- Have the guardians inform the child's school or day
  care center of the infection/infestation. The child
  should stay home during the incubation period.
- Use commercially-prepared oral rehydration therapy when the child
  experiences diarrhea. Foods and fluids to avoid include the following.
  ○ Fruit juices, carbonated sodas, and gelatin, which have high
    carbohydrate content, low electrolyte content, and high osmolality
  ○ Caffeine, due to its mild diuretic effect
  ○ Chicken or beef broth, which have high sodium
    content and inadequate carbohydrates
- Follow prevention measures, including immunization for rotavirus
  and methods to prevent further spread of the disease.
- Provide frequent skin care to prevent skin breakdown.
- Reinforce with the family how to avoid the
  spread of infectious diseases.
- Change bed linens and underwear daily for several days.
  Avoid shaking linens to prevent the spread of disease.
- Cleanse toys and child care areas thoroughly to
  prevent further spread or reinfestation.
- Shower frequently.
- Avoid undercooked or under-refrigerated food.
- Perform proper hand hygiene after toileting
  and after changing diapers.
- Do not share dishes and utensils. Wash them in
  hot, soapy water or in the dishwasher.
- Clip nails, and discourage nail-biting and thumb-sucking.
- Clean toilet areas.

Ⓝ *NCLEX® Connection: Physiological Adaptation, Alterations in*
Body Systems

CHAPTER 22
Gastrointestinal Structural and Inflammatory Disorders

Gastrointestinal structural disorders include cleft lip and palate, gastroesophageal reflux disease, hypertrophic pyloric stenosis, Hirschsprung's disease, and intussusception.

Inflammatory disorders include appendicitis and Meckel's diverticulum.

Cleft lip and palate

- Cleft lip (CL) results from the incomplete fusion of the oral cavity during intrauterine life. Cleft palate (CP) results from the incomplete fusion of the palates during intrauterine life.
- Although a CL and CP can occur together, either defect can occur alone. The defects can be unilateral (one-sided) or bilateral (two-sided). **(22.1)**

DATA COLLECTION

RISK FACTORS

- Genetic syndromes
- Combination of maternal and environmental factors
- Family history of cleft lip or palate
- Exposure to alcohol, cigarette smoke, anticonvulsants, retinoids, or taking steroids during pregnancy
- Folate deficiency during pregnancy; folic acid supplements during pregnancy can prevent clefting

EXPECTED FINDINGS

- Cleft lip is a visible separation from the upper lip toward the nose.
- Cleft palate is a visible or palpable opening of the palate connecting the mouth and the nasal cavity.

PATIENT-CENTERED CARE

NURSING CARE

- Support and encourage guardians in the general care of their child.
- Promote guardian-infant bonding.
- Promote healthy self-esteem throughout the child's development.

THERAPEUTIC PROCEDURES

Cleft lip
- Repair is typically performed between 2 and 3 months of age.
- Additional surgeries are usually required to the lip and nose in severe defects to improve aesthetic outcome.

Cleft palate
- Repair is typically performed between 6 to 12 months of age.
- Most require additional surgeries to improve speech quality and aesthetic outcome.

PREOPERATIVE NURSING ACTIONS

- Obtain baseline weight.
- Observe interaction between the family and infant.
- Determine emotional needs of the family and provide support.
- Recommend applicable support groups.
- Consult with social services to provide needed services (financial, insurance) for the family and infant.
- Instruct guardians about proper feeding and care.
- Determine ability to feed.
- Initiate strategies for successful feeding.
  - **For isolated cleft lip**
    - Encourage breast feeding.
    - Use a wide-based nipple for bottle feeding.
    - Squeeze the infant's cheeks together during feeding to decrease the gap.
  - **For cleft palate or cleft lip and palate**
    - Position the infant upright while cradling the head during feeding.
    - Use a specialized bottle with a one-way valve and a specially cut nipple.
    - Burp the infant frequently.
    - Syringe feeding can be necessary for the infant who is unsuccessful with other methods.

22.1 Cleft palate

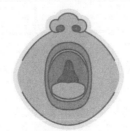

incomplete cleft palate

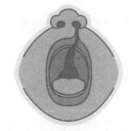

unilateral complete lip and palate

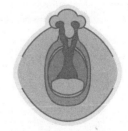

bilateral complete lip and palate

POSTOPERATIVE NURSING ACTIONS

- Perform standard postoperative care, including obtaining vital signs, oxygen saturation, and performing pain management using an age-appropriate tool.
- Keep the infant pain-free to decrease crying and stress on repair.
- Administer analgesics as prescribed.
- Examine operative sites for manifestations of crusting, bleeding, and infection.
- Avoid having the infant suck on a nipple or pacifier.
- Avoid spoons, forks, and other objects the infant might bring to the mouth that could damage the incision site.
- Monitor I&O and weigh daily.
- Observe the family's interaction with the infant.
- Determine emotional needs of the family and provide support.
- **For cleft lip**
  - Monitor the integrity of the postoperative protective device.
  - Position the infant on the back and upright, or on the side during the immediate postoperative period to maintain the integrity of the repair.
  - Apply elbow restraints to keep the infant from injuring the repair site.
  - Use sterile normal saline, sterile water, or diluted hydrogen peroxide to clean the incision site. Apply antibiotic ointment if prescribed.
  - Gently aspirate secretions of mouth and nasopharynx to prevent respiratory complications.
- **For cleft palate**
  - Change the infant's position frequently to facilitate drainage and breathing.
  - Place the infant in a side-lying position to facilitate drainage of secretions and prevent aspiration.
  - Maintain IV fluids until the infant is able to eat and drink.
  - The infant is usually NPO for 4 hr then allowed liquids only for the first 3 to 4 days, then progressed to a soft diet.
  - Avoid placing a straw, tongue depressor, hard pacifier, rigid utensils, hard-tipped sippy cups, or suction catheters in the infant's mouth after cleft palate repair.
  - Close observation for manifestations of airway obstruction, hemorrhage, and laryngeal spasm.
  - Use a face mask to deliver oxygen.

CLIENT EDUCATION

- Reinforce teaching about the proper use of the restraints.
- Reinforce guidelines for postoperative diet and feeding techniques.
- Reinforce teaching on proper care of the operative site.

INTERPROFESSIONAL CARE

Care of the child who has CL and CP requires care from members of various disciplines (plastic surgeon, orthodontist, otolaryngologist, speech-language pathologist, pediatrician, nursing, audiologist, social worker and psychologist).

COMPLICATIONS

Ear infections and hearing loss

Related to altered structure and recurrent otitis media

NURSING ACTIONS

- Feed the infant in an upright position.
- Monitor temperature.
- Insertion of pressure-equalizing tubes to facilitate fluid drainage from the ears and prevent middle ear effusion and otitis media can be required.

CLIENT EDUCATION: Observe for manifestations of ear infections and seek treatment early.

Speech and language impairment

More common with cleft palate

NURSING ACTIONS: Refer guardians to a speech therapist for intervention as early as possible.

Dental problems

Teeth might not erupt normally, and orthodontia is usually necessary later in life.

CLIENT EDUCATION

- Promote healthy dental hygiene.
- Seek early dental care.

Gastrointestinal reflux disease

- Gastroesophageal reflux (GER) occurs when gastric contents reflux back up into the esophagus, making esophageal mucosa vulnerable to injury from gastric acid.
- Gastroesophageal reflux disease (GERD) is tissue damage from GER.
- GER is self-limiting and usually resolves by 1 year of age.

DATA COLLECTION

RISK FACTORS

GER: Prematurity, bronchopulmonary dysplasia, neurologic impairments, asthma, cystic fibrosis, cerebral palsy, scoliosis

GERD: Neurologic impairments, hiatal hernia, morbid obesity

EXPECTED FINDINGS

INFANTS

- Spitting up or forceful vomiting, irritability, excessive crying, blood in vomitus, arching of back, stiffening
- Respiratory problems
- Failure to thrive
- Apnea

CHILDREN: Heartburn, abdominal pain, difficulty swallowing, chronic cough, noncardiac chest pain

DIAGNOSTIC PROCEDURES

- Upper GI endoscopy to detect GI structural abnormalities
- 24-hr intraesophageal pH study to measures the amount of gastric acid reflux into the esophagus
- Endoscopy with biopsy to detect esophagitis and strictures
- Scintigraphy to identify the cause of gastric content aspiration

PATIENT-CENTERED CARE

NURSING CARE

GER
- Depends on the severity of the findings.
- Offer small, frequent meals.
- Thicken infants formula with 1 tsp to 1 tbsp rice cereal per 1 oz formula.
- Avoid foods that cause reflux (caffeine, citrus, peppermint, spicy or fried foods).
- Assist with weight control.
- Position the child with the head elevated after meals.
- Place infants supine to sleep, rather than prone, side-lying, or sitting upright.

GERD: Initiate interventions for GER, plus administering a proton pump inhibitor (omeprazole, esomeprazole, pantoprazole and rabeprazole), or an H_2-receptor antagonist (cimetidine or famotidine).

THERAPEUTIC PROCEDURES

Nissen fundoplication
- Laparoscopic surgical procedure that wraps the fundus of the stomach around the distal esophagus to decrease reflux
- Used for clients who have severe cases of GERD

COMPLICATIONS

Recurrent pneumonia, weight loss, and failure to thrive
Repeated reflux of stomach contents can lead to erosion of the esophagus or pneumonia if stomach contents are aspirated.

NURSING ACTIONS
- Evaluate the prescribed treatment plan.
- Monitor for manifestations of pneumonia and failure to thrive.

CLIENT EDUCATION
- Reinforce the plan of care with the family.
- Observe for manifestations for pneumonia.

Hypertrophic pyloric stenosis

- Hypertrophic pyloric stenosis is the thickening of the pyloric sphincter, which creates an obstruction.
- Usually occurs the first few weeks of life.

DATA COLLECTION

RISK FACTORS

Genetic predisposition

EXPECTED FINDINGS

- Vomiting that often occurs following a feeding, but can occur up to several hours following a feeding and becomes projectile as obstruction worsens
- Nonbilious vomitus can be blood-tinged
- Constant hunger
- Olive-shaped mass in the right upper quadrant of the abdomen and possible peristaltic wave that moves from left to right when lying supine
- Failure to gain weight and manifestations of dehydration (pallor, cool lips, dry skin and mucous membranes, decreased skin turgor, diminished urinary output, concentrated urine, thirst, rapid pulse, sunken eyes).

LABORATORY TESTS

Blood electrolytes

DIAGNOSTIC PROCEDURES

Ultrasound reveals an elongated mass surrounding an elongated pyloric canal.

PATIENT-CENTERED CARE

NURSING CARE

Prepare the child for surgery.

THERAPEUTIC PROCEDURES

Pyloromyotomy

Performed by laparoscope

PREOPERATIVE NURSING ACTIONS
- IV fluids for correction of dehydration and electrolyte imbalances
- Insert a nasogastric (NG) tube for decompression.
- NPO
- I&O
- Daily weights

POSTOPERATIVE NURSING ACTIONS
- Obtain routine postoperative vital signs.
- Provide IV fluids.
- Monitor daily weights and I&O.
- Administer analgesics for pain.
- Check for manifestations of infection.
- Start clear liquids 4 to 6 hr after surgery. Advance to breast milk or formula as tolerated 24 hr after surgery.
- Document tolerance to feedings.

Hirschsprung's disease

Hirschsprung's disease (congenital aganglionic megacolon) is a structural anomaly of the GI tract caused by lack of ganglionic cells in segments of the colon resulting in decreased motility and mechanical obstruction.

DATA COLLECTION

RISK FACTORS

Family history of Hirschsprung's disease

EXPECTED FINDINGS

Newborn
- Failure to pass meconium within 24 to 48 hr after birth
- Episodes of vomiting bile
- Refusal to eat
- Abdominal distention

Infant
- Failure to thrive
- Constipation
- Vomiting
- Episodes of diarrhea and vomiting

Child
- Undernourished, anemic appearance
- Abdominal distention
- Visible peristalsis
- Palpable fecal mass
- Constipation
- Foul-smelling, ribbonlike stool

LABORATORY TESTS

- Blood electrolytes
- CBC

DIAGNOSTIC PROCEDURES

Rectal biopsy to confirm the absence of ganglion cells

PATIENT-CENTERED CARE

NURSING CARE

- Prepare family and client for surgery.
- Assist family with improving nutritional status until surgery.
  - High-protein, high-calorie, low-fiber diet
  - Total parenteral nutrition in some cases

THERAPEUTIC PROCEDURES

- Surgical removal of the aganglionic section of the bowel.
- Temporary colostomy can be required.

PREOPERATIVE NURSING ACTIONS
- Prepare the child and family for surgery using developmentally appropriate techniques.
- Administer electrolyte and fluid replacement.
- Monitor for enterocolitis.
- Bowel prep with saline enemas and oral antibiotics.

POSTOPERATIVE NURSING ACTIONS
- Check respiratory status and maintain airway.
- Provide supplemental oxygen.
- Obtain vital signs.
- Administer analgesics for pain.
- Examine surgical site for bleeding or other abnormalities.
- Provide Foley catheter care.
- Determine bowel sounds and bowel function.
- Provide ostomy care if appropriate.
- Make appropriate referrals.

CLIENT EDUCATION
- Perform ostomy care if indicated.
- Practice incisional care and to monitor for infection.
- Observe for manifestations of dehydration.

COMPLICATIONS

Enterocolitis (inflammation of the bowel)

Treatment focuses on resolving inflammation, preventing bowel perforation, maintaining hydration, initiating antibiotic therapy, and performing surgery for colostomy or ileostomy if there is extensive bowel involvement.

NURSING ACTIONS
- Monitor vital signs.
- Obtain abdominal girth.
  - Measure girth with a paper tape at the level of the umbilicus or at the widest point of the abdomen.
  - Mark the area with a pen to ensure continuity of future measurements.
- Monitor for manifestations of sepsis, peritonitis, or shock caused by enterocolitis.
- Monitor and manage fluid, electrolyte, and blood product replacement.
- Administer antibiotics as prescribed.

Anal stricture and incontinence

- Bowel-retraining therapy
- Can require further procedures (dilatation)

Intussusception

- Proximal segment of the bowel telescopes into a more distal segment, resulting in lymphatic and venous obstruction causing edema in the area. With progression, ischemia and increased mucus into the intestine will occur.
- Common in infants and children ages 3 months to 6 years.

DATA COLLECTION

EXPECTED FINDINGS

- Sudden episodic abdominal pain
- Screaming with drawing knees to chest during episodes of pain
- Abdominal mass (sausage-shaped)
- Stools mixed with blood and mucus that resemble the consistency of red currant jelly
- Vomiting
- Fever
- Tender, distended abdomen

DIAGNOSTIC PROCEDURES

Ultrasound

PATIENT-CENTERED CARE

NURSING CARE

- Reinforce teaching with the family and child about the nonsurgical procedure.

THERAPEUTIC PROCEDURES

Air enema

- With or without contrast
- Performed by a radiologist

COMPLICATIONS

Reoccurring intussusception

Surgery is required for reoccurring cases.

Appendicitis

- Inflammation of the vermiform appendix caused from an obstruction of the lumen of the appendix.
- Average client age is 10 years.

DATA COLLECTION

EXPECTED FINDINGS

- Abdominal pain in the right lower quadrant
- Rigid abdomen
- Decreased or absent bowel sounds
- Fever
- Diarrhea or constipation
- Lethargy
- Tachycardia
- Rapid, shallow breathing
- Anorexia
- Possible vomiting

LABORATORY TESTS

- CBC
- Urinalysis

DIAGNOSTIC PROCEDURES

Computed tomography scan shows an enlarged diameter of appendix, as well as thickening of the appendiceal wall.

PATIENT-CENTERED CARE

NURSING CARE

- Prepare the child and family for surgery using developmentally appropriate techniques.
- Avoid applying heat to the abdomen.
- Avoid enemas or laxatives.

THERAPEUTIC PROCEDURES

Removal of the nonruptured appendix

Laparoscopic surgery

POSTOPERATIVE NURSING ACTIONS

- Monitor respiratory status and maintain airway.
- Provide supplemental oxygen as prescribed.
- Obtain vital signs.
- Ensure the administration of analgesics for pain.
- Monitor surgical site for bleeding or any other abnormalities.
- Check bowel sounds and bowel function.

Removal of the ruptured appendix

Laparoscopic or open surgery

POSTOPERATIVE NURSING ACTIONS
- Check respiratory status, and maintain airway.
- Provide supplemental oxygen.
- Obtain vital signs.
- Administer analgesics for pain.
- Examine surgical site for bleeding or other abnormalities.
- Check bowel sounds and bowel function.
- Assist with administering IV fluids and antibiotics.
- Maintain NPO status.
- Maintain NG tube to low continuous suction.
- Provide wound irrigation care for open surgical sites with antibacterial solution or saline-soaked gauze.
- Provide drain care.
- Check for peritonitis.
  - Fever
  - Sudden relief from pain after perforation, followed by a diffuse increase in pain
  - Irritability
  - Rigid abdomen
  - Abdominal distention
  - Tachycardia
  - Rapid, shallow breathing
  - Pallor
  - Chills

CLIENT EDUCATION
- Follow instructions for incision care.
- Observe for manifestations of infection.

COMPLICATIONS

Peritonitis (inflammation in the peritoneal cavity)

NURSING ACTIONS
- Check for peritonitis.
- Provide pain management.
  - Determine pain level using a developmentally appropriate tool.
  - Administer analgesics.
- Manage IV fluid therapy.
- Assist with administering IV antibiotics.
- Manage NG tube suction.
- Provide preoperative and postoperative nursing care.
- Provide surgical wound care with wound irrigation and/or dressings if delayed wound closure is necessary.
- Provide psychosocial support for the child and family.

CLIENT EDUCATION
- Preoperative care (the need to maintain NPO status and the need for pain medication)
- Postoperative care (early ambulation, advancement of diet, wound care, and monitoring for infection)

Meckel's diverticulum

Meckel's diverticulum is a complication resulting from failure of the omphalomesenteric duct to fuse during embryonic development.

DATA COLLECTION

EXPECTED FINDINGS
- Rectal bleeding, usually painless
- Abdominal pain
- Bloody, mucus stools

LABORATORY TESTS

CBC and metabolic panel

DIAGNOSTIC EVALUATION

RADIONUCLIDE SCAN: Meckel's scan is the most effective diagnostic test

PATIENT-CENTERED CARE

NURSING CARE

Prepare the child and family for surgery using developmentally appropriate techniques.

THERAPEUTIC PROCEDURES

Surgical removal of the diverticulum

PREOPERATIVE NURSING ACTIONS
- Provide oxygen as prescribed.
- Administer antibiotics.
- Maintain bed rest.
- Closely monitor blood loss in stools.

POSTOPERATIVE NURSING ACTIONS
- Check respiratory status and maintain airway.
- Provide supplemental oxygen.
- Obtain vital signs.
- Administer analgesics for pain.
- Examine surgical site for bleeding or any other abnormalities.
- Check bowel sounds and bowel function.
- Maintain NPO status.
- Assist with administering IV fluid and antibiotics.
- Maintain NG tube to low continuous suction.

CLIENT EDUCATION: Observe for manifestations of infection.

COMPLICATIONS

GI hemorrhage and bowel obstruction (for untreated Meckel's diverticulum)

Application Exercises

1. A nurse is collecting data from an infant who has hypertrophic pyloric stenosis. Which of the following manifestations should the nurse expect? (Select all that apply.)

   A. Projectile vomiting

   B. Dry mucus membranes

   C. Currant jelly stools

   D. Sausage-shaped abdominal mass

   E. Constant hunger

2. A nurse is caring for a child who has Hirschsprung's disease. Which of the following actions should the nurse take?

   A. Encourage a high-fiber, low-protein, low-calorie diet.

   B. Prepare the family for surgery.

   C. Place an NG tube for decompression.

   D. Initiate bed rest.

3. A nurse is assisting with the care of an infant who has just returned from PACU following cleft lip and palate repair. Which of the following actions should the nurse take?

   A. Remove the packing in the mouth.

   B. Place the infant in an upright position.

   C. Offer a pacifier with sucrose.

   D. Observe the mouth with a tongue blade.

4. A nurse is collecting data from a child who has Meckel's diverticulum. Which of the following manifestations should the nurse expect? (Select all that apply.)

   A. Abdominal pain

   B. Fever

   C. Mucus and blood in stools

   D. Vomiting

   E. Rapid, shallow breathing

5. A nurse is reinforcing teaching with the guardian of an infant about gastrointestinal reflux disease. Which of the following instructions should the nurse include? (Select all that apply.)

   A. Offer frequent feedings.

   B. Thicken formula with rice cereal.

   C. Use a bottle with a one-way valve.

   D. Position baby upright after feedings.

   E. Use a wide-based nipple for feedings.

Active Learning Scenario

A nurse is assisting with the care of a child who is postoperative following an open appendectomy for a perforated appendix. Use the ATI Active Learning Template: System Disorder to complete this item.

NURSING CARE: List postoperative nursing interventions.

Application Exercises Key

1. A. **CORRECT:** A client who has a pyloric stricture has thickening of the pyloric sphincter, resulting in projectile vomiting.
    B. **CORRECT:** A client who has pyloric stricture is unable to consume adequate food and fluid, resulting in dehydration. Dry mucous membranes is a manifestation of hypertrophic pyloric stenosis.
    C. A client who has intussusception has bloody mucus stools, resulting in currant jelly stools.
    D. A client who has intussusception has telescoping intestine, resulting sausage shaped abdominal mass.
    E. **CORRECT:** A client who has pyloric stricture is unable to consume adequate food and fluid, resulting in constant hunger.

    Ⓝ *NCLEX® Connection: Physiological Adaptation, Basic Pathophysiology*

2. A. A client who has Hirschsprung's disease is encouraged to eat a low-fiber, high-protein, high-calorie diet.
    B. **CORRECT:** A client who has Hirschsprung's disease requires surgery to remove the affected segment of the intestine. Preparing the family for surgery is an appropriate action for the nurse to take.
    C. A client who has Hirschsprung's disease is managed nutritionally. Placing an NG tube for decompression is not an appropriate action for the nurse to take.
    D. A client who has Meckel's diverticulum is placed on bed rest to prevent further bleeding.

    Ⓝ *NCLEX® Connection: Physiological Adaptation, Basic Pathophysiology*

3. A. The packing in the mouth should stay in place for 2 to 3 days.
    B. **CORRECT:** Placing the infant in an upright position will facilitate drainage and prevent aspiration.
    C. Objects in the mouth could injure the surgical site and should be avoided.
    D. Objects in the mouth could injure the surgical site and should be avoided.

    Ⓝ *NCLEX® Connection: Reduction of Risk Potential, Potential for Complications from Surgical Procedures and Health Alterations*

4. A. **CORRECT:** Abdominal pain is a manifestation of Meckel's diverticulum.
    B. Fever is a manifestation of appendicitis.
    C. **CORRECT:** Mucus and bloody stools are a manifestation of Meckel's diverticulum.
    D. Vomiting is a manifestation of appendicitis.
    E. Rapid, shallow breathing is a manifestation of appendicitis.

    Ⓝ *NCLEX® Connection: Physiological Adaptation, Basic Pathophysiology*

5. A. **CORRECT:** Frequent feeding will assist in decreasing the amount of vomiting episodes.
    B. **CORRECT:** Thickened formula will assist in decreasing the amount of vomiting episodes.
    C. A bottle with a one-way valve is used for an infant who has cleft lip and palate.
    D. **CORRECT:** Positioning the infant in an upright position following feedings will assist in decreasing the amount of vomiting episodes.
    E. A wide-based nipple is used for an infant who has cleft lip and palate.

    Ⓝ *NCLEX® Connection: Physiological Adaptation, Alterations in Body Systems*

Active Learning Scenario Key

Using the ATI Active Learning Template: System Disorder

NURSING CARE
- Check respiratory status and maintain airway.
- Provide supplemental oxygen as prescribed.
- Obtain vital signs.
- Administer analgesics for pain as prescribed.
- Examine surgical site for bleeding or any other abnormalities.
- Check bowel sounds and bowel function.
- Assist with administering IV fluids and antibiotics as prescribed.
- Maintain NPO status.
- Maintain NG tube to low continuous suction.
- Provide wound care for open surgical sites with antibacterial solution or saline as prescribed.
- Provide drain care.
- Examine for peritonitis.

Ⓝ *NCLEX® Connection: Potential for Complications of Diagnostic Tests/Treatments/Procedures, Potential for Complications from Surgical Procedures and Health Alterations*

NCLEX® Connections

When reviewing the following chapters, keep in mind the relevant topics and tasks of the NCLEX outline, in particular:

Basic Care and Comfort

ELIMINATION: Identify the client at risk for impaired elimination.

MOBILITY/IMMOBILITY: Maintain correct client body alignment.

Pharmacological Therapies

DOSAGE CALCULATIONS: Perform calculations needed for medication administration.

EXPECTED ACTIONS/OUTCOMES
Reinforce education to client regarding medications.

Identify client expected response to medication.

Reduction of Risk Potential

LABORATORY VALUES: Notify primary health care provider about client laboratory test results.

Physiological Adaptation

ALTERATIONS IN BODY SYSTEMS
Provide care to correct client alteration in body system.

Reinforce education to the client regarding care and condition.

BASIC PATHOPHYSIOLOGY
Identify signs and symptoms related to an acute or chronic illness.

Consider general principles of the client's disease process when providing care.

Apply knowledge of pathophysiology to monitoring client for alterations in body systems.

POTENTIAL FOR COMPLICATIONS OF DIAGNOSTIC TESTS/ TREATMENTS/PROCEDURES: Use precautions to prevent injury and/or complications associated with a procedure or diagnosis.

CHAPTER 23 *Enuresis and Urinary Tract Infections*

Enuresis is uncontrolled or unintentional urination that occurs after a child is beyond an age at which bladder control is achieved.

A urinary tract infection (UTI) is an infection in any portion of the urinary tract.

Enuresis

Inappropriate urination during the day or night at least twice a week for at least 3 months should be evaluated for children who have a developmental or chronological age of at least 5-years old.

Rule out other causes of incontinence (medication adverse effects, medical conditions) prior to diagnosis of enuresis.

Primary enuresis: A child has never been free of bed-wetting for any extended periods of time.

Secondary enuresis: A child who started bed-wetting after development of urinary control.

DATA COLLECTION

RISK FACTORS

- Family history of enuresis
- Disorders associated with bladder dysfunction
- Males
- Emotional events (new sibling, divorce)
- Behavioral disorders

EXPECTED FINDINGS

- History of alterations in toilet training, voiding behaviors, and bowel movement patterns QPCC
- History of chronic or acute illness (UTI, diabetes mellitus, sickle cell disease, neurologic deficits)
- Fluid intake, especially in the evening
- Restlessness, urinary frequency and urgency

DIAGNOSTIC EVALUATION

- Functional bladder capacity screening: child is instructed to hold off urinating for as long as possible and then instructed to urinate into a container. The urine output is then measured. The expected bladder capacity (in ounces) is the child's age plus 2.
- Record of enuresis pattern.

PATIENT-CENTERED CARE

NURSING CARE

- Evaluate the child's self-esteem.
- Evaluate the child's coping strategies and available support systems.
- Evaluate the family's coping.
- Evaluate peer and family support groups.
- Reinforce education with the child and family regarding the management of enuresis.
  - Have the child urinate prior to bedtime.
  - Restrict fluids at least 2 hr prior to bedtime.
  - Avoid caffeinated or carbonated drinks.
  - Use positive reinforcement. Avoid punishing, scolding, or teasing the child following an incident.
  - Assist the child/caregivers in keeping a calendar of wet and dry days.
  - Have the child change the bed linens and clothing following an incident.
  - Wake the child up at scheduled intervals during the night to void.
  - Administer prescribed medications.
  - Offer support to the child and the family.

THERAPEUTIC MEASURES

Conditioning therapy: Placing an alarm sensor on the bed that rings/alarms when the child voids to awaken the child to get up to use the bathroom

Kegel/pelvic exercises

Retention control measures: Have the child consume a large amount of fluid to stretch the bladder, if not contraindicated.

MEDICATIONS

Antidiuretic hormone

Desmopressin acetate reduces the volume of urine.

NURSING ACTIONS
- Can be prescribed either orally or intranasal.
- Monitor I&O.

CLIENT EDUCATION
- Restrict the child's fluid intake after dinner. QEBP
- Administer the medication at bedtime.
- Possible adverse reactions include headaches, nausea. Nasal spray can cause nasal irritation.

Tricyclic antidepressants

Imipramine hydrochloride inhibits urination.

NURSING ACTIONS
- Monitor children for an increase in suicidality.
- Monitor for therapeutic effectiveness.
- Length of treatment is 6 to 8 weeks. Then, plan to taper the medication gradually.
- Administer with food.

CLIENT EDUCATION
- Administer the mediation 1 hr before bedtime.
- Observe for possible adverse reactions.
- Avoid sun exposure.
- Avoid using with over-the-counter medications.

Anticholinergics

Oxybutynin chloride reduces bladder contractions.

NURSING ACTIONS: Monitor for effectiveness of therapy.

CLIENT EDUCATION: Observe for possible adverse reactions.

COMPLICATIONS

Emotional problems (low self-esteem, altered body image, social isolation, fears)

NURSING ACTIONS
- Support the child and family by listening to concerns and correcting misperceptions.
- Involve the child in the reinforced teaching and management.
- Assist with referrals to appropriate resources (support groups, counseling) as necessary.

CLIENT EDUCATION: Assist the child and family to understand the emotional aspects of the disorder. Early interventions can alleviate long-term emotional issues.

Urinary tract infections

Bacteriuria: bacteria in the urine
- Asymptomatic bacteriuria: bacteriuria with no manifestations of UTI
- Symptomatic bacteriuria: bacteriuria with manifestations of UTI

Recurrent UTI: multiple occurrences of asymptomatic or symptomatic bacteriuria

Persistent UTI: bacteriuria that does not resolve with antibiotic therapy

Febrile UTI: symptomatic bacteriuria with fever
- Urosepsis: febrile UTI with systemic manifestations.

Cystitis: inflammation of the bladder

Urethritis: inflammation of the urethra

Pyelonephritis: inflammation of the upper urinary tract and the kidneys

DATA COLLECTION

RISK FACTORS

- Urinary stasis
- Urinary tract anomalies
- Reflux within the urinary tract system
- Constipation
- Onset of toilet training
- Inadequate hygiene of an uncircumcised penis
- Females (urethra in close proximity to rectum)
- Underwear that is tight or made from synthetic fabric
- Bubble baths
- Sexual activity

EXPECTED FINDINGS
- INFANTS
  - Poor feeding, vomiting, or failure to gain weight
  - Increase in thirst
  - Frequent urination
  - Straining or screaming with urination
  - Foul-smelling urine
  - Fever
  - Diaper rash
  - Dehydration
  - Seizure
  - Pallor
- CHILDREN
  - Abdominal or back pain
  - Pain with urination
  - Poor appetite
  - Vomiting
  - Slowed growth
  - Increase in thirst
  - Enuresis, frequent urination, dysuria
  - Swelling of the face
  - Seizures
  - Pallor
  - Fatigue
  - Blood in the urine
  - Edema
  - Hypertension
  - Tetany

LABORATORY TESTS

Urinalysis and urine culture and sensitivity

- Sterile catheterization and suprapubic aspiration are the most accurate methods for obtaining urine for urinalysis and culture in children less than 2 years of age.
- Obtain a clean-catch urine sample from children who are able to cooperate.

NURSING ACTIONS
- Before performance of a suprapubic aspiration occurs, assist with confirming that informed consent has been obtained.
- To prevent a falsely low bacterial count, avoid having the child drink a large amount of fluids prior to obtaining a urine specimen.
- Send the specimen for culture to the laboratory without delay.
- Perform urinary dipstick for preliminary screening due to the length of time for culture results.
- Review findings indicative of UTI.
  - Urine culture: Positive for infecting organisms (*Escherichia coli, Proteus, Pseudomonas, Klebsiella, Enterococcus, Staphylococcus aureus*)
  - Gram stain: Positive for causative bacteria
  - Urinalysis
    - pH: acidic
    - Protein: positive
    - Glucose: positive
    - Ketones: positive
    - Leukocytes: positive
    - Nitrites: positive
    - RBC: Positive

DIAGNOSTIC PROCEDURES

Locate the primary infection site or anatomic defects
- Radioisotope renography
- Bladder wash outs
- Ultrasonography
- Voiding cystourethrogram (VCUG)
- IV pyelogram (IVP)
- Dimercaptosuccinic acid scan (DMSA)

NURSING ACTIONS
- Reinforce teaching with the child and family about the procedure for the diagnostic test prescribed.
- Determine if the child has an allergy to iodine or shellfish.
- Assist with the sedation of infants and young children as required. Encourage an older child to remain quiet during the examinations.
- Maintain the child on NPO status after midnight in preparation for a cystoscopy and IVP. IVP requires bowel preparation.
- Prepare the child if catheterization is necessary.
- Monitor the child after the procedure, according to facility protocol.

PATIENT-CENTERED CARE

NURSING CARE

- Encourage frequent voiding and complete emptying of the bladder.
- Encourage fluids.
- Monitor urine output.
- Prepare the child for diagnostic tests.
- Administer a mild analgesic (acetaminophen) for pain management.

MEDICATIONS

- Antibiotics based on findings of urine culture and sensitivity testing (penicillins, sulfonamide, cephalosporins, and nitrofurantoin).
- Antibiotics can be prescribed PO or IV depending on the severity.

NURSING ACTIONS: Monitor for potential allergic response.

CLIENT EDUCATION: Complete all prescribed antibiotics, even if manifestations are no longer present.

CLIENT EDUCATION

- Watch for manifestations of recurrence of UTIs (dysuria, frequency, urgency).
- Provide instruction to prevent recurrence.
  - For females, wipe the perineal area from front to back.
  - For uncircumcised clients, ensure foreskin is retracted prior to performing hygiene and replaced afterward.
  - Change infant's diapers frequently.
  - Keep underwear dry.
  - Use cotton underwear.
  - Maintain adequate hydration with caffeine-free beverages.
  - Avoid bubble baths.
  - Void frequently.
  - Empty bladder completely.
  - Avoid constipation by increasing fiber intake and avoid straining with bowel movements.
  - If sexually active, void immediately after intercourse.
  - If child has a history of recurrent UTIs, the child will need a repeat urinalysis 7 days after treatment.

COMPLICATIONS

Progressive kidney injury

Pyelonephritis

Urosepsis

NURSING ACTIONS: Monitor for findings of UTIs.

CLIENT EDUCATION: Reinforce teaching about prevention, early identification, and treatment of UTIs.

Active Learning Scenario

A nurse is assisting a nurse educator with preparing an in-service for a group of newly-hired nurses about caring for children who have enuresis. What should the nurse plan to include in the presentation? Use the ATI Active Learning Template: System Disorder to complete this item

ALTERATION IN HEALTH (DIAGNOSIS)

CLIENT EDUCATION: List at least 10 points to review.

Active Learning Scenario Key

Using the ATI Active Learning Template: System Disorder

ALTERATION IN HEALTH (DIAGNOSIS): Inappropriate urination must occur at least twice a week for at least 3 months, and the child must be at least 5 years of age before there's consideration about diagnosing enuresis.

CLIENT EDUCATION
- Have the child empty the bladder prior to bedtime.
- Encourage fluids during the day, and restrict fluids 2 hr before bedtime.
- Avoid fruit and fruit drinks.
- Avoid caffeinated or carbonated drinks.
- Use positive reinforcement. Avoid punishing, scolding, or teasing the child following an incident.
- Assist the child in keeping a calendar of wet and dry days.
- Have the child change bed linens and clothing following an incident.
- Wake the child at scheduled intervals during the night to void.
- Ensure the child takes all medications as prescribed.
- Use conditioning therapy, retention control measures, and reinforce Kegel/pelvic floor exercises.

Ⓝ *NCLEX® Connection: Physiological Adaptation, Alterations in Body Systems*

Application Exercises

1. A nurse is reinforcing teaching with the guardian of a child who has a urinary tract infection. Which of the following instructions should the nurse include? (Select all that apply.)

   A. Wear nylon underpants.

   B. Avoid bubble baths.

   C. Empty bladder completely with each void.

   D. Watch for manifestations of infection.

   E. Wipe perineal area back to front.

2. A nurse is contributing to the plan of care for a child who has a urinary tract infection. Which of the following interventions should the nurse include?

   A. Administer an antidiuretic.

   B. Restrict fluids.

   C. Evaluate the child's self-esteem.

   D. Encourage frequent voiding.

3. A nurse is caring for a child who has enuresis. The nurse should identify that which of the following conditions is a complication of enuresis?

   A. Urinary tract infections

   B. Emotional problems

   C. Urosepsis

   D. Progressive kidney disease

4. A nurse is collecting data from an infant who has a suspected urinary tract infection. Which of the following findings should the nurse expect? (Select all that apply.)

   A. Increase in hunger

   B. Irritability

   C. Decrease in urination

   D. Vomiting

   E. Fever

5. A nurse is collecting data from a child who has a urinary tract infection. Which of the following findings should the nurse expect? (Select all that apply.)

   A. Night sweats

   B. Swelling of the face

   C. Pallor

   D. Pale-colored urine

   E. Fatigue

Application Exercises Key

1. A. Discuss the use of underwear from natural fibers (cotton).
   B. **CORRECT:** Discuss avoiding bubble baths.
   C. **CORRECT:** Discuss the need to completely empty the bladder with each void.
   D. **CORRECT:** Review the manifestations of infection.
   E. Discuss the importance of wiping the perineal area from front to back.

   (N) NCLEX® Connection: Physiological Adaptation, Alterations in Body Systems

2. A. An antidiuretic is indicated for a child who has enuresis.
   B. Encourage fluids to a child who has a urinary tract infection.
   C. Evaluate self-esteem in children who have enuresis.
   D. **CORRECT:** It's important to encourage frequent voiding. This assists in flushing the bacteria through the urinary system.

   (N) NCLEX® Connection: Coordinated Care, Collaboration with Interdisciplinary Team

3. A. Urinary tract infections can occur in children; however, they are not a complication of enuresis.
   B. **CORRECT:** Emotional problems are a complication of enuresis.
   C. Urosepsis is a complication of urinary tract infections.
   D. Progressive kidney disease is a complication of urinary tract infections.

   (N) NCLEX® Connection: Physiological Adaptation, Basic Pathophysiology

4. A. An increase in thirst is a manifestation in an infant who has a urinary tract infection.
   B. **CORRECT:** Irritability is a manifestation in an infant who has a urinary tract infection.
   C. An increase in urination is a manifestation in an infant who has a urinary tract infection.
   D. **CORRECT:** Vomiting is a manifestation in an infant who has a urinary tract infection.
   E. **CORRECT:** Fever is a manifestation in an infant who has a urinary tract infection.

   (N) NCLEX® Connection: Physiological Adaptation, Alterations in Body Systems

5. A. Night sweats are not a manifestation in a child who has a urinary tract infection.
   B. **CORRECT:** Swelling of the face is a manifestation in child who has a urinary tract infection.
   C. **CORRECT:** Pallor is a manifestation in child who has a urinary tract infection.
   D. Bloody urine is a manifestation in child who has a urinary tract infection.
   E. **CORRECT:** Fatigue is a manifestation in child who has a urinary tract infection.

   (N) NCLEX® Connection: Physiological Adaptation, Alterations in Body Systems

CHAPTER 24 *Structural Disorders of the Genitourinary Tract and Reproductive System*

Various structural disorders can be evident at birth and can affect normal genitourinary and reproductive function.

Children become aware of and are very interested in the genital area, normality of genital function, and sex differences between 3 and 6 years of age. Due to this, repair of structural defects ideally should be done between 6 to 12 months of age, but before 3 years of age, to minimize impact on body image and to promote healthy development.

DATA COLLECTION

RISK FACTORS

Can have a genetic link

EXPECTED FINDINGS

OBSTRUCTIVE DEFECTS: Obstructive uropathy
- Hydronephrosis can be present if the ureteropelvic junction becomes obstructed and the renal pelvis and calyces become dilated, and might be detected during a fetal ultrasound.
- Partial obstructions can go undetected.
- Oligohydramnios can be a prenatal indicator of poor renal function or a severe obstruction in the infant.
- Urinary tract infections.
- Increased urine flow.

PATIENT-CENTERED CARE

NURSING CARE

Nursing care should focus on education and support of the family and child.
- Evaluate the family's perception of the child's defect, family support, and coping.
- Assist guardians to identify ways to help the child maintain a positive self-image.
- Promote healthy growth and development.
- Assist child with maintaining self-image.

DEFECTS OF THE GENITOURINARY TRACT

Obstructive uropathy

Structural or functional obstruction in the urinary system

THERAPEUTIC PROCEDURE: Surgical procedures that divert the flow of urine to bypass the obstruction

Chordee

Ventral curvature of the penis

THERAPEUTIC PROCEDURE: Surgical release of the fibrous band

Bladder exstrophy

- Eversion of the posterior bladder through the anterior bladder wall and lower abdominal wall
- Exposed bladder, urethra, and ureteral orifices through the suprapubic area
- Epispadias present

NURSING ACTIONS: Bladder exstrophy
- Cover the exposed bladder with sterile, nonadherent dressing.
- Prepare the newborn for immediate surgery.

Hypospadias

- Urethral opening located just below the glans penis, behind the glans penis, or on the ventral surface of the penile shaft
- Meatus opening below the glans penis
- Meatus opening along the ventral surface of the penis, scrotum, or perineum
- Possible chordee present

Epispadias

MALE
- Widened pubic symphysis
- Urethra opened on dorsal surface of the penis
- Possible exstrophy of the bladder

FEMALE
- Wide urethra
- Bifid clitoris
- Possible exstrophy of the bladder

THERAPEUTIC PROCEDURES
- Surgery performed during the first year of life.

Phimosis

- Narrowing of the preputial opening of the foreskin.
- Inability to retract foreskin of penis.
- Normal finding in infants and young boys and usually disappears as the child grows.

NURSING ACTION: Proper hygiene for phimotic foreskin is external cleansing during routine bathing; the foreskin should not be forcibly retracted.

Cryptorchidism

- Undescended testes
- Inability to palpate testes within the scrotum

THERAPEUTIC PROCEDURE

- Surgical orchiopexy
- Surgery performed at 6 and 24 months of age

Hydrocele

- Fluid in the scrotum
- Enlarged scrotal sac
- Can resolve spontaneously

THERAPEUTIC PROCEDURE: Surgical repair if not resolved in 1 year

Varicocele

Elongation, dilation, and tortuosity of the veins of the spermatic cord superior to the testicle. Some males experience discomfort during sexual stimulation.

THERAPEUTIC PROCEDURE: Varicocelectomy

Testicular torsion

Testis hangs free from its vascular structures.

Pain is acute in onset, and abdominal pain can also be reported.

THERAPEUTIC PROCEDURE: Manual detorsion can be attempted, followed by immediate surgery if unsuccessful.

Ambiguous genitalia

- Erroneous or abnormal sexual differentiation.
- Karyotyping is performed to determine the infant's chromosomal pattern and gonadal function tested. Adrenal function should also be tested because of the high-risk for adrenal insufficiency.
- Genetic counseling can help the family understand the cause.

THERAPEUTIC PROCEDURES

Structural defects will be treated with surgical intervention. The goal of most structural defect repairs is to preserve or create normal urinary and sexual function. Early intervention will minimize emotional trauma.

PREOPERATIVE NURSING ACTIONS

- Provide education to the child and family related to the procedure and expectations for postoperative care.
- Provide emotional support to the child and family.
- Encourage parent to express concerns and fears related to the surgical procedure and outcomes.
- If NPO status is necessary, explain the parameters to the family and/or child.

POSTOPERATIVE NURSING ACTIONS

- Collect data regarding pain using an age-appropriate pain scale or data collection tool.
- Administer pain medication. Anticholinergics can be administered to decrease spasms of the bladder.
- Monitor I&O.
- Monitor urinary catheters, drains, tubes, or stents.
- Provide wound and/or dressing care.
- Monitor for findings of infection (redness, warmth, drainage, or edema at surgical site, fever, lethargy, and foul-smelling urine).

CLIENT EDUCATION

- Perform measures to prevent infection including good hand hygiene, and care of wounds, drains, and urinary catheters and drainage bags.
- Surgery is not a punishment, and it will not mutilate the body.
- Do not provide tub baths for at least 1 week or as prescribed.
- Limit activity as prescribed.

COMPLICATIONS

Infection

NURSING ACTIONS: Observe for findings of infection including fever, skin inflammation, foul urine odor, cloudy urine, and/or urinary frequency.

CLIENT EDUCATION

- Observe for findings of infection.
- Report any findings of infection immediately.

Emotional problems

Poor self-esteem, altered body image, social isolation, fears

NURSING ACTIONS

- Support the child and family by listening to concerns and correcting misperceptions.
- Use play therapy for toddlers and preschoolers.
- Encourage peer-to-peer social networking for older children.

CLIENT EDUCATION: Consider attending support groups. Qpcc

Application Exercises

1. A nurse is caring for an infant who has a hydrocele. Which of the following actions should the nurse take?

   A. Prepare the infant for surgery.

   B. Explain to the guardians that the issue generally self-resolves.

   C. Retract the foreskin and cleanse several times daily.

   D. Refer the family for genetic counseling.

2. A nurse is caring for a male infant who has an epispadias. Which of the following findings should the nurse expect? (Select all that apply.)

   A. Bladder exstrophy

   B. Inability to retract foreskin

   C. Widened pubic symphysis

   D. Urethral opening on the dorsal side of the penis.

   E. Pain

3. A nurse is caring for an infant who has ambiguous genitalia. Which of the following actions should the nurse take? (Select all that apply.)

   A. Prepare the infant for surgery.

   B. Test the infant's adrenal function.

   C. Cover the genitals with a sterile dressing.

   D. Refer the family for genetic counseling.

   E. Explain the need for a chromosomal analysis.

4. A nurse is caring for an infant who has obstructive uropathy. Which of the following findings should the nurse expect? (Select all that apply.)

   A. Decreased urine flow

   B. Urinary tract infection

   C. History of maternal polyhydramnios

   D. Concentrated urine

   E. Hydronephrosis

Active Learning Scenario

A nurse is discussing structural disorders of the genitourinary tract and reproductive system with a newly licensed nurse. What should the nurse include in the teaching? Use the ATI Active Learning Template: Basic Concept to complete this item.

RELATED CONTENT: Describe six structural disorders of the genitourinary tract and reproductive system.

Application Exercises Key

1. A. Hydroceles are surgically repaired if they have not resolved spontaneously in 1 year.
   B. **CORRECT:** Hydrocele is fluid in the scrotum and resolves spontaneously in the majority of cases.
   C. Retracting foreskin and cleansing several times each day is done when an infant has phimosis.
   D. A referral for genetic counseling is recommended for families who have an infant with ambiguous genitalia.

   Ⓝ *NCLEX® Connection: Physiological Adaptation, Alterations in Body Systems*

2. A. **CORRECT:** Bladder exstrophy is a possible expected finding of a male infant who has epispadias.
   B. Inability to retract foreskin is a manifestation of phimosis.
   C. **CORRECT:** Widened pubic symphysis is an expected finding for a male infant who has epispadias.
   D. **CORRECT:** Presence of the urethral opening on the dorsal side of the penis is an expected finding for a male infant who has epispadias.
   E. Pain is a manifestation of testicular torsion, varicocele, and hydrocele.

   Ⓝ *NCLEX® Connection: Physiological Adaptation, Basic Pathophysiology*

3. A. **CORRECT:** Infants who have ambiguous genitalia will need surgery. Preparing the family for surgery is an appropriate action to take.
   B. **CORRECT:** Plan to test the infant's adrenal function to rule out adrenal insufficiency.
   C. Cover the bladder with a sterile dressing for bladder exstrophy.
   D. **CORRECT:** Families with an infant who has ambiguous genitalia will need ongoing support. Referring to genetic counseling is an appropriate action to take.
   E. **CORRECT:** Chromosomal analysis is used for sex assignment, and is therefore an appropriate action to take.

   Ⓝ *NCLEX® Connection: Health Promotion and Maintenance, Aging Process*

4. A. Increased urine flow is a manifestation of obstructive uropathy.
   B. **CORRECT:** Urinary tract infection is a manifestation of obstructive uropathy.
   C. History of maternal oligohydramnios is an indication of possible urinary obstruction in the fetus.
   D. Inability to concentrate urine is a manifestation of obstructive uropathy.
   E. **CORRECT:** Hydronephrosis is a manifestation of obstructive uropathy.

   Ⓝ *NCLEX® Connection: Physiological Adaptation, Basic Pathophysiology*

Active Learning Scenario Key

Using the ATI Active Learning Template: Basic Concept

RELATED CONTENT

- Obstructive uropathy: Structural or functional obstruction in the urinary system.
- Chordee: Ventral curvature of the penis.
- Bladder exstrophy: Eversion of the posterior bladder through the anterior bladder wall and lower abdominal wall.
- Hypospadias: Urethral opening located just below the glans penis, behind the glans penis, or on the ventral surface of the penile shaft.
- Epispadias: Meatal opening located on the dorsal surface of the penis.
- Phimosis: Narrowing of the preputial opening of the foreskin.
- Cryptorchidism: Undescended testes.
- Hydrocele: Fluid in the scrotum.
- Varicocele: Elongated, dilated, and tortuosity of the veins superior to the testicle.
- Testicular torsion: Testicle hangs free from the vascular structures.
- Ambiguous genitalia: Erroneous or abnormal sexual differentiation.

Ⓝ *NCLEX® Connection: Physiological Adaptation, Basic Pathophysiology*

CHAPTER 25 *Kidney Disorders*

This chapter includes acute glomerulonephritis, nephrotic syndrome, hemolytic uremic syndrome (HUS), acute kidney injury (AKI), and chronic kidney disease (CKD).

Acute glomerulonephritis

- Benign inflammation of the glomeruli which causes intravascular coagulation that lasts about 1 to 2 weeks.
- Common features are oliguria, edema, hypertension and circulatory congestion, hematuria, and proteinuria.
- Acute post-streptococcal glomerulonephritis (APSGN) is an antibody-antigen disease that occurs as a result of certain strains of the group A beta-hemolytic streptococcal infection and is most commonly seen in children between the ages of 5 and 7 years.

DATA COLLECTION

RISK FACTORS

- Acute post-streptococcal glomerulonephritis
- Recent upper respiratory infection or streptococcal infection

EXPECTED FINDINGS

- Cloudy, tea-colored urine
- Decreased urine output
- Hematuria
- Proteinuria
- Irritability
- Ill appearance
- Lethargy
- Anorexia
- Vague reports of discomfort (headache, abdominal pain, dysuria)
- Periorbital edema
- Facial edema that is worse in the morning but then spreads to extremities and abdomen with progression of the day
- Mild to severe hypertension
- Low grade fever
- Vomiting
- Encephalopathy (headache, irritability, seizures)
- Genitalia and gonadal swelling

LABORATORY TESTS

Throat culture: to identify possible streptococcus infection (usually negative by the time of diagnosis)

Urinalysis: proteinuria, smoky or tea-colored urine, hematuria, increased specific gravity

Kidney function: elevated BUN and creatinine. Decreased glomerular filtration rates.

Antistreptolysin O (ASO) titer: positive indicator for the presence of streptococcal antibodies

Antihyaluronidase (AHase)

Antideoxyribonuclease B (Anti-DNase B)

Anti-streptokinase (ASKase)

Antinicotyladenine dinucleotidase (ANADase)

Blood complement (C3): decreased initially; increases as recovery takes place; returns to normal at 8 to 10 weeks post glomerulonephritis

DIAGNOSTIC PROCEDURES

Kidney biopsy

PATIENT-CENTERED CARE

NURSING CARE

- Clients who have normal blood pressure and urine output can be managed at home.
- Monitor I&O.
- Monitor urine volume and character.
- Weigh the child on the same scale with the same amount of clothing daily.
- Monitor vital signs.
- Monitor neurologic status and observe for behavior changes, especially in children who have edema, hypertension, and gross hematuria. Implement seizure precautions if condition indicates.
- Encourage adequate nutritional intake.
  - Possible restriction of sodium and fluid.
  - Restrict foods high in potassium during periods of oliguria.
  - Restrict protein for severe azotemia.
- Manage fluid restrictions as prescribed. Fluids can be restricted during periods of edema and hypertension.
- Determine activity tolerance. Provide frequent rest periods and cluster care tasks.
- Provide for age-appropriate diversional activities.
- Monitor and prevent infection.

MEDICATIONS

Diuretics and antihypertensives

To remove accumulated fluid and manage hypertension

NURSING ACTIONS
- Monitor blood pressure.
- Monitor I&O.
- Monitor for electrolyte imbalances (hypokalemia).
- Observe for adverse effects of medications.

CLIENT EDUCATION
- Dizziness can occur with the use of antihypertensives.
- Take the medication as prescribed and notify the provider if adverse effects occur. Continue the medication unless instructed otherwise.

Antibiotics

Treat streptococcal infections

Phosphate binders

Sodium polystyrene sulfonate

Corrects hyperkalemia

INTERPROFESSIONAL CARE

Obtain a dietary consult.

CLIENT EDUCATION

- Encourage the child to verbalize feelings related to body image.
- Educate the child regarding appropriate dietary management.
- Encourage adequate rest.
- Inform the family about the need for follow-up care.
- Reinforce teaching with the family on how to monitor blood pressure and daily weight.
- Instruct the family about administration and adverse effects of diuretics and antihypertensive medications.
- Encourage the child and family to avoid contact with others who might be ill.

COMPLICATIONS

- Hypertensive encephalopathy
- Circulatory overload
- Anemia
- Hyperkalemia
- Seizures
- Cardiac failure
- Acute kidney injury

Nephrotic syndrome

- Alterations in the glomerular membrane allow proteins (especially albumin) to pass into the urine, resulting in decreased blood osmotic pressure, which leads to proteinuria, hyperlipidemia, and edema.
- It can be primary, secondary, or congenital.

DATA COLLECTION

RISK FACTORS

Minimal change nephrotic syndrome (MCNS)
- Peak incidence is between 2 and 3 years of age.
- Cause is unknown, but it can have a multifactorial etiology (metabolic, biochemical, or physiochemical disturbance in the basement membrane of the glomeruli).

Secondary nephrotic syndrome: occurs after or is associated with glomerular damage due to a known cause

Congenital nephrotic syndrome: an inherited disorder

EXPECTED FINDINGS

- Weight gain over a period of days or weeks
- Facial and periorbital edema: decreased throughout the day
- Ascites
- Edema to lower extremities and genitalia
- Muehrcke lines on fingernails (white lines parallel to the lunula)
- Pallor
- Anorexia
- Diarrhea
- Irritability
- Lethargy
- Dyspnea
- Vomiting
- Decreased, frothy urine
- Blood pressure within expected reference range or slightly below. Hypertension can be rare finding in MCNS.

LABORATORY TESTS

Urinalysis/24-hr urine collection

- Proteinuria: present; up to 15 grams of protein in a 24-hr specimen
- Hyaline casts
- Few RBCs
- Oval fat bodies
- Increased specific gravity

Blood chemistry

Hypoalbuminemia: reduced blood protein and albumin

Hyperlipidemia: elevated blood lipid levels

Hemoconcentration: elevated Hgb, Hct, and platelets

Possible hyponatremia: reduced sodium level

Glomerular filtration rate: normal or high

Total calcium: decreased

Erythrocyte sedimentation rate (ESR): increased

DIAGNOSTIC PROCEDURES

Kidney biopsy is indicated only if nephrotic syndrome is unresponsive to steroid therapy. Biopsy will show damage to the epithelial cells lining the basement membrane of the kidney.

MRI: Scarring of the kidneys' glomeruli

PATIENT-CENTERED CARE

NURSING CARE

Outcome of therapy and interventions is to decrease the excretion of protein by the kidneys.
- Provide rest.
- Maintain strict I&O. Weigh infant diapers for recording output.
- Monitor urine for protein.
- Monitor vital signs.
- Monitor daily weights; weigh the child on the same scale with the same amount of clothing.
- Monitor edema and measure abdominal girth daily. Measure at the widest area, usually at or above the umbilicus. Monitor degree of pitting, color, and texture of skin.
- Elevate legs and feet to relieve edema.
- Monitor and prevent infection (increased Risk for upper respiratory infection).
- Encourage nutritional intake within restriction guidelines. Salt can be restricted during the edematous phase.
- Cluster care to provide for rest periods.
- Examine skin for breakdown areas.
- Provide support to families and make appropriate referrals as needed. Relapses can cause physical, emotional, and financial stress for the client and family.

MEDICATIONS

Corticosteroid: prednisone

NURSING ACTIONS
- 60 mg/m²/day for 4 to 6 weeks followed by 40 mg/m² every other day for 2 to 5 months with taper. **Q**EBP
- Monitor for adverse effects (hirsutism, slowed linear growth, hypertension, GI bleeding, infection, and hyperglycemia).
- Administer with meals.

CLIENT EDUCATION
- Avoid large crowds (to decrease the risk of infection).
- Using corticosteroids can increase appetite, cause weight gain (especially in the face), and cause mood swings.
- Adhere to the medication regime.
- Observe for adverse effects and notify the provider if necessary.

Diuretic: furosemide

Eliminates excess fluid from the body

NURSING ACTIONS
- Encourage the child to eat foods that are high in potassium.
- Monitor blood electrolyte levels periodically (hypokalemia).

Plasma expanders: 25% albumin

Increases plasma volume and decreases edema

NURSING ACTIONS
- Administer per protocol.
- Monitor I&O.
- Monitor for anaphylaxis.

Immunosuppressant: cyclophosphamide

Administer for children who cannot tolerate prednisone or who have repeated relapses of MCNS.

NURSING ACTIONS: Monitor for leukopenia.

INTERPROFESSIONAL CARE

Obtain a dietary consult.

CLIENT EDUCATION
- Encourage the client to verbalize feelings related to body image.
- Manage diet appropriately.
- Take all immunizations as scheduled (pneumococcal). Use caution with live vaccines while taking steroids.
- Allow adequate rest.
- Follow-up with the provider as instructed for continued monitoring of the child's response to therapy.
- Strategies to decrease the risk of infection include good hand hygiene, up-to-date immunizations, avoidance of infected people.
- Monitor blood pressure, daily weight, and protein in urine. Notify the provider if manifestations worsen, which indicates relapse.
- Be aware of proper administration and adverse effects of medication.

COMPLICATIONS

Sepsis/infection
- Steroid therapy increases the risk for infection.
- Monitor for findings of infection.
- CLIENT EDUCATION
  - Even if the child improves, complete the full dose of antibiotic.
  - To prevent infection, perform frequent hand hygiene.
  - Contact the provider for any manifestations of infection.
  - Keep the child away from potential infection sources.

Hemolytic uremic syndrome

- HUS is an acute kidney injury characterized by acute kidney failure, hemolytic anemia and thrombocytopenia.
- HUS represents one of the main causes of acute kidney injury in early childhood.
- Breakdown of red blood cells clog the kidneys.
- Toxins enter the bloodstream and destroy red blood cells

DATA COLLECTION

RISK FACTORS

- Peak incidence 6 months to 4 years
- Predominantly in Caucasian children, and prevalent in South Africa, Argentina, and west coasts of North and South America.

Diarrhea-positive (D+) HUS
- Responsible for 90% of cases; caused by ingestion of Shiga toxin producing *Escherichia coli*, *E. coli* 0157:H7 is common pathogen

Diarrhea-negative (D-) or atypical HUS: Can be due to nonenteric infections, disturbances in the complement system, malignancies, or genetic disorders

EXPECTED FINDINGS

- Occurs after prodromal period of diarrhea and vomiting
- Occasionally occurs after an upper respiratory infection, varicella, measles, or a UTI
- Loss of appetite
- Irritable
- Lethargy
- Stupor
- Hallucinations
- Edema
- Pallor
- Bruising, purpura, or rectal bleeding
- Anuric and hypertensive in severe form
- Urinary output can be reduced or increased

LABORATORY TESTS

- CBC: Decreased hemoglobin and hematocrit
- Elevated reticulocyte count
- Urine: Positive for blood, protein, and casts
- Elevated BUN and blood creatinine
- Fibrin split products in blood and urine (thrombocytopenia)

PATIENT-CENTERED CARE

NURSING CARE

SUPPORTIVE MEASURES
- Monitor I&O.
- Obtain daily weights.
- Administer fluid replacement.
- Treat hypertension.
- Correct acidosis and electrolyte imbalances.
- Monitor CNS for seizure activity and stupor.
- Initiate seizure precautions.
- Blood transfusions with fresh, washed packed cells for severe anemia: used with caution.
- Recommendations for a child who is anuric for 24 hr or is experiencing oliguria with uremia or hypertension and seizures include:
  - Hemodialysis.
  - Peritoneal dialysis.
  - Continuous hemofiltration.

NUTRITION
- Once vomiting and diarrhea resolves, enteral nutrition is initiated.
- Parenteral nutrition is provided for children who have severe, persistent colitis and marked tissue catabolism.

MEDICATIONS

- No evidence that heparin, corticosteroids, or fibrinolytic agents are beneficial.
- Plasma infusion is under study and can be useful.

INTERPROFESSIONAL CARE

Obtain a dietary consult.

CLIENT EDUCATION

- Instruct the family to avoid undercooked meat, especially ground beef. Internal temperature of meat should be at least 74° C (165° F).
- Avoid unpasteurized apple juice and unwashed raw vegetables.
- Avoid alfalfa sprouts.
- Avoid public pools.
- Do not use antimotility medications for diarrhea.
- Support the child and family regarding severity of the illness.

Acute kidney injury

- AKI is the inability of the kidneys to excrete waste material, concentrate urine, and conserve electrolytes.
- The disorder can be acute or chronic and affects most of the systems of the body.
- Causes are classified as prerenal, intrinsic renal, and postrenal. Prerenal are most common cause of AKI.

DATA COLLECTION

RISK FACTORS

Prerenal
- Dehydration secondary to diarrheal disease or persistent vomiting.
- Surgical shock and trauma (including burns)
- Accidental poisoning
- Prolonged anesthesia

Intrinsic renal: Damage to the glomeruli, tubules, or kidney vasculature from disease or nephrotoxicity

Postrenal: Obstruction of the urinary system

EXPECTED FINDINGS

- Oliguria: in reversible AKI there is a period of severe low urinary output
- Abrupt diuresis: with return to normal urine volumes
- Edema
- Drowsiness
- Circulatory congestion
- Cardiac arrhythmia: from hyperkalemia (irregular, weak pulse, abdominal cramps, weakness)
- Seizures: from hyponatremia or hypocalcemia (tetany)
- Tachypnea: from metabolic acidosis
- CNS manifestations: from continued oliguria

LABORATORY/DIAGNOSTIC TESTS

Monitor kidney function related to preexisting kidney disease.
- Hyperkalemia
- Hyponatremia
- Metabolic acidosis
- Hypocalcemia
- Anemia
- Azotemia
- Elevated phosphorus
- Elevated plasma creatinine
- Elevated BUN
- ECG for cardiac arrhythmias
- IVP and MRI evaluate kidney function

PATIENT-CENTERED CARE

NURSING CARE

- Treat underlying cause of AKI.
- Admit to pediatric intensive care unit.
- Monitor strict I&O.
- Determine fluid and electrolyte balance.
- Limit fluid intake.
- Obtain daily weights.
- Monitor vital signs for hypertension complication.
- Maintain neutral temperature.
- Provide replacement IV fluids slowly.
- Monitor central venous pressure.
- Maintain urinary catheterization.
- Limit activity.
- Check for behavior changes or seizure activity.
- Implement seizure precautions if indicated.
- Examine for infection.

MEDICATIONS

Mannitol and furosemide to provoke a flow of urine in child who has oliguria and no lower tract obstruction

Calcium gluconate 0.5 mL/kg IV every 2 to 4 min with continuous ECG monitoring to reduce blood potassium levels

Sodium bicarbonate, 2 to 3 mEq/kg IV every 30 to 60 min, elevates blood pH and causes a transient fluid shift to reduce blood potassium levels by shifting potassium into the cells.

Glucose and insulin IV causes glucose and potassium to move into cells. Insulin facilitates entry of glucose into cells and helps to reduce blood potassium levels by moving potassium into the cells.

Sodium polystyrene sulfonate
- 1 g/kg orally or rectally to bind potassium and excrete it from body

Labetalol or sodium nitroprusside IV (with close monitoring) hypertension if encephalopathy threat present.

Hydralazine, clonidine, or verapamil can be given IV for hypertension in less urgent situations.

Captopril, hydralazine, minoxidil, propranolol, nifedipine, or furosemide can be give orally for hypertension.

THERAPEUTIC PROCEDURES

Dialysis or continuous hemofiltration can be required to correct hyperkalemia.

NUTRITION

- Ingest concentrated foods without fluids.
- Maintain calories while minimizing tissue catabolism, metabolic acidosis, hyperkalemia, and uremia.
- When nourishment is via IV route, prevent fluid overload.

INTERPROFESSIONAL CARE

Support the child and family.

CLIENT EDUCATION

- Get adequate rest.
- Adhere to the therapeutic regimen.
- Attend follow-up care.
- Monitor urinary output.

Chronic kidney disease

- CKD or insufficiency begins when the diseased kidneys can no longer maintain the normal chemical structure of body fluids under normal conditions, and there is extensive irreversible damage to the nephrons.
- A variety of diseases and disorders can result in CKD.

DATA COLLECTION

RISK FACTORS

- Most common causes before 5 years of age are congenital, renal, and urinary tract malformations and vesicoureteral reflux.
- Glomerular and hereditary renal disease predominate in the 5- to 15-year-old age group.

EXPECTED FINDINGS

- Loss of energy
- Increase fatigue on exertion
- Pallor
- Occasional elevated blood pressure
- Delayed growth
- Anorexia
- Nausea and vomiting
- Decrease interest in activities
- Decreased or increased urinary output and compensatory increase in fluid intake
- Uremic odor to breath
- Headache
- Muscle cramps
- Weight loss
- Puffiness to face
- Malaise
- Bone or joint pain
- Itchy, bruised skin
- Amenorrhea in adolescent girls
- Circulatory overload manifested by hypertension, congestive heart failure and pulmonary edema
- Neurologic involvement (tremors, muscle twitching, confusion, seizures, coma).

LABORATORY/DIAGNOSTIC TESTS

- Blood electrolytes: hyperkalemia, hypocalcemia, hyperphosphatemia
- CBC: anemia
- Blood creatinine and BUN: elevated
- Arterial blood gases: metabolic acidosis

PATIENT-CENTERED CARE

NURSING CARE

- Provide rest.
- Monitor I&O. Initiate fluid restriction if edema present.
- Monitor vital signs.
- Monitor daily weights.
- Manage hypertension.
- Monitor for infection.
- Maintain sodium restriction.
- Encourage reduction of dietary phosphorus.
- Encourage guardians to maintain dialysis schedule.
- Reinforce teaching with the family regrading medication compliance and adherence.
- Keep family informed of child's progress.

MEDICATIONS

- Thiazides or furosemide for hypertension
- Beta blockers and vasodilators for severe hypertension
- Phosphorus binding agent to prevent retention of phosphorus
- Calcium supplements
- Vitamin D: active form
- Water-soluble vitamins
- Sodium bicarbonate and potassium citrate to alleviate acidosis
- Folic acid and recombinant human erythropoietin for anemia
- Recombinant growth hormone for children who have growth retardation
- Antimicrobials for infection
- Antiepileptic for seizures
- Diphenhydramine for pruritus
- Packed RBCs to correct anemia. Administer slowly.

NUTRITION

- Goal is to provide adequate calories and protein for growth.
- Restrict dietary phosphorus intake.
- Potassium is restricted if oliguria or anuria.
- Limit protein intake to the RDA for the child's age.
- Dietary sources of folic acid and iron.

INTERPROFESSIONAL CARE

- Obtain a dietary consult.
- Encourage regular dental visits.

CLIENT EDUCATION

- Increase rest.
- Adhere to therapeutic regimen.
- Encourage the child to remain active, and attend school.
- Child should participate in meal planning according to dietary restrictions.

COMPLICATIONS

- End-stage kidney disease
- Progressive deterioration
- Irreversible progress of renal insufficiency
- Increased susceptibility to infections (pneumonia)

Application Exercises

1. A nurse is collecting data from a child who has nephrotic syndrome. Which of the following findings should the nurse expect? (Select all that apply.)

   A. Urine dipstick +2 protein

   B. Edema in the ankles

   C. Hyperlipidemia

   D. Polyuria

   E. Anorexia

2. A nurse is caring for a school-age child who has acute glomerulonephritis. Which of the following findings should the nurse report to the provider?

   A. BUN 8 mg/dL

   B. Blood creatinine 1.3 mg/dL

   C. Blood pressure 100/74 mm Hg

   D. Urine output 550 mL in 24 hr

3. A nurse is caring for a preschooler who has nephrotic syndrome. Which of the following findings should the nurse report to the provider?

   A. Blood protein 5.0 g/dL

   B. Hgb 14.5 g/dL

   C. Hct 40%

   D. Platelet 200,000 mm³

4. A nurse is collecting data from a child who has chronic kidney disease. Which of the following findings should the nurse expect?

   A. Flushed face

   B. Hyperactivity

   C. Weight gain

   D. Delayed growth

5. A nurse is collecting data from a child who has acute post-streptococcal glomerulonephritis (APSGN). Which of the following manifestations should the nurse expect? (Select all that apply.)

   A. Pale urine

   B. Periorbital edema

   C. Ill appearance

   D. Decreased creatinine

   E. Hypertension

Active Learning Scenario

A nurse is reinforcing teaching with the guardian of a child who has a new prescription for prednisone for nephrotic syndrome. Use the Active Learning Template: Medication to complete this item.

NURSING INTERVENTIONS: List three.

CLIENT EDUCATION: List four teaching points.

Application Exercises Key

1. A. **CORRECT:** A client who has nephrotic syndrome will exhibit proteinuria of due to the kidneys' inability to filter urine.
   B. **CORRECT:** A client who has nephrotic syndrome will exhibit edema in the ankles due to the decreasing colloidal osmotic pressure in the capillaries.
   C. **CORRECT:** A client who has nephrotic syndrome will exhibit hyperlipidemia due to the increased hepatic synthesis of proteins and lipids.
   D. A client who has nephrotic syndrome will exhibit decreased urinary output.
   E. **CORRECT:** A client who has nephrotic syndrome will exhibit anorexia due to the edema of the intestinal mucosa.

   Ⓝ *NCLEX® Connection: Physiological Adaptation, Basic Pathophysiology*

2. A. A BUN of 8 mg/dL is within the expected reference range for a school-age child.
   B. **CORRECT:** Blood creatinine 1.3 mg/dL is above the expected reference range for school-age child, and should be reported to the provider.
   C. Blood pressure of 100/74 mm Hg is within the expected reference range for a school-age child.
   D. Urine output of 550 mL over 24 hr is within the expected reference range for a school-age child.

   Ⓝ *NCLEX® Connection: Reduction of Risk Potential, Laboratory Values*

3. A. **CORRECT:** Blood protein 5.0 g/dL is out of the expected reference range for a preschooler and should be reported to the provider.
   B. Hgb 14.5 g/dL is within the expected reference range for a preschooler.
   C. Hct 40% is within the expected reference range for a preschooler.
   D. Platelets 200,000 mm³ is within the expected reference range for a preschooler.

   Ⓝ *NCLEX® Connection: Reduction of Risk Potential, Laboratory Values*

4. A. Expect the child to exhibit pallor, not flushing.
   B. Expect the child to be fatigued, not hyperactive.
   C. Expect the child to have weight loss from anorexia, nausea, and vomiting.
   D. **CORRECT:** Expect the child to exhibit delayed growth.

   Ⓝ *NCLEX® Connection: Physiological Adaptation, Basic Pathophysiology*

5. A. A client who has APSGN will exhibit cloudy, tea-colored urine due to blood and protein in the urine.
   B. **CORRECT:** A client who has APSGN will exhibit periorbital edema due to decrease in plasma filtration.
   C. **CORRECT:** A client who has APSGN will exhibit an ill appearance due to the manifestations experienced from the inadequate functioning of the kidneys.
   D. A client who has APSGN will exhibit increased creatinine due to impaired glomerular filtration of the kidneys.
   E. **CORRECT:** A client who has APSGN will exhibit hypertension due to inadequate function of the kidneys and possibly edema.

   Ⓝ *NCLEX® Connection: Physiological Adaptation, Basic Pathophysiology*

Active Learning Scenario Key

Using the Active Learning Template: Medication

NURSING INTERVENTIONS

- Administer 2 mg/kg/day for 6 weeks followed by 1.5 mg/kg every other day for 6 weeks.
- Monitor for adverse effects (hirsutism, slowed linear growth, hypertension, GI bleeding, infection, and hyperglycemia).
- Administer with meals.

CLIENT EDUCATION

- Avoid large crowds (to decrease the risk of infection).
- Using corticosteroids can increase appetite, cause weight gain (especially in the face), and cause mood swings.
- Adhere to the medication regimen.
- Monitor for adverse effects and notify the provider.

Ⓝ *NCLEX® Connection: Pharmacological Therapies, Medication Administration*

ⓝ NCLEX® Connections

When reviewing the following chapters, keep in mind the relevant topics and tasks of the NCLEX outline, in particular:

Basic Care and Comfort

MOBILITY/IMMOBILITY: Provide care to an immobilized client based on need.

Pharmacological Therapies

EXPECTED ACTIONS/OUTCOMES: Apply knowledge of pathophysiology when addressing client pharmacological agents.

Reduction of Risk Potential

POTENTIAL FOR COMPLICATIONS OF DIAGNOSTIC TESTS/ TREATMENTS/PROCEDURES: Use precautions to prevent injury and/or complications associated with a procedure or diagnosis.

POTENTIAL FOR COMPLICATIONS FROM SURGICAL PROCEDURES AND HEALTH ALTERATIONS: Assist with care for client before and after surgical procedure.

THERAPEUTIC PROCEDURES: Assist with the performance of a diagnostic or invasive procedure.

Physiological Adaptation

ALTERATIONS IN BODY SYSTEMS: Reinforce education to the client regarding care and condition.

BASIC PATHOPHYSIOLOGY
Identify signs and symptoms related to an acute or chronic illness.

Consider general principles of client disease process when providing care.

Apply knowledge of pathophysiology to monitoring client for alterations in body systems.

FLUID AND ELECTROLYTE IMBALANCES
Identify signs and symptoms of client fluid and/or electrolyte imbalances.

Provide care for a client with a fluid and electrolyte balance.

CHAPTER 26

CHAPTER 26 *Fractures*

A fracture occurs when the resistance between a bone and an applied stress results in a disruption to the integrity of the bone. Bone healing and remodeling is faster in children than in adults, due to a thicker periosteum and good blood supply.

Epiphyseal plate injuries can result in altered bone growth. Radiographic evidence of previous fractures in various stages of healing or in infants can be the result of physical maltreatment or osteogenesis imperfecta.

DATA COLLECTION

RISK FACTORS
- Obesity
- Poor nutrition
- Developmental characteristics, ordinary play activities, and recreation that place children at risk for injury (falls from climbing or running; trauma to bones from skateboarding, skiing, or playing soccer or basketball)

EXPECTED FINDINGS
- Pain
- Crepitus
- Deformity
- Edema
- Ecchymosis
- Warmth or redness
- Decreased use of affected area

COMMON TYPES OF FRACTURES IN CHILDREN
- **Plastic deformation (bend):** The bone is bent no more than 45° without breakage.
- **Buckle (torus):** Compression of the bone resulting in a bulge or raised area at the fracture site.
- **Greenstick:** Incomplete fracture of the bone.
- **Transverse:** Break is straight across the bone. Q EBP
- **Oblique:** Break is diagonal across the bone.
- **Spiral:** Break spirals around the bone.
- **Physeal (growth plate):** Injury to the end of the long bone on the growth plate.
- **Stress:** Small fractures/cracks in the bone due to repeated muscle contractions.
- **Complete:** Bone fragments are separated.
- **Incomplete:** Bone fragments are still attached.
- **Closed or simple:** The fracture occurs without a break in the skin.

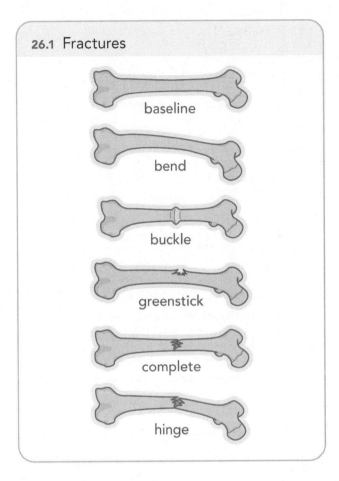

26.1 Fractures

- baseline
- bend
- buckle
- greenstick
- complete
- hinge

- **Open or compound:** The fracture occurs with an open wound and bone protruding.
- **Complicated fracture:** The fracture results in injury to other organs and tissues.
- **Comminuted:** The fracture includes small fragments of bone that lie in surrounding tissue.

DIAGNOSTIC PROCEDURES

Radiograph

Used to confirm diagnosis and determine the positioning of the bone

NURSING ACTIONS: Instruct and assist the client to remain still during the procedure.

CLIENT EDUCATION
- Be aware of what to expect during the procedure.
- Provide emotional support.

PATIENT-CENTERED CARE

NURSING CARE

Provide emergency care at the time of injury.
- Obtain a history of how the injury occurred.
- Maintain ABCs.
- Monitor vital signs, pain, and neurologic status.
- Position the child in a supine position for injuries to the distal arm, pelvis, and lower extremities.
- Position the child in a sitting position for injuries to the shoulder or upper arm.
- Remove jewelry or objects that can cause constriction on the affected extremity.
- Stabilize the injured area, avoiding unnecessary movement.
- Provide splinting at the joint above and below the injured area.
- If a pelvic fracture is suspected, monitor urine for blood and for development of hypovolemic shock
- Elevate the affected limb and apply ice packs (not to exceed 20 min).
- Administer analgesics as prescribed.
- Keep the child warm.

GENERAL NURSING INTERVENTIONS
- Determine pain level frequently using an age-appropriate pain tool. Use appropriate pain management, both pharmacological and nonpharmacological.
- Maintain proper alignment.
- Promote range of motion of fingers, toes, and unaffected extremities.
- Instruct the client and family regarding activity restrictions.
- Reassure and provide comfort to the caregivers and child.
- Increase calcium intake if not contraindicated.

NEUROVASCULAR STATUS
- **Sensation:** Examine extremity for numbness or tingling sensation. Loss of sensation can indicate nerve damage.
- **Skin temperature:** Determine the temperature of the extremity. It should be warm, not cool, to touch.
- **Skin color:** Determine the color of the affected extremity. Check distal to the injury and look for changes in pigmentation.
- **Capillary refill:** Press the nail beds of the affected extremity until blanching occurs. Blood return should be within 3 seconds.
- **Pulses:** Pulses should be palpable and strong. Pulses should also be equal to the pulses of the unaffected extremity.
- **Movement:** The client should be able to move the joints distal to the injury (fingers or toes).

MEDICATIONS

Analgesics

Administer analgesics for pain.

Opioid analgesia

NURSING ACTIONS: Monitor for respiratory depression and constipation.

CLIENT EDUCATION: Be aware of the need for adequate pain relief.

Immunizations

Administer tetanus for open fractures.

Antibiotics

Administer for open fractures.

THERAPEUTIC PROCEDURES

Casting

TYPES OF CASTS: long-leg, short-leg, bilateral long-leg, long-arm, short-arm, shoulder spica, 1 1/2 spica, full spica, and single spica
- Plaster of Paris casts are heavy, not water-resistant, and can take 10 to 72 hr to dry. Synthetic fiberglass casts are light, water-resistant, and dry quickly (5 to 20 min).
- Prior to casting, the skin area should be observed for integrity, cleaned, and dried. Bony prominences should be padded to prevent skin breakdown. The provider then applies the casting material.

NURSING ACTIONS
- Provide atraumatic care prior to cast application by showing the procedure on a doll or toy.
- Elevate the cast above the level of the heart during the first 24 to 48 hr to prevent swelling.
- Apply ice for the first 24 hr to decrease swelling.
- Turn and position the child at least once every 2 hr so that dry air circulates around and under the cast for faster drying. This also will prevent pressure from changing the shape of the cast. Do not use heat lamps or warm hair dryers.
- Turn the child frequently while supporting all extremities and joints.
- Instruct the child to keep the affected extremity supported (with a sling) or elevated on a pillow when sitting.
- Check for increased warmth or hot spots on the cast surface, which could indicate infection.
- Monitor for drainage on the cast. Outline any drainage on the outside of the cast with a pen (and note date and time) so it can be monitored for any additional drainage.
- Examine the general skin condition and the area around the cast edges.
- Provide routine skin care and thorough perineal care to maintain skin integrity.

- For plaster casts, use palms of hands to avoid denting, and expose the case to air to promote drying.
- Use moleskin to petal the edges over any rough area of the cast that can rub against the client's skin.
- Cover areas of the cast with plastic to avoid soiling from urine or feces.
- Assist with proper crutch fitting, and reinforce proper use.

CLIENT EDUCATION
- Reinforce teaching with the child and parents that when the cast is applied it will feel warm, but it will not burn the client.
- Instruct the guardians and child to report pain that is extremely severe or is not relieved 1 hr after the administration of pain medication.
- Reinforce instructions for the proper use of crutches for lower-extremity casts.
- Reinforce skin and perineal care with a spica cast.
- Instruct the child not to place any foreign objects inside the cast to avoid trauma to the skin.
- Reinforce use of proper restraints when transporting the client in any vehicle.
- Reinforce teaching with the child and guardians about cast removal and cast cutter.
- Notify provider immediately of any hot or soft spots on the cast, change in sensation or increased pain.
- Cleanse with damp cloth if becomes soiled.
- Instruct the client to soak the extremity in warm water and then apply lotion after the cast has been removed.

Traction care

Traction involves the use of a pulling force to reduce a fracture, maintain alignment, and provide muscle rest. The type of traction used depends on the fracture, age of the client, and associated injuries.
- **Skin traction** uses a pulling force that is applied by weights. Using tape and straps applied to the skin along with boots and/or cuffs, weights are attached by a rope to the extremity (Buck, Russell, Bryant traction).
- **Skeletal traction** uses a continuous pulling force that is applied directly to the skeletal structure and/or specific bone. It is used when more pulling force is needed than skin traction can withstand. A pin or rod is inserted through or into the bone. Force is applied through the use of weights attached by rope. The weights are never to be removed by the nurse.
- **Halo traction (cervical traction)** uses a halo-type bar that encircles the head. Screws are inserted into the outer skull. The halo is attached to either bed traction or rods that are secured to a vest worn by the client.

NURSING ACTIONS
- Maintain body alignment.
- Provide pharmacological and nonpharmacological interventions for the management of pain and muscle spasms.
- Notify the provider if the client experiences severe pain from muscle spasms that is unrelieved with medications or repositioning.
- Monitor neurovascular status.
- Routinely monitor skin integrity and document findings. Ⓠpcc

- Check pin sites for pain, redness, swelling, drainage, or odor. Provide pin care per facility protocol.
- Monitor for changes in elimination, and maintain usual patterns of elimination.
- Ensure that all the hardware is tight and that the bed is in the correct position.
- Ensure the weights hang freely and the knots do not touch the pulley. Do not lift or remove weights unless prescribed and supervised by the provider.
- Consult with the provider for an overbed trapeze to assist the child to move in bed.
- Provide range of motion and encourage activity of nonimmobilized extremities to maintain mobility and prevent contractures.
- Encourage deep breathing and use of the incentive spirometry.
- Promote frequent position changing within restrictions of traction to prevent skin breakdown.
- Remove sheets from the head of the bed to the foot of the bed, and remake the bed in the same manner.

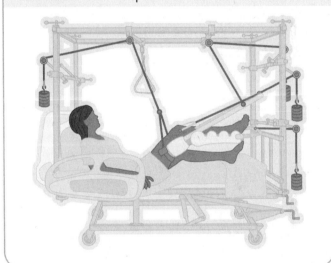

26.2 Balanced suspension skeletal traction

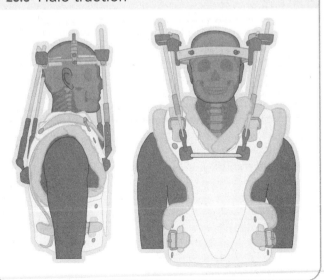

26.3 Halo traction

FOR THE CLIENT IN A HALO DEVICE

- Ensure that the wrench to release the rods is readily available when using halo traction in the event that CPR is necessary.
- Assist with moving the child in halo traction as a unit without applying pressure to the rods. This will prevent loosening of the pins and pain.
- Inspect the pins regularly to ensure loosening does not occur.
- Monitor integrity of the skin beneath the halo vest.

CLIENT EDUCATION

- Provide adequate hydration and nutrition while in traction.
- Utilize stool softeners as necessary.
- Reinforce teaching with the child and guardians how to provide pin site care.
- Identify manifestations of infection.
- Report manifestations of compartment syndrome immediately.
- Instruct the client and guardians that powder is not to be used under the halo vest.

COMPLICATIONS

Compartment syndrome

- Compression of nerves, blood vessels, and muscle inside a confined place, resulting in neuromuscular ischemia; most commonly occurring in relation to tibial fractures or fractures involving the forearm.
- If untreated, deformity of the extremity, paralysis and infection can result.

Volkmann contracture: a permanent contracture of the forearm and hand

CAUSES: tight dressing or cast, hemorrhage, burns, surgery, massive IV infiltration

Renal calculi

Occurs with non-weight-bearing injuries. Ensure adequate nutrition and hydration.

Embolism

Fat embolism: Fat breaks away from the bone marrow of the injured one and enters the blood stream.

Pulmonary embolism: Clot develops, forms at the injury site, and travels to the lungs.

FINDINGS (REMEMBER THE 5 P'S) Qs

- **Pain** that is unrelieved with elevation or analgesics; increases with passive movement
- **Paresthesia** or numbness (early finding)
- **Pulselessness** distal to the fracture (late finding)
- **Paralysis** or an inability to move digits (nerve damage)
- **Pale**, cold skin and cyanosis to nail beds

NURSING ACTIONS

- Check the extremity every hour for the first 24 hr.
- The space between the skin and the cast should allow for one finger to be placed.
- Notify the provider if compartment syndrome is suspected.
- Place the affected extremity at heart level.
- Loosen the dressing or assist with opening the cast.
- Assist with preparing for fasciotomy.
- Complete dressing changes or maintain negative pressure wound therapy.

CLIENT EDUCATION: Report pain that is not relieved by analgesics, pain that continues to increase in intensity, numbness or tingling, or a change in color of the extremity.

Osteomyelitis

Infection within the bone secondary to a bacterial infection from an outside source (with an open fracture [endogenous] or from a bloodborne bacterial source [hematogenous])

MANIFESTATIONS

- Irritability
- Fever
- Tachycardia
- Edema
- Pain is constant but increases with movement
- Not wanting to use the affected extremity
- Site of infection tender, swollen, and warm to touch

NURSING ACTIONS

- Assist in diagnostic procedures (obtaining skin, blood, and bone cultures).
- Assist with joint or bone biopsy.
- Administer IV and oral antibiotic therapy.
- Monitor hepatic, hematologic, and renal function.
- Monitor for the development of superinfection (candidiasis, *C. difficile* infection).
- Immobilize and elevate the extremity.
- Administer pain medication as prescribed.
- Consult with the guardians and provider regarding home care needs.

CLIENT EDUCATION

- Reinforce teaching with the child and guardians about the length of treatment that can be needed and long-term antibiotic therapy.
- Monitor hearing due to ototoxicity of some antibiotics.
- Limit movement of the affected limb and avoid bearing any weight until cleared by the provider.
- Provide for diversional activities consistent with the client's level of development.
- Ensure proper nutrition.

Application Exercises

1. A nurse is caring for a child who is in a plaster spica cast. Which of the following actions should the nurse take?

   A. Use a heat lamp to facilitate drying.

   B. Avoid turning the child until the cast is dry.

   C. Assist the client with crutch walking after the cast is dry.

   D. Apply moleskin to the edges of the cast.

2. A nurse is reinforcing teaching with a group of caregivers about fractures. Which of the following information should the nurse include?

   A. "Children need a longer time to heal from a fracture than an adult."

   B. "Epiphyseal plate injuries can result in altered bone growth."

   C. "A greenstick fracture is a complete break in the bone."

   D. "Bones are unable to bend, so they break."

3. A nurse is caring for a child who sustained a fracture. Which of the following actions should the nurse take? (Select all that apply.)

   A. Place a heat pack on the site of injury.

   B. Elevate the affected limb.

   C. Check neurovascular status frequently.

   D. Encourage ROM of the affected limb.

   E. Stabilize the injury.

4. A nurse is caring for a child who has a fracture. Which of the following findings should the nurse expect? (Select all that apply.)

   A. Crepitus

   B. Edema

   C. Pain

   D. Fever

   E. Ecchymosis

5. A nurse is caring for a child who is in skeletal traction. Which of the following actions should the nurse take? (Select all that apply.)

   A. Remove the weights to reposition the client.

   B. Check the child's position frequently.

   C. Monitor pin sites every 4 hr.

   D. Ensure the weights are hanging freely.

   E. Ensure the rope's knot is in contact with the pulley.

Active Learning Scenario

A nurse is reinforcing teaching about compartment syndrome to a group of newly licensed nurses. Use the ATI Active Learning Template: System Disorder to complete this item.

EXPECTED FINDINGS: List five.

NURSING CARE: List three nursing actions.

CLIENT EDUCATION: List one teaching point.

Application Exercises Key

1. A. A cool fan can be used to facilitate drying of a plaster cast.
   B. The child should be turned every 2 hr to expose all areas of the cast to facilitate drying.
   C. A client who has a spica cast is non-weight-bearing until the cast is removed.
   D. **CORRECT:** Apply moleskin to the edges of the cast to prevent the cast from rubbing on the client's skin.

   Ⓝ *NCLEX® Connection: Physiological Adaptation, Alterations in Body Systems*

2. A. Children heal from fractures quicker than adults due to a thicker periosteum and good blood supply.
   B. **CORRECT:** Detection and early treatment are crucial for an epiphyseal plate injury to prevent altered bone growth.
   C. A greenstick fracture is a partial break in the bone.
   D. Children's bones are soft and pliable, and can bend up to 45° before breaking.

   Ⓝ *NCLEX® Connection: Physiological Adaptation, Basic Pathophysiology*

3. A. Place a cold pack on the site of injury to decrease swelling.
   B. **CORRECT:** Elevating the affected limb can decrease swelling at the injury site.
   C. **CORRECT:** Monitoring neurovascular status assists in determining if the affected limp has adequate blood supply.
   D. Encourage ROM of the nonaffected limb.
   E. **CORRECT:** Stabilizing the injury will prevent further injury and damage.

   Ⓝ *NCLEX® Connection: Physiological Adaptation, Alterations in Body Systems*

4. A. **CORRECT:** A fracture can leave bone fragments that will exhibit a grating sound. Crepitus is a manifestation of a fracture.
   B. **CORRECT:** Swelling at the site occur related to the trauma. Edema is a manifestation of a fracture.
   C. **CORRECT:** A child who has a fracture will experience pain from the trauma.
   D. A child who has a fracture will not exhibit a fever related to the fracture.
   E. **CORRECT:** Bleeding under the skin can occur related to the trauma. Ecchymosis is a manifestation of a fracture.

   Ⓝ *NCLEX® Connection: Physiological Adaptation, Basic Pathophysiology*

5. A. The weights should only be removed by the provider or in an emergency situation.
   B. **CORRECT:** Monitor the child's position frequently to ensure proper alignment is present. This avoids putting stress on the pinned areas and other areas of the body causing pain.
   C. **CORRECT:** Pin sites should be checked frequently to monitor for the development of infection or loosening of the pins. Pin site care should be administered per facility policy.
   D. **CORRECT:** Ensure that the weights are hanging freely to allow for prescribed traction.
   E. The knot in the rope should not touch the pulley as this will alter the weight of the traction.

   Ⓝ *NCLEX® Connection: Basic Care and Comfort, Mobility/ Immobility*

Active Learning Scenario Key

Using the ATI Active Learning Template: System Disorder

EXPECTED FINDINGS
- Pain that is unrelieved with elevation or analgesics; increases with passive movement
- Paresthesia or numbness (early finding)
- Pulselessness distal to the fracture (late finding)
- Paralysis or an inability to move digits (nerve damage)
- Pale, cold skin and cyanosis to nail beds

NURSING CARE
- Check the extremity every hour for the first 24 hr.
- The space between the skin and the cast should allow for one finger to be placed.
- Notify the provider if compartment syndrome is suspected.
- Place the affected extremity at heart level.
- Loosen the dressing or open and bivalve the cast.
- Prepare the child for fasciotomy.
- Complete dressing changes or maintain negative pressure wound therapy.

CLIENT EDUCATION: Report pain that is not relieved by analgesics, pain that continues to increase in intensity, numbness or tingling, or a change in color of the extremity.

Ⓝ *NCLEX® Connection: Reduction of Risk Potential, Potential for Complications from Surgical Procedures and Health Alterations*

CHAPTER 27 *Musculoskeletal Congenital Disorders*

Musculoskeletal congenital disorders might be identified at birth or might not be present until later in infancy, childhood, or adolescence. These disorders can involve a specific area of the child's body or affect the child's entire musculoskeletal system. Careful data collection and interprofessional management assist in promoting the child's growth, development, and mobility.

Clubfoot

- A complex deformity of the ankle and foot
- Can affect one or both feet, occur as an isolated defect, or in association with other disorders (cerebral palsy and spinal bifida).
- Categorized as **positional** clubfoot (occurs from intrauterine crowding), **syndromic** (occurs in association with other syndromes), and **congenital** (idiopathic)

DATA COLLECTION

RISK FACTORS: presence of other syndromes, hereditary factors

EXPECTED FINDINGS
- The affected foot (feet) is shorter and smaller.
- Heel pad empty with plantar crease visible at mid-foot
- If deformity is unilateral, calf atrophy is visible.

DIAGNOSTIC PROCEDURES: Prenatal ultrasound provides data for identification of the deformity.

PATIENT-CENTERED CARE

NURSING CARE
- Encourage guardians to hold and cuddle the child.
- Encourage guardians to meet the developmental needs of the child.
- Assist with performing neurovascular and skin integrity checks.

THERAPEUTIC PROCEDURES: **Ponseti method**
- Series of castings beginning with the first month of life and continuing until maximum correction is accomplished (approximately 5 to 8 weeks).
- Weekly manipulation of the foot to stretch the muscles with subsequent placement of a long-leg cast. ⓠEBP
- Following casting, a heel cord tenotomy is usually performed followed by a long leg cast for 3 weeks.
- After casting is complete, a Denis Browne bar that connects Ponseti sandals, placed in abduction, is applied to maintain correction and prevent recurrence.
- The abduction brace is maintained at bedtime for approximately 3 to 5 years.

NURSING CARE
- Monitor neurovascular status.
- Perform cast care.

CLIENT EDUCATION
- Proper cast care.
- Importance of regular cast changes.
- Change diapers frequently.
- Check for indications of ischemia (pain, pallor, pulselessness, paralysis) and notify the provider.

COMPLICATIONS

Growth and development delays related to immobility
- NURSING CARE: Monitor growth and development.
- CLIENT EDUCATION: Use strategies to enhance normal growth and development.

Effects of casting
- Skin breakdown
- Neurovascular alterations

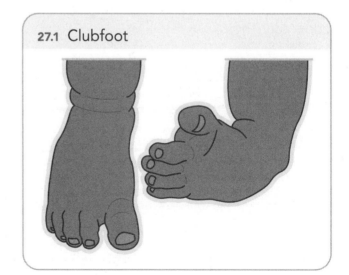

27.1 Clubfoot

Legg-Calve-Perthes disease

Aseptic necrosis of the femoral head can be unilateral or bilateral. Stages include: synovitis, necrotic, fragmentation, reconstruction.

DATA COLLECTION

RISK FACTORS

- Age: Affects children 2 to 12 years but more common between ages 4 to 8 years
- Sex: More common in boys
- Trauma, decreased circulation, inflammation to the femoral head

EXPECTED FINDINGS

- Intermittent painless limp
- Hip stiffness
- Limited ROM
- Hip, thigh, knee pain
- Shortening of the affected leg
- Muscle wasting

DIAGNOSTIC PROCEDURES: Radiograph of the hip and pelvis, MRI

PATIENT-CENTERED CARE

NURSING CARE

- Treatment varies with the child's age and the appearance of the femoral head.
- Administer NSAIDs as prescribed.
- Maintain rest and limited weight bearing.
  - Abduction brace or casts
  - Physical therapy
  - Traction
- Advance to active motion as prescribed.

SURGICAL INTERVENTIONS: Osteotomy of the hip or femur

CLIENT EDUCATION

- Understand the prescribed limited weight bearing treatment.
- Understand appropriate strategies for learning and activities during the limited weight bearing periods. Qpcc

COMPLICATIONS

- Joint degeneration
- Permanent disability

Developmental dysplasia of the hip (DDH)

A variety of disorders resulting in abnormal development of the hip structures that can affect infants or children

- **Acetabular dysplasia:** delay in acetabular development (acetabular roof is shallow and oblique)
- **Subluxation:** incomplete dislocation of the hip
- **Dislocation:** femoral head does not have contact with the acetabulum

DATA COLLECTION

RISK FACTORS

- Birth order (firstborn)
- Female sex
- Family history
- Breech intrauterine position
- Delivery type
- Joint stability
- Oligohydramnios
- Large for gestational age

EXPECTED FINDINGS

INFANT

- Asymmetry and unequal number of skin folds on the posterior thigh
- Limited hip abduction
- Shortening of the femur
- Widened perineum
- Positive Ortolani test performed by provider (hip is reduced by abduction)
- Positive Barlow test performed by provider (hip is dislocated by adduction)

CHILD

- One leg shorter than the other
- Walking on toes on one foot
- Walk with a limp

DIAGNOSTIC PROCEDURES

Ultrasound: performed at 2 weeks of age to determine the cartilaginous head of the femur

X-ray: can diagnose DDH in infants older than 4 months of age

PATIENT-CENTERED CARE

NURSING CARE

- Treatment starts as soon as DDH is diagnosed and depends on the child's age and the extent of the dysplasia.
- Encourage guardians to hold and cuddle the infant/child.
- Encourage guardians to meet the developmental needs of the infant/child.

Newborn to 6 months

Pavlik harness (chest harness that abducts legs)
- Maintain harness placement for to 12 weeks.
- Check straps every 1 to 2 weeks for adjustment.
- Assist with performing neurovascular and skin integrity checks.
- Removing the harness is dependent on the client.

CLIENT EDUCATION
- Do not adjust the straps.
- If removal is prescribed, understand how to place the harness. Qs
- Reinforce the importance of skin care with the family (use an undershirt, wear knee socks, check skin, gently massage skin under straps, avoid lotions and powders, place diaper under the straps).
- Check skin under the straps.

When adduction contracture is present

Bryant traction
- Skin traction
- Hips flexed at a 90° angle with the buttock raised off of the bed

NURSING ACTIONS
- Assist with performing neurovascular checks.
- Maintain traction (ropes, boots, pulleys, and weights).
- Ensure the client maintains alignment.
- Perform skin care.

Hip spica cast (maintains external rotation of the hip)
Needs to be changed to accommodate growth
NURSING ACTIONS
- Maintain the hip spica cast.
- Assist with performing frequent neurovascular checks.
- Perform range of motion with the unaffected extremities.
- Perform frequent monitoring of skin integrity, especially in the diaper area.
- Determine pain using an age-appropriate pain tool. Intervene as indicated. Qpcc
- Monitor hydration status frequently.
- Monitor elimination status daily.

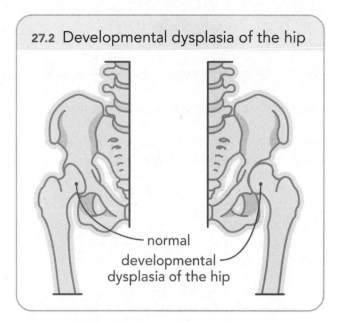

27.2 Developmental dysplasia of the hip

— normal
developmental —
dysplasia of the hip

CLIENT EDUCATION
- Understand proper positioning, turning, neurovascular monitoring, and care of the cast.
- Position casts on pillows. Qebp
- Keep the casts elevated until dry.
- Change position frequently to allow for drying.
- Handle the casts with the palm of the hand until dry.
- Note color and temperature of toes on casted extremity.
- Give sponge baths to avoid wetting the cast.
- Use a waterproof barrier around the genital opening of spica cast to prevent soiling with urine or feces.
- After discharge, use appropriate care and equipment (stroller, wagon, car seat; accommodate large cast) for maintaining mobility.

6 months to 2 years

Surgical closed reduction with placement of hip spica cast

NURSING ACTIONS
- Prepare family and client for surgery.
- Assist with performing neurovascular checks.
- Manage postoperative pain.
- Perform skin care.
- Perform cast care.

CLIENT EDUCATION: Understand spica cast and home care management.

Older children

- Surgical reduction with presurgical traction
- Femoral osteotomy, reconstruction, and tenotomy are often needed

COMPLICATIONS

Postoperative complications: Atelectasis, ileus, infection

Effects of immobilization: Decreased muscle strength, bone demineralization, altered bowel motility

Effects of casting: Skin breakdown, neurovascular alterations

Infection

Infection can be caused by bacteria (*Staphylococcus aureus*).

NURSING ACTIONS

- Monitor vital signs. Observe changes in temperature that could be associated with complications of infection.
- Keep the cast dry and intact.
- Monitor for changes in neurovascular status (numbness; tingling; decreased mobility, sensation, or capillary refill).
- Reposition the child frequently.
- Maintain a high-fiber diet and promote adequate hydration.
- Monitor bowel and bladder elimination. Report any changes, especially the decrease or absence of bowel sounds or distention.
- Report any foul odor from cast or urine.
- Observe changes in behavior, especially increasing irritability in infants.

CLIENT EDUCATION

- Discuss possible complications of specific treatment or procedure with the child and/or family.
- Reinforce the need to notify the provider with any concerns or indications of complications.
- Educate the child and family about follow-up.

Osteogenesis imperfecta

An inherited connective tissue condition that results in bone fractures and deformity along with restricted growth

DATA COLLECTION

RISK FACTORS: Parent who has osteogenesis imperfecta (OI)

EXPECTED FINDINGS: Classic manifestations
- Multiple bone fractures
- Blue sclera
- Early hearing loss
- Small, discolored teeth

DIAGNOSTIC PROCEDURES: **Bone biopsy**

NURSING ACTIONS
- Prepare the child for the procedure.
- Assist with positioning the child.

PATIENT-CENTERED CARE

NURSING CARE: Treatment is supportive.

MEDICATION: **Pamidronate (bisphosphonate therapy)**
- Increase bone density
- Prevent fractures

NURSING ACTIONS
- Administered IV by the RN.
- Monitor for adverse effects (hypokalemia, hypomagnesemia, hypocalcemia, hypophosphatemia, thrombocytopenia, neutropenia, dysrhythmias, kidney failure, general malaise).
- Monitor for respiratory infections.

CLIENT EDUCATION
- Vaccines containing live viruses are not recommended.
- Observe for adverse effects and call the provider if necessary.
- Antibiotics will be needed prior to some dental work.
- Understand low-impact exercises.
- Adhere to the medication regime as prescribed.
- Consult with physical therapy.
- Assist with braces and splints as prescribed.
- Assist client with meeting developmental milestones.
- Understand limitations during recovery.
- Attend support groups.

SURGICAL INTERVENTIONS
- For severe cases
- Correct bone deformities, placement of rods
- Bone marrow transplant

COMPLICATIONS

Disuse osteoporosis
- Limit time in casts.
- Encourage activity.

Hearing loss

Permanent deformities

Scoliosis

- Scoliosis is a complex deformity of the spine that also affects the ribs.
- Characterized by a lateral curvature of the spine and spinal rotation that causes rib asymmetry.
- Idiopathic or structural scoliosis is the most common form of scoliosis and can be seen in isolation or associated with other conditions.

DATA COLLECTION

RISK FACTORS
- Genetic tendency
- Sex: more common in females
- Age: highest incidence between 8 to 15 years of age

EXPECTED FINDINGS
- Asymmetry in scapula, ribs, flanks, shoulders, and hips
- Improperly fitting clothing (one leg shorter than the other)

DIAGNOSTIC PROCEDURES
- Screen during preadolescence for boys and girls.
  - Observe the child, who should be wearing only underwear, from the back.
  - Have the child bend over at the waist with arms hanging down and observe for asymmetry of ribs and flank.
  - Measure spinal curvature with a scoliometer.
- Radiography
  - Use the Cobb technique to determine the degree of curvature.
  - Use the Risser scale to determine the skeletal maturity.
  - MRI and CT scans can be used.

PATIENT-CENTERED CARE

NURSING CARE

Treatment depends on the degree, location, and type of curvature.

THERAPEUTIC PROCEDURES

Bracing: Customized braces slow the progression of the curve. Types of braces include Milwaukee, TLSO, Wilmington, and Charleston.

NURSING ACTIONS
- Assist with fitting the client with a brace.
- Examine skin.
- Promote the client's positive self-image. Qpcc

CLIENT EDUCATION
- Understand how to apply the brace.
- Wear brace for 23 hr per day only remove for personal hygiene (showering).

Surgical interventions

Spinal fusion with rod placement: Used for curvatures greater than 45°

PREOPERATIVE NURSING ACTIONS
- Inform and assist the adolescent to obtain autologous (self-donated) blood donations.
- Obtain routine laboratory studies, including a type and cross match for blood as prescribed.
- Orient the adolescent and family to the ICU.
- Inform the adolescent and family about what can be expected during the postoperative period (monitoring equipment, NG tube, chest tubes, indwelling urinary catheters, and self-administering analgesic pumps).

POSTOPERATIVE NURSING ACTIONS
- Adolescent will be monitored initially in the intensive care unit.
- Perform standard postoperative care to prevent complications.
- Monitor pain using an age-appropriate pain tool.
- Reinforce education about administering analgesia using a patient-controlled analgesic (PCA) pump as prescribed.
- Assist with performing frequent neurovascular checks.
- Use a log rolling technique when turning the adolescent to prevent damage to the spinal fusion.
- Monitor skin for pressure areas, especially if a brace has been prescribed. Qs
- Provide skin care by keeping skin clean and dry.
- Monitor surgical and drain sites for indications of infection. Provide wound care as prescribed.
- Check bowel sounds and monitor, observing for paralytic ileus.
- Monitor for decreases in Hgb and Hct. Observe for indications of bleeding.
- Assist the RN with blood transfusion. The adolescent can have self-donated blood available for transfusion.
- Encourage mobility as soon as tolerated. Ambulation by 2nd or 3rd day.
- Monitor for infection.
- Perform range of motion on unaffected extremities.
- Provide age-appropriate activities and opportunities to visit with friends and family during the hospital stay. Qpcc

CLIENT EDUCATION

PREOPERATIVE
- Reinforce teaching (use of incentive spirometer, turning, coughing, deep breathing) to prevent complications.
- Reinforce preoperative teaching to educate the adolescent and family and to promote cooperation and participation in recovery.
- Review demonstrations of the use of a PCA pump if age-appropriate.
- Reinforce log rolling that will be used after surgery.
- Reinforce the demonstration of the respiratory therapy techniques that will be used postoperatively to reduce complications of anesthesia.
- Discuss medical terms that are unfamiliar to the adolescent and/or family.

POSTOPERATIVE
- Emphasize the importance of physical therapy and proper positioning of the spine.
- Encourage independence following surgery for the adolescent who has a brace.
- Encourage the adolescent to contact friends when able.
- Emphasize the necessity of follow-up care.

CARE AFTER DISCHARGE
- Reinforce the expected course of treatment and recovery.
- Suggest that the family arrange the environment to facilitate the adolescent's ability to be as independent as possible (keep favorite items within reach).
- Emphasize the necessity of follow-up care.

COMPLICATIONS

Breathing difficulties (with severe curvatures)

Spine or nerve damage

Lowered self-esteem: Assist the client with age-appropriate actions to promote positive self-esteem.

Small bowel obstruction

Infection following surgery
- Infection can be caused by bacteria (*Staphylococcus aureus*).

NURSING ACTIONS
- Monitor vital signs. Observe changes in temperature that could be associated with complications of infection.
- Monitor for changes in neurovascular status (numbness; tingling; decreased mobility, sensation, or capillary refill).
- Reposition the child frequently.
- Maintain a high-fiber diet and promote adequate hydration.

CLIENT EDUCATION
- Discuss possible complications of specific treatment or procedure with the child and family.
- Reinforce the need to notify the provider with any concerns or indications of complications.
- Reinforce with the child and family about the importance of follow-up.

Active Learning Scenario

A nurse is caring for a child in a hip spica cast. What should the nurse recommend for inclusion in the care of this client? Use the ATI Active Learning Template: Therapeutic Procedure to complete this item.

NURSING INTERVENTIONS: List at least five actions the nurse should include in the child's care.

CLIENT EDUCATION: List at least six instructional points the nurse should include for the client and the client's guardians.

Application Exercises

1. A nurse is caring for a toddler who has hip dysplasia and has been placed in a hip spica cast. The child's guardian asks the nurse why a Pavlik harness is not being used. Which of the following responses should the nurse make?
   - A. "The Pavlik harness is used for children with scoliosis, not hip dysplasia."
   - B. "The Pavlik harness is used for school-age children."
   - C. "The Pavlik harness cannot be used for your child because their condition is too severe."
   - D. "The Pavlik harness is used for infants less than 6 months of age."

2. A nurse is reinforcing preoperative teaching with an adolescent client who is scheduled to receive spinal instrumentation for scoliosis. Which of the following information should the nurse include?
   - A. "You will go home the same day of surgery."
   - B. "You will have minimal pain."
   - C. "You will need to receive blood."
   - D. "You will not be able to eat until the day after surgery."

3. A nurse is caring for a child who is suspected of having Legg-Calve-Perthes disease. The nurse should prepare the child for which of the following diagnostic procedures?
   - A. Bone biopsy
   - B. Genetic testing
   - C. CT scan
   - D. Radiographs

4. A nurse is collecting data from a child who has Legg-Calve-Perthes disease. Which of the following findings should the nurse expect? (Select all that apply.)
   - A. Longer affected leg
   - B. Hip stiffness
   - C. Back pain
   - D. Limited ROM
   - E. Limp with walking

5. A nurse is caring for an infant and notices an audible click in their left hip. Which of the following diagnostic test should the nurse expect the provider to perform? (Select all that apply.)
   - A. Barlow test
   - B. Babinski reflex
   - C. Manipulation of foot and ankle
   - D. Ortolani test
   - E. Ponseti method

Application Exercises Key

1. A. The Pavlik harness is for infants who have hip dysplasia.
   B. The Pavlik harness is for infants who have hip dysplasia.
   C. The Pavlik harness is for infants who have hip dysplasia.
   D. **CORRECT:** The Pavlik harness is a soft brace designed for infants less than 6 months of age. A toddler is too large to fit into the brace.

   Ⓝ *NCLEX® Connection: Physiological Adaptation, Alterations in Body Systems*

2. A. Clients who have spinal instrumentation for scoliosis are hospitalized for approximately 1 week.
   B. Clients who have spinal instrumentation for scoliosis experience intense pain that requires a PCA pump.
   C. **CORRECT:** Clients who have spinal instrumentation for scoliosis have a lengthy surgery with blood loss and require blood replacements.
   D. Clients who have spinal instrumentation for scoliosis are allowed to advance the diet as tolerated.

   Ⓝ *NCLEX® Connection: Reduction of Risk Potential, Potential Complications from Surgical Procedures and Health Alterations*

3. A. A bone biopsy is used to diagnose cancer, infection, and other bone disorders. It is not indicated to diagnose Legg-Calve-Perthes.
   B. Legg-Calve-Perthes is necrosis of the femoral head and is not genetic. Genetic testing is not indicated to diagnose Legg-Calve-Perthes.
   C. An MRI is used to visualize structures inside the body. Legg-Calve-Perthes is necrosis of the femoral head. An MRI is not indicated to diagnose Legg-Calve-Perthes.
   D. **CORRECT:** A child who has Legg-Calve-Perthes exhibits necrosis of the femoral head and can be diagnosed by radiographs of the hip and pelvis.

   Ⓝ *NCLEX® Connection: Reduction of Risk Potential, Therapeutic Procedures*

4. A. A child who has Legg-Calve-Perthes exhibit shortening of the affected leg.
   B. **CORRECT:** A child who has Legg-Calve-Perthes exhibits hip stiffness due to the necrosis of the femoral head.
   C. **CORRECT:** A child who has Legg-Calve-Perthes exhibits a painless intermittent limp.
   D. **CORRECT:** A child who has Legg-Calve-Perthes exhibits limited ROM due to the necrosis of the femoral head.
   E. **CORRECT:** E. A child who has Legg-Calve-Perthes exhibits a limp with walking due to the necrosis of the femoral head.

   Ⓝ *NCLEX® Connection: Physiological Adaptation, Basic Pathophysiology*

5. A. **CORRECT:** The RN can use a Barlow test to assess developmental dysplasia of the hip for infants. The provider will flex the infants hip and knees to a right angle position.
   B. Babinski reflex is when the provider strokes the lateral portion of the foot to assess for neurologic deficits.
   C. Manipulation of the foot and ankle by the provider is a test that assesses for clubfoot.
   D. **CORRECT:** The Ortolani test assesses developmental dysplasia of the hip for infants. The provider will flex the infants hip and knees to a right angle position.
   E. Ponseti method is used to treat clubfoot of the newborn.

   Ⓝ *NCLEX® Connection: Reduction of Risk Potential, Potential for Alterations in Body Systems*

Active Learning Scenario Key

Using the ATI Active Learning Template: Therapeutic Procedure

NURSING INTERVENTIONS
- Maintain the hip spica cast.
- Assist with performing frequent neurovascular checks.
- Assist with performing range of motion with the unaffected extremities.
- Perform frequent monitoring of skin integrity, especially in the diaper area.
- Determine pain control using an age-appropriate pain tool. Intervene as indicated.
- Monitor hydration status frequently.
- Check elimination status daily.

CLIENT EDUCATION
- Reinforce teaching regarding positioning, turning, neurovascular assessments, and care of the cast.
- Position casts on pillows.
- Keep the casts elevated until dry.
- Encourage frequent position changes to allow for drying.
- Handle the casts with the palm of the hand until dry.
- Note color and temperature of toes on casted extremity.
- Give sponge baths to avoid wetting the cast.
- Use a waterproof barrier around the genital opening of spica cast to prevent soiling with urine or feces.
- Reinforce teaching regarding care after discharge with emphasis on using appropriate equipment (stroller, wagon, car seat) for maintaining mobility.

Ⓝ *NCLEX® Connection: Reduction of Risk Potential, Potential for Complications of Diagnostic Tests/Treatments/Procedures*

UNIT 2   SYSTEM DISORDERS
SECTION: MUSCULOSKELETAL DISORDERS

CHAPTER 28 *Chronic Neuromusculoskeletal Disorders*

Chronic problems associated with mobility can be reflective of a problem with the musculoskeletal system or the result of a disorder related to the neural pathway extending from the brain's cortex to the neuromuscular junction.

Cerebral palsy

- Cerebral palsy (CP) is a nonprogressive impairment of motor function, especially that of muscle control, coordination, and posture.
- CP can cause abnormal perception and sensation; visual, hearing, and speech impairments; seizures; and cognitive disabilities.
- CP manifests differently in each child. Developmental outcomes vary and are dependent on the severity of the injury.

DATA COLLECTION

RISK FACTORS

The exact cause of CP is not known. Prenatal, perinatal, and postnatal risk factors known to be associated with CP include the following.
- Existing brain anomalies, cerebral infections, head trauma (shaken baby syndrome), or anoxia to the brain
- Maternal chorioamnionitis
- Maternal infection
- Premature birth
- Multiple births
- Very low birth weights in newborns
- Inability of the placenta to provide the developing fetus with oxygen and nutrients
- Interruption of oxygen delivery to the fetus during birth
- Direct injury to the neonate during birth
- Maternal nutritional deficiencies or drug use

EXPECTED FINDINGS

- Guardians report difficulty meeting developmental milestones
- Persistent primitive reflexes (Moro or tonic neck)
- Gagging or choking with feeding, poor suck reflex
- Tongue thrust
- Poor head control

- Rigid posture and extremities, abnormal posturing
- Asymmetric crawl
- Hyperreflexia
- Vision, speech, or hearing impairments
- Seizures
- Impaired social relationships
- Early hand preference
- Toe walking
- Arching back
- Strabismus
- Difficulty diapering baby

Spastic CP (pyramidal)
- Hypertonicity (muscle tightness or spasticity); increased deep tendon reflexes; clonus; and poor control of motion, balance, and posture.
- Impairments of fine and gross motor skills.
- Can present in all four extremities (tetraplegia); all extremities affected, lower more than upper (diplegia); three limbs (triplegia); one limb (monoplegia); or one side of the body (hemiplegia).
- Gait can appear crouched with a scissoring motion of the legs with feet plantar flexed.
- Babinski reflex.

Dyskinetic CP (non-spastic, extrapyramidal)
- Athetoid: Findings include involuntary jerking movements that appear slow, writhing, and wormlike. These movements involve the extremities, trunk, neck, face, and tongue.
- Dystonic: Slow, twisting movements affect the trunk or extremities with abnormal posturing from muscle contractions. Drooling and speech impairment related to involvement of the muscles of pharynx, larynx, and oral regions.

Ataxic CP (non-spastic, extrapyramidal)
- Evidence of wide-based gait and difficulty with coordination
- Poor ability to do repetitive movements
- Lack of coordination with purposeful movements, such as reaching for an object

DIAGNOSTIC PROCEDURES

Complete neurologic data collect

Metabolic and genetic testing

General movements data collection in children older than 2 years and younger than 5 years of age

MRI: Used to evaluate structures or abnormal areas

NURSING ACTIONS
- Assist the child to remain still during the procedure.
- Assist with sedation if prescribed.
CLIENT EDUCATION: Provide emotional support.

EEG

Skull x-ray

Ultrasound

PATIENT-CENTERED CARE

NURSING CARE

- Individualize care to meet client needs.
- Monitor developmental milestones.
- Determine the need for hearing and speech evaluations.
- Promote independence with self-care activities as much as possible. Assist the client to maintain a positive self-image and a high level of self-esteem.
- Determine the extent of family coping and support.
- Determine the family's awareness of available resources.
- Determine the client's developmental level.
- Structure interventions and communications around the client's developmental level, rather than chronological age.
- Communicate with the child directly, but include caregivers as needed. Qᴘᴄᴄ
- Help the child to use augmented communication (electronic devices for speech and other types of communication tools [flash cards, picture boards, touch screen computers]).
- Include the family in physical care during hospitalization.
  - Ask the family about routine care, and encourage them to provide it if appropriate.
  - Encourage the family to help verify the client's needs if communication is impaired.
- Maintain an open airway by elevating the head of the child's bed. (This is especially important if the child has increased oral secretions.) Qs
- Ensure suction equipment is available if required.
- Monitor for pain (especially with muscle spasms) using a developmentally appropriate pain tool.
- Administer medication for pain and/or spasms as prescribed.
- Ensure adequate nutrition.
  - Check for the possibility of aspiration for children who are severely disabled.
  - Position upright after feeding.
  - Determine the child's ability to take oral nutrition.
  - Ascertain the correct positioning for feeding the child. Use head positioning and manual jaw control methods as needed.
  - Provide foods that are similar to foods eaten at home when possible. Administer supplements as prescribed.
  - Encourage foods high in fiber to prevent constipation.
  - Administer feedings by gastric tube as prescribed.
  - Maintain weight/height chart.
- Provide skin care.
  - Examine skin under splints and braces if applicable.
  - Maintain skin integrity by turning the child to keep pressure off bony prominences.
  - Keep skin clean and dry.
- Provide rest periods as needed.

MEDICATIONS

Baclofen

Used as a centrally acting skeletal muscle relaxant that decreases muscle spasm and severe spasticity

NURSING ACTIONS

- Administer orally or intrathecally via a specialized, surgically implanted pump.
- Monitor effectiveness of the medication.
- Monitor for muscle weakness, increased fatigue, or less-common adverse effects (diaphoresis, headaches, nausea, constipation).
- Monitor for hepatotoxicity.

CLIENT EDUCATION

- Observe for expected responses of medications.
- Reinforce with the family the adverse effects of medications and when to call the provider.
- With the pump, medication is replaced every 4 to 6 weeks.

Diazepam

Skeletal muscle relaxant used to decrease muscle spasms and severe spasticity

NURSING ACTIONS

- Use in older children and adolescents.
- Monitor for drowsiness and fatigue.
- Monitor for hepatotoxicity.

CLIENT EDUCATION

- Observe for expected responses to medications.
- Monitor for adverse effects of the medication and call the provider.

Botulinum toxin A

- Administered IM
- Reduces spasticity in specific muscle groups
- Used primarily for children who have spasticity only in the lower extremities
- Decreases muscle movement by inhibiting the release of acetylcholine

NURSING ACTIONS: Monitor for temporary weakness and pain at the injection site.

CLIENT EDUCATION: Onset of the medication is 24 to 72 hr, with a peak of 2 weeks, lasting 3 to 6 months.

Antiepileptics

- Examples: Valproic acid, gabapentin, carbamazepine
- Controls seizure activity

Dopaminergics

- Example: Carbidopa
- Promotes the relaxation of muscles

Alternative therapies

- Chinese herbs
- Acupuncture
- Hyperbaric oxygen

INTERPROFESSIONAL CARE

- Participate in care with other professionals (speech, physical and occupational therapists, and education and/or medical specialists).
- Assist with referral for technical aids that can assist with coordination, speaking, mobility, and an increased level of independence. Some children can benefit from the use of a voice-activated wheelchair.
- Surgical intervention is indicated for tendon release to correct contractures or other spastic deformities.

Physical therapy (PT)

- Orthotic devices: Braces, splints
- Adaptive equipment: Scooters, wheelchairs

Occupational therapy (OT)

- Feeding utensils
- Aids for ADLs

Speech therapy

- Special intervention programs
- Increase socialization

Surgical intervention

Indicated for progressive deformities; correct contractures

Tendon lengthening

Dorsal rhizotomy

CLIENT EDUCATION

- Adhere to therapeutic plan of care.
- Provide time for rest periods.
- Adhere to feeding schedule and utilize feeding techniques if changes were made during hospitalization.
- Adhere to medication regimen.
- Practice proper dental care.
- Assist with providing developmental stimulation.
- Understand proper wound care if needed.
- Understand ankle-foot orthoses if prescribed.
- Understand self-urinary catheterization if needed.
- Utilize pulmonary hygiene techniques.
- Attend interprofessional team meetings.
- Identify resources needed (respite care).
- Consider participation in a support group for CP.

COMPLICATIONS

Aspiration

NURSING ACTIONS
- Keep the child's head elevated.
- Keep suction available if copious oral secretions are present or the child has difficulty with swallowing foods or fluids. Qs

CLIENT EDUCATION
- Perform appropriate feeding techniques to decrease the risk of aspiration.
- Take CPR classes.

Potential for injury

NURSING ACTIONS
- Make sure the child's bed rails are raised to prevent falls from the bed.
- Pad side rails and wheelchair arms to prevent injury.
- Secure the child in mobility devices (wheelchairs).
- Encourage the child to receive adequate rest to prevent injury at times of fatigue.
- Encourage the use of helmets, seat belts, and other safety equipment.

CLIENT EDUCATION: Perform appropriate safety precautions.

Spina bifida

Spinal bifida is a neural tube defect (NTD) present at birth and is characterized by failure of the osseous spine to close with CNS effects.

Spina bifida occulta: Mostly affects the lumbosacral area and is not visible externally. Surface of the vertebral bone is missing; no spinal cord involvement.

Spina bifida cystica: Protrusion of the sac is visible
- Meningocele: The sac contains spinal fluid and meninges. Increased risk for infection if ruptures. No neurologic deficits.
- Myelomeningocele (most common): The sac contains spinal fluid, meninges, and nerves. Failure of the neural tube to close causes decreased motor and sensory function.

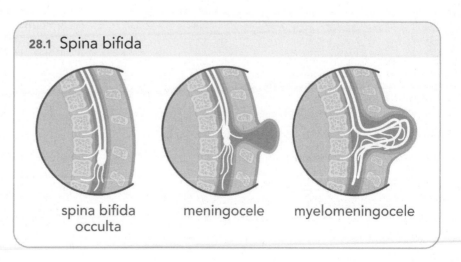

28.1 Spina bifida

spina bifida occulta   meningocele   myelomeningocele

DATA COLLECTION

RISK FACTORS

- Medications/substances taken during pregnancy
- Maternal malnutrition
- Insufficient folic acid intake during pregnancy
- Exposure to radiation or chemicals during pregnancy

EXPECTED FINDINGS

SUBJECTIVE FINDINGS

- Presence of risk factors in prenatal history
- Family history of neural tube defects

Occulta

- Dimpling in the lumbosacral area (occulta)
- Port wine angioma
- Dark hair tufts
- Subcutaneous lipoma

Cystica

- Flaccid muscles
- Lack of bowel control
- Prolapse of the rectum
- Spinal curvature abnormalities (scoliosis, kyphosis)
- Protruding sac midline of the osseous spine

LABORATORY TESTS

MATERNAL BLOOD TESTS: Blood alpha-fetoprotein during the second trimester of gestation indicate possible NTD.

INFANT BLOOD TESTS: Blood cultures to determine causative pathogen if appropriate.

DIAGNOSTIC PROCEDURES

PRENATAL

- **Ultrasound** can show visual defect.
- **Amniocentesis** is done following elevated alpha-fetoprotein levels to detect anencephaly or myelomeningocele.
- **Chorionic villus sampling**

INFANT FOLLOWING BIRTH: MRI, ultrasonography, and CT to evaluate spinal cord and brain, myelography, spinal x-ray (Occulta)

PATIENT-CENTERED CARE

NURSING CARE

- Determine infant-guardian attachment.
- Examine the sac.
- Complete a routine newborn data collection.
- Determine the level of neurologic involvement.
- Obtain accurate output measurements.
- Check head circumference and fontanels.
- Maintain measures to prevent infection.
- Observe neurologic data collection.
- Reinforce teaching with the guardians about intermittent bladder catheterizations if needed.

INTERPROFESSIONAL CARE

Neurosurgery, neurology, urology, orthopedics, pediatrics, physical therapy, occupational therapy, and social services

THERAPEUTIC PROCEDURES

Closure of a myelomeningocele sac is done as soon as possible to prevent complications of injury and infection. Risk for the development of hydrocephalus.

PREOPERATIVE NURSING ACTIONS

- Assist with preparing the family for surgery (within the first 24 to 72 hr after birth).
- Protect the sac from injury.
- Place infant in an incubator if needed, without clothing.
- Apply a sterile, moist, non-adhering dressing with 0.9% sodium chloride on the sac, changing it every 2 hr. Q EBP
- Do not remove dressing if becomes dry; add more solution (sodium chloride).
- Inspect the sac closely for leaks, irritation, abrasions and localized indications of infection.
- Monitor for systemic indications of infection (fever, irritability, and lethargy).
- Maintain infant in the prone position with hips flexed, legs abducted.
- Ensure delivery of IV antibiotic therapy.
- Avoid rectal temperatures.
- Avoid cuddling or putting pressure on the sac.
- Measure head circumference to establish a baseline measurement.
- Report leakage of fluid.

PREOPERATIVE CLIENT EDUCATION: There will be decreased motor and sensory functions of lower extremities.

POSTOPERATIVE NURSING ACTIONS

- Monitor vital signs.
- Monitor I&O.
- Monitor for indications of infection.
- Provide pain management.
- Provide incision care. Keep clean. Do not allow urine or feces to contaminate incision.
- Monitor for manifestations of increased intracranial pressure.
- Use paper tape.
- Monitor for indications of CSF leakage.
- Maintain prone position until other positions are prescribed.
- Resume oral feedings.
- Provide range of motion (ROM) to extremities.

POSTOPERATIVE CLIENT EDUCATION

- Understand proper postoperative care at home.
- Understand ROM techniques depending on disability.

ONGOING CARE

- Check head circumference.
- Monitor skin integrity.
- Monitor for allergies (latex allergy).
- Monitor cognitive development.
- Monitor bladder and bowl functioning.

- Reinforce teaching with the caregivers about intermittent bladder catheterizations if needed.
- Monitor motor development.
- Monitor for infections.
- Address body image concerns.
- Offer support to the family.
- Assist the client with independence through the lifespan.
- Assist the family with obtaining medical equipment/services needed at home.

COMPLICATIONS

Skin ulceration

Caused by prolonged pressure in one area

NURSING ACTIONS
- Monitor skin for breakdown.
- Reposition frequently to prevent pressure on bony prominences.
- Monitor skin under splints and braces.

CLIENT EDUCATION: Monitor skin integrity.

Latex allergy

The child is at an increased risk for a latex allergy. Allergy responses range from urticaria to wheezing, which can progress to anaphylaxis. A latex allergy is linked to allergies to certain foods (bananas, avocados, kiwi, and chestnuts).

NURSING ACTIONS
- Assist with testing for allergy.
- Reduce exposure.

CLIENT EDUCATION
- Avoid exposing the child to latex.
- Be aware of household items that can contain latex (water toys, pacifiers, plastic storage bags).
- Observe for indications of allergic reaction and report them to the provider.
- Understand proper use of epinephrine. Qs

Increased intracranial pressure

- Caused by shunt malfunction or hydrocephalus.
- Prepare for surgery for shunt or shunt revision.

MANIFESTATIONS
- INFANTS: high-pitched cry, lethargy, vomiting, bulging fontanels, widening cranial suture lines, increased head circumference
- CHILDREN: headache, lethargy, nausea, vomiting, double vision, decreased school performance of learned tasks, decreased level of consciousness, seizures

NURSING ACTIONS
- Use gentle movements when performing ROM exercises.
- Minimize environmental stressors (noise, frequent visitors).
- Determine pain level and manage pain.

CLIENT EDUCATION: Observe for manifestations of shunt malfunction and hydrocephalus, and notify the provider if necessary.

Bladder issues

The child who has myelomeningocele is at an increased risk for bladder dysfunction (either spasms or flaccidity).

NURSING ACTIONS
- Monitor for indications of bladder dysfunction.
- Monitor for indications of bladder infection.
- Monitor for blood in the urine.
- Administer antispasmodics or perform intermittent catheterizations as needed.
- Prepare the family and client for surgery if needed.

CLIENT EDUCATION: Perform proper care of stoma (vesicostomy) if applicable.

Orthopedic issues

Corrections of associated potential problems (clubfoot, scoliosis, and other malformations of the feet and legs)

NURSING ACTIONS
- Monitor for indications of infection.
- Administer pain medications.
- Prepare the family and client for surgery if needed.
- Provide cast care if cast is present.
- Monitor for neurologic deficits.
- Perform passive ROM exercises, position, and stretching exercises.

CLIENT EDUCATION
- Reinforce teaching with the family about indications of infection.
- Reinforce teaching with the family about cast and splint care if indicated.

Bowel control measures

- Increased risk for constipation.
- Administer laxatives and fiber supplements.
- Administer antegrade continence enemas (ACE) every 1 to 2 days as needed for older children.

Juvenile idiopathic arthritis

- Juvenile idiopathic arthritis (JIA) is a chronic autoimmune inflammatory disease affecting joints and other tissues.
- The chronic inflammation of the synovium of the joints leads to wearing down and damage to the articular cartilage.
- JIA is rarely life-threatening, and it can subside over time, but it can result in residual joint deformities and altered joint function.
- There are multiple classifications of JIA with or without a rheumatoid factor.

DATA COLLECTION

RISK FACTORS

- Immunogenic susceptibility
- Environmental triggers
- Genetic predisposition

EXPECTED FINDINGS

- Joint swelling, stiffness, redness, and warmth that tend to be worse in the morning or after inactivity
- Mobility limitations
- Fever
- Rash
- Limp in the morning
- Delayed growth

LABORATORY TESTS

- Elevated C-reactive protein can be present.
- Erythrocyte sedimentation rate (ESR) can be elevated.
- CBC with differential can show elevated WBCs, especially during exacerbations.
- Antinuclear antibodies (ANA) indicate an increased risk for uveitis.
- Rheumatoid factor is rarely detected in children.

DIAGNOSTIC PROCEDURES

- Radiographic studies can be used for baseline comparison. X-rays can demonstrate increased synovial fluid in the joint, which causes soft tissue swelling or widening of the joint. Later findings can include narrowed joint spaces.
- Slit lamp eye examination is used to diagnosis uveitis.
- It can be performed every 6 months for adolescents with pauciarticular arthritis.

PATIENT-CENTERED CARE

NURSING CARE

- Care is primarily in an outpatient setting.
- Goal is to control pain, minimize damage from inflammation, preserve joint functioning, and promote normal growth and development.
- Assist the client with an exercise program.
- Reinforce teaching about relaxation techniques and nonpharmacological pain management.
- Monitor the child's pain and response to prescribed analgesics.
- Encourage attending a support group.
- Encourage the child to participate in a physical therapy program to increase mobility and prevent deformities.
- Encourage activity as tolerated.
- Encourage full ROM exercises.
- Apply heat or warm moist packs to the child's affected joints prior to exercise.
- Promote appropriate exercises (swimming).
- Encourage warm baths (paraffin [hands] or whirlpools).
- Identify alternate ways for the child to meet developmental needs, especially during periods of exacerbation.
- Encourage self-care by allowing adequate time for completion. Qpcc
- Encourage a well-balanced diet with adequate fluid intake.
- Encourage participation in school and contact with peers.
- Collaborate with the school nurse and teachers to arrange for care during the school day (medication administration, in-school physical therapy, extra sets of books, split days).

CLIENT EDUCATION

- Practice relaxation techniques and nonpharmacological pain management.
- Exacerbation worsens with illnesses.
- Schedule routine follow up with provider and regular eye exams.

MEDICATIONS

Nonsteroidal anti-inflammatory medications

Ibuprofen, naproxen, diclofenac, indomethacin, and tolmetin control pain and inflammation.

CLIENT EDUCATION

- Administer nonsteroidal anti-inflammatory medications (NSAIDs) as prescribed.
- NSAIDs should be taken with food to minimize gastric irritation.
- Report changes in stool and GI discomfort or increase in bruising immediately.
- Take as directed. Often prescribed 4 times a day for 6 to 8 weeks (even if feeling better).

Methotrexate

A cytotoxic disease-modifying antirheumatic drug (DMARD) that slows joint degeneration and progression of rheumatoid arthritis when NSAIDs do not work alone. Administered weekly in a low dose.

NURSING ACTIONS: Monitor liver function tests and CBC regularly. Medication can cause bone marrow suppression and liver toxicity, and is teratogenic and carcinogenic.

CLIENT EDUCATION

- Avoid alcohol.
- Utilize effective birth control to avoid birth defects while taking this medication.
- Take at bedtime to prevent nausea.
- If pregnant, decrease contact with medication due to the teratogenic effects on fetus.

Corticosteroids

Prednisone provides relief of inflammation and pain. They are reserved for life-threatening complications, severe arthritis, pericarditis, and uveitis.

NURSING ACTIONS

- Administer as eye solution, orally, or IV. An injection directly into the intra-articular space of the affected joint can provide effective pain relief.
- Administer at the lowest effective dose for short-term therapy and then discontinue by tapering the dose.

CLIENT EDUCATION

- Weight gain, especially in the face, is a common adverse effect.
- Monitor height and weight.
- An alteration in growth is a possible long-term complication of corticosteroids.
- Avoid exposure to potentially infectious agents.
- Practice healthy eating habits.

Etanercept

Etanercept is a tumor necrosis factor alpha-receptor inhibitor, another DMARD that is used when methotrexate is not effective for immunosuppressive action and decrease the inflammatory response.

NURSING ACTIONS

- Infliximab can be administered in an outpatient setting.
- Administer a tuberculin skin test prior to starting etanercept and yearly while taking the medication.
- Administer etanercept once or twice each week by subcutaneous injection.
- Monitor for lymphomas.

CLIENT EDUCATION

- Observe for allergic reactions.
- Avoid exposure to infectious agents.

THERAPEUTIC PROCEDURES

- Often delayed until growth is complete
- Synovectomy after all other interventions fail
- Joint replacement in older children

INTERPROFESSIONAL CARE

Physical therapist, occupational therapist, ophthalmologist, dentist, dietitian, social worker, school nurse, counselors, and psychologists

COMPLICATIONS

Joint deformity and functional disability

NURSING ACTIONS

- Reinforce the individualized therapeutic plan of care.
- Advocate for the child when treatments are not producing expected results.

CLIENT EDUCATION

- Encourage the child and family to adhere to the treatment regimen.
- Encourage self-care and active participation in an exercise program.

Muscular dystrophy

Muscular dystrophy (MD) is a group of inherited disorders with progressive degeneration of symmetric skeletal muscle groups causing progressive muscle weakness and wasting, which can lead to disability and deformity.

Onset of disease, pace of progression, and muscle group affected depend on the type of MD.

- **Duchenne (pseudohypertrophic) muscular dystrophy** (DMD) is the most common form of MD. Inherited as an X-linked recessive trait, DMD has an onset between 3 and 5 years of age. Progressive disease with life expectancy with current technology for DMD reaches into early adulthood. Fat tissue replace muscles in lower limbs (gastrocnemius).
- **Facioscapulohumeral muscular dystrophy** is an autosomal dominant inherited disorder with the age of onset occurring during early adolescence. Progression is slow with normal life span. Characterized by facial weakness and inversion of the shoulders.
- **Limb-girdle muscular dystrophy** is an autosomal dominant and recessive, heterogeneous disorder. It appears later in childhood with a slow progression.

DATA COLLECTION

RISK FACTORS

Family genetic history

EXPECTED FINDINGS

- Fatigue
- Muscle weakness beginning in the lower extremities
- Unsteady gait, with a waddle
- Lordosis
- Delayed motor skill development
- Frequent falling
- Gowers' sign: Difficulty getting out of bed, rising from a seated position, or climbing stairs
- Gowers' sign: Child walks hands up legs for support while going to a standing position
- Learning difficulties
- Mild cognitive delays that do not worsen with disease progression
- Progressive difficulty walking with possible loss of ability to walk
  - Often occurs by the age of 12 years (DMD)
- Progressive muscle atrophy of face, chest, and neck
- Respiratory and cardiac difficulties as the disease progresses

LABORATORY TESTS

- Blood polymerase chain reaction to detect the dystrophin gene mutation
- Blood creatine kinase: elevated and can be elevated prior to manifestations
- Genetic analysis

DIAGNOSTIC PROCEDURES

- Muscle biopsy
- EMG

PATIENT-CENTERED CARE

NURSING CARE

- Encourage and assist with providing for genetic counseling.
- Monitor the following.
  - Ability to perform ADLs
  - Respiratory function, including depth, rhythm, and rate of respirations during sleep and daytime hours
  - Cardiac function
  - The child and caregivers' understanding of long-term effects
  - The child and caregivers' coping and support system
- Maintain optimal physical function for as long possible.
  - Encourage the child to be independent for as long as possible and to perform ADLs.
  - Perform ROM exercises and provide appropriate physical activity (stretching exercises, strength and muscle training, breathing exercises). Q EBP

- Maintain proper body alignment and encourage the child to reposition self frequently to avoid skin breakdown.
- Assist with orthoses and braces as prescribed.
- Maintain respiratory functioning.
  - Encourage the use of incentive spirometry.
  - Position the child to enhance expansion of lungs.
  - Provide oxygen as prescribed.
  - Assist with providing noninvasive ventilation as prescribed.
- Encourage adequate fluid intake.
- Monitor and encourage adequate nutritional intake.
  - Low calorie, high protein and fiber
- Encourage routine physical exams and immunizations.
- Facilitate discussion of end-of-life decisions when appropriate.

CLIENT EDUCATION: Understand proper use of a mechanical cough device.

MEDICATIONS

Corticosteroids

Prednisone increases muscle strength

NURSING ACTIONS
- Monitor for infection.
- Monitor for adverse effects.

CLIENT EDUCATION
- Avoid potentially infectious agents.
- Practice healthy eating habits.
- Observe for adverse effects and notify the provider if necessary.
- Medications must be taken on a regular scheduled basis.

INTERPROFESSIONAL CARE

Neurologist; genetic counselor; physical, occupational, and respiratory therapists; dietitian; social worker; nurses, school teacher
- Encourage guardians to consider assistance with care as disease progresses (respite care, long-term care, palliative care, and home-health care).
- Recommend a referral for the child and guardians to support groups for MD.

THERAPEUTIC PROCEDURES

Surgery can be indicated for release or repair of contractures or for insertion of a gastrostomy tube or tracheostomy.

COMPLICATIONS

- Obesity
- Contractures
- Scoliosis
- Infections

Respiratory compromise

Progressive weakening of respiratory muscles decrease the child's ability to maintain adequate respirations.

NURSING ACTIONS
- Help the child turn hourly or more frequently.
- Have the child use deep breathing and coughing.
- Suction as needed.
- Administer oxygen.
- Use intermittent positive pressure ventilation and mechanically-assisted cough devices if indicated.
- Administer antibiotics.

CLIENT EDUCATION: Discuss mechanical ventilation options with the child and guardians.

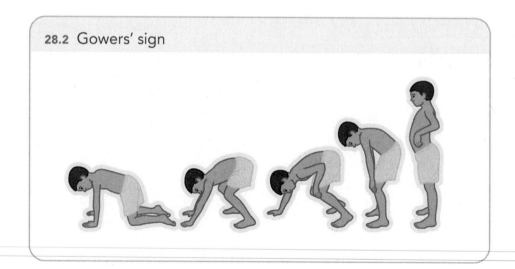

28.2 Gowers' sign

Application Exercises

1. A nurse is caring for a child who has cerebral palsy and is experiencing muscle spasms. Which of the following medications should the nurse expect the provider to prescribe? (Select all that apply.)

   A. Baclofen

   B. Diazepam

   C. Oxybutynin

   D. Methotrexate

   E. Prednisone

2. A nurse is contributing to the plan of care for a toddler who has cerebral palsy. Which of the following interventions should the nurse include?

   A. Structure interventions according to the toddler's chronological age.

   B. Determine the toddler's need for an evaluation of hearing ability.

   C. Monitor the toddler's pain level routinely using a numeric rating scale.

   D. Provide total care for daily hygiene activities.

3. A nurse is reinforcing discharge teaching with the guardians of a school-age child who has juvenile idiopathic arthritis. Which of the following instructions should the nurse include? (Select all that apply.)

   A. Provide extra time for completion of ADLs.

   B. Use cold compresses for joint pain.

   C. Take ibuprofen on an empty stomach.

   D. Remain home during periods of exacerbation

   E. Perform range-of-motion exercises.

4. A nurse is collecting data from a child who has muscular dystrophy. Which of the following findings should the nurse expect? (Select all that apply.)

   A. Purposeless, involuntary, abnormal movements

   B. Spinal defect and saclike protrusion

   C. Muscular weakness in lower extremities

   D. Unsteady, wide-based or waddling gait

   E. Upward slant to the eyes

5. A nurse is assisting with the care of an infant who has a myelomeningocele. Which of the following actions should the nurse take?

   A. Encourage the guardian to cuddle the infant.

   B. Monitor the infant's temperature rectally.

   C. Maintain the infant in a supine position.

   D. Apply a sterile, moist dressing on the sac.

Active Learning Scenario

A nurse is caring for a child who has a new prescription for baclofen. Use the ATI Active Learning Template: Medication to complete this item.

THERAPEUTIC USES

MEDICATION ADMINISTRATION

COMPLICATIONS: List several adverse effects of baclofen.

CLIENT EDUCATION: Include two actions the nurse should take.

Application Exercises Key

1. A. **CORRECT:** Baclofen is a centrally acting skeletal muscle relaxant that decreases muscle spasm and severe spasticity.
   B. **CORRECT:** Diazepam is a skeletal muscle relaxant that decreases muscle spasms and severe spasticity.
   C. Oxybutynin is an antispasmodic, anticholinergic medication that decreases bladder spasms.
   D. Methotrexate is a cytotoxic disease-modifying antirheumatic drug that slows joint degeneration and progression of rheumatoid arthritis. It is used for children who have juvenile idiopathic arthritis (JIA).
   E. Prednisone is a corticosteroid that increases muscle strength for children who have muscular dystrophy. It decreases inflammation in children who have JIA.

   Ⓝ NCLEX® Connection: Pharmacological Therapies, Expected Actions/Outcomes

2. A. Structure interventions according to the toddler's developmental level, rather than chronological age.
   B. **CORRECT:** Recognize that the toddler who has CP has an increased risk for hearing impairment; therefore, determine the toddler's need for an evaluation of hearing ability.
   C. Routinely monitor the toddler's pain level using a developmentally appropriate pain tool (a FACES pain rating scale). The numeric rating scale is appropriate for children as young as 5 years of age who have a concept of numbers.
   D. Though a preschooler requires assistance and supervision with hygiene activities, promote as much independence as possible.

   Ⓝ NCLEX® Connection: Coordinated Care, Collaboration with the Interdisciplinary Team

3. A. **CORRECT:** Providing extra time for the completion of ADLs promotes independence in the client and provides a means to maintain mobility.
   B. Using a warm compresses or moist packs can provide comfort and relieve stiffness.
   C. Ibuprofen should be taken with food to prevent GI distress.
   D. The client should be encouraged to attend school, even during periods of exacerbation when pain is increased.
   E. **CORRECT:** Range of motion will assist in maintaining function of the joints.

   Ⓝ NCLEX® Connection: Physiological Adaptation, Alterations in Body Systems

4. A. A child who has cerebral palsy exhibits purposeless, involuntary, abnormal movements.
   B. An infant who has the spinal defect myelomeningocele will exhibit a saclike protrusion.
   C. **CORRECT:** A child who has MD will exhibit muscular weakness in the lower extremities as one of the first manifestations.
   D. **CORRECT:** A child who has MD will exhibit an unsteady, wide-based, or waddling gait due to the progressive muscle weakness.
   E. A child who has Down syndrome can exhibit an upward slant to the eyes.

   Ⓝ NCLEX® Connection: Physiological Adaptation, Basic Pathophysiology

5. A. Cuddling the infant could cause pressure on the sac, which could cause rupture. This should not be in the preoperative plan of care.
   B. Rectal temperatures could cause irritation or rectal prolapse. This should not be in the preoperative plan of care.
   C. Placing the infant in supine position could cause pressure on the sac, which could cause rupture. This should not be in the preoperative plan of care.
   D. **CORRECT:** A sterile, moist, nonadhering dressing is placed on the sac to keep it moist until surgery. This should be in the preoperative plan of care.

   Ⓝ NCLEX® Connection: Physiological Adaptation, Basic Pathophysiology

Active Learning Scenario Key

Using the ATI Active Learning Template: Medication

THERAPEUTIC USES: Used as a centrally acting skeletal muscle relaxant that decreases muscle spasm and severe spasticity. Indicated for the treatment of cerebral palsy.

NURSING ADMINISTRATION
- Administer orally or assist with intrathecal administration via a specialized, surgically implanted pump.
- Monitor effectiveness of the medication.

COMPLICATIONS
- Muscle weakness
- Increased fatigue
- Less-common adverse effects (diaphoresis, constipation)

CLIENT EDUCATION
- Reinforce teaching with the family about expected responses of medications.
- Reinforce adverse effects of medications with the family and inform when to call the provider.

   Ⓝ NCLEX® Connection: Pharmacological Therapies, Medication Administration

NCLEX® Connections

When reviewing the following chapters, keep in mind the relevant topics and tasks of the NCLEX outline, in particular:

Pharmacological Therapies

MEDICATION ADMINISTRATION
Administer medication by ear, eye, nose, inhalation, rectum, vagina, or skin route.

Collect required data prior to medication administration.

Reinforce client teaching on client self administration of medications.

Reduction of Risk Potential

LABORATORY VALUES: Monitor diagnostic or laboratory test results.

Physiological Adaptation

ALTERATIONS IN BODY SYSTEMS
Identify signs and symptoms of an infection.

Provide care to correct client alteration in body system.

Reinforce education to client regarding care and condition.

BASIC PATHOPHYSIOLOGY
Identify signs and symptoms related to an acute or chronic illness.

Consider general principles of client disease process when providing care.

Apply knowledge of pathophysiology to monitoring the client for alterations in body systems.

FLUID AND ELECTROLYTE IMBALANCES: Provide care for a client with a fluid and electrolyte balance.

MEDICAL EMERGENCIES: Notify primary health care provider about client unexpected response/emergency situation.

UNIT 2 **SYSTEM DISORDERS**

SECTION: INTEGUMENTARY DISORDERS

CHAPTER 29 *Skin Infections and Infestations*

Skin infections are bacterial, viral, or fungal. Arthropod bites and stings are caused by flies, mosquitoes, chiggers, bees, fire ants, mites, ticks, spiders, and scorpions. Skin infestations include scabies and lice.

Skin infections

- Bacterial infections include impetigo contagiosa, pyoderma, folliculitis, furuncle, carbuncle, cellulitis, and staphylococcal scalded skin syndrome.
- Viral infections include verruca, verruca plantaris, herpes simplex virus, varicella zoster virus, and molluscum contagiosum.
- Fungal infections include tinea capitis, tinea corporis, tinea cruris, tinea pedis, and candidiasis.

DATA COLLECTION

RISK FACTORS

BACTERIAL
- Contact with infected person
- Congenital or acquired immunodeficiency disorders
- Immunosuppression

VIRAL: Contact with infected person

FUNGAL
- Contact with infected person
- Geographic area

EXPECTED FINDINGS

History of causative agent/exposure
- Bacterial **(29.1)**
- Viral **(29.2)**
- Fungal **(29.3)**

LABORATORY TESTS

Cultures (bacterial, viral, fungal)

29.1 Bacterial skin infections

	CAUSATIVE ORGANISM	MANIFESTATIONS	MANAGEMENT
Impetigo contagiosa	Staphylococcus	Reddish macule becomes vesicular	Topical bactericidal or triple antibiotic ointment
		Erupts easily leaving moist erosion on the skin, secretions dry forming honey-colored crusts	Oral or parenteral antibiotics for severe cases
		Spreads peripherally and by direct contact	
		Pruritus common	
Pyoderma	Staphylococcus Streptococcus	Deeper infection into the dermis	Cleanse with soap and water
		Possible systemic effects (fever, lymphangitis)	Bathe using antibacterial soap
			Launder washcloths and towels separately to prevent bacterial spread
			Apply mupirocin to lesions
			Systemic antibiotics
Folliculitis (pimple)	*Staphylococcus aureus* Methicillin-resistant *Staphylococcus aureus* (MRSA)	Infection of a hair follicle	Apply warm moist compresses
			Clean skin often
			Topical antibiotic medications
			Systemic antibiotics for severe cases
Furuncle (boil)	*Staphylococcus aureus* MRSA	Larger swollen, red lesion of a single hair follicle	Incision, draining, and irrigation of severe lesions
Carbuncle (multiple boils)	*Staphylococcus aureus* MRSA	More extensive swollen, red lesions involving multiple hair follicles	For MRSA infections, soak in diluted bleach solution
Cellulitis	Streptococcus Staphylococcus *Haemophilus influenzae*	Firm, swollen, red area of the skin and subcutaneous tissue	Oral or parenteral antibiotics
		Possible systemic effects (fever, malaise)	Rest and immobilize affected area
			Acute care for systemic manifestations
Staphylococcal scalded skin syndrome	*Staphylococcus aureus*	Rough-textured skin with macular erythema	Systemic antibiotics
		Epidermis becomes wrinkled within 2 days with large bullae appearing	Burow's solution or saline for gentle cleansing
			Compresses of 0.25% silver nitrate

29.2 Viral skin infections

	CAUSATIVE ORGANISM	MANIFESTATIONS	MANAGEMENT
Verruca (warts)	Human papillomavirus	Elevated, rough, gray-brown firm papules Can occur anywhere on the skin Can be single or in groups	Individualized destructive therapy (surgical removal, electrocautery, cryotherapy, laser)
Verruca plantaris (plantar warts)		Flat warts on the plantar surface of the feet Possibly surrounded by hyperkeratosis	Caustic solution applied to wart Wear insoles with holes to decrease pressure for 2 to 3 days Soak affected area for 20 min Repeat treatment until wart falls off
Cold sore, fever blister	Herpes simplex virus type 1	Near a mucocutaneous area (lips, nose, buttock, genitalia) Group of vesicles that itch and burn	Apply Burrow solution during weeping stage Oral antiviral (acyclovir) to reduce duration
Genital herpes	Herpes simplex virus type 2	After drying, form a crusty area followed by exfoliation Healing occurs in 8 to 10 days Possible lymphadenopathy	Oral antiviral (valacyclovir) for genital herpes
Herpes zoster *Shingles*	Varicella zoster virus	Neurologic pain, hyperesthesias, or itching Same virus as chicken pox	Use oral or topical analgesics Apply moist compresses Oral antiviral (acyclovir)
Molloscum contagiosum	Poxvirus	Flesh-colored papules on stalks (extremities, face, trunk)	Resolves spontaneously in 18 months Complicated cases: remove pox chemically or with curettage, cryotherapy or electrodessication

29.3 Fungal skin infections

	CAUSATIVE ORGANISM	MANIFESTATIONS	MANAGEMENT
Tinea capitis (ringworm of the scalp)	Trichophyton tonsurans Microsporum audouinii Microsporum canis	Scaly, circumscribed lesion with alopecia on the scalp Pruritic	Use of selenium sulfide shampoos Oral griseofulvin Kerion-griseofulvin and oral corticosteroids for 2 weeks Complicated cases: oral ketoconazole Treat infected pets (especially cats), if necessary
Tinea corporis (ringworm of the body)	Trichophyton rubrum Trichophyton mentagrophytes Microsporum canis	Round or oval erythematous scaling patch Spreads peripherally and unilaterally and clears centrally	Oral griseofulvin Topical antifungal (tolnaftate, clotrimazole) Apply wet compresses or take sitz bath
Tinea cruris (jock itch)	Epidermophyton floccosum Trichophyton rubrum Trichophyton mentagrophytes	Medial and proximal aspect of the thigh and crural folds May include the scrotum Pruritic Round erythematous scaling patch Spreads peripherally and clears centrally	Wear light-colored socks, well-ventilated shoes Treat infected pets (Tinea corporis) *Clotrimazole or ciclopirox twice a day for 2 to 4 weeks*
Tinea pedis (athlete's foot)	Trichophyton rubrum Trichophyton interdigitale Epidermophyton floccosum	Between toes or on the plantar surface of the feet Maceration and fissuring lesions between the toes and patches with tiny vesicles on the plantar surface of the foot	Ciclopirox or clotrimazole Griseofulvin for severe infections
Candidiasis (moniliasis)	Candida albicans	Found in moist areas of the skin surface White exudate, peeling inflamed areas that bleed easily Pruritic	Topical antifungal ointment (miconazole, nystatin)

29.4 Arthropod bites and stings

	MANIFESTATIONS	MANAGEMENT
Mosquitoes, fleas, flies	Variable, from no reaction to hypersensitivity reaction Papular urticaria Firm papules	Use antipruritic agent. Administer oral and topical antihistamines. Take baths.
Bees, wasps, hornets, fire ants, yellow jackets	Local reaction: small red itchy wheal that is warm to the touch Systemic reaction (mild to severe): generalized edema, pain, nausea and vomiting, confusion, respiratory problems, and shock	Scrape or pull out stinger as quickly as possible. Cleanse with soap and water. Apply cool compresses. Apply home products (baking soda, lemon juice). Administer topical and oral antihistamines. Epinephrine and corticosteroids for severe cases.
Chiggers	Bites on warm parts of the body Variable, from no reaction to hypersensitivity reaction Papular urticaria Firm papules	Systemic steroids for severe cases
Ticks	Attaches to the skin with head embedded Firm, discrete, pruritic nodule at site Possible urticaria or persistent localized edema	Remove by pulling straight up with steady, even pressure with tweezers to remove the tick. Remove any remaining parts using a sterile needle. Cleanse site with soap and disinfectant.
	Lyme disease: tick infected with *Borrelia burgdorferi* Can appear in any of these stages: Stage 1: 3 to 30 days following bite Erythema migrans at site Chills, fever, itching, headache, fainting, stiff neck, muscle weakness, bull's eye rash at the site of the bite Stage 2: occurs 3 to 10 weeks following bite Systemic involvement begins (neurologic, cardiac, and musculoskeletal) Paralysis or weakness in the face, muscle pain, swelling in large joints (knees), fever, fatigue, splenomegaly Stage 3: 2 to 12 months following bite Systemic involvement is advanced (musculoskeletal pain that includes the muscles, tendons, bursae, and synovia); possible arthritis, deafness, cardiac complications, and encephalopathy. Abnormal muscle movement and weakness, numbness and tingling, speech problems	Observe clients bitten by a tick for 30 days Antibiotic (single dose) for clients who meet criteria Antibiotic (2- to 3-week course) for clients who have confirmed disease Doxycycline for children older than 8 years and amoxicillin or cefuroxime for children under 8 years. Cefuroxime for children who have an allergy to penicillin
Brown recluse spiders	Mild sting leads to transient erythema and blister Pain 2 to 8 hr following bite Star-shaped purple area in 3 to 4 days Necrotic ulceration in 7 to 14 days	Cool compresses Antibiotic, corticosteroids Analgesic for pain Possible skin graft
Black widow spiders	Mild sting leads to swollen, painful, and erythematous site Dizziness, weakness, and abdominal pain Possible delirium, paralysis, seizures, and death	Cleanse bite with antiseptic. Apply cool compresses. Administer antivenin. Administer muscle relaxant. Administer analgesics.
Scorpions	Intense pain Erythema, burning, numbness Restlessness and vomiting Ascending paralysis: seizures, weakness, increase in pulse, thirst, salivation, dysuria, pulmonary edema leading to coma and death Death for children less than age 4 in the first 24 hr	Position site in dependent position. Keep child calm. Administer antivenin. Analgesic for pain. Admit to intensive care unit for close monitoring.

PATIENT-CENTERED CARE

NURSING CARE

- Check the general condition of the affected area.
- Monitor for evidence of associated infection.
- Assist in preventing the child to touch or scratch the affected areas.
- Reinforce teaching about the importance of proper hand hygiene.
  BACTERIAL (29.1)
  VIRAL (29.2)
  FUNGAL (29.3)

CLIENT EDUCATION

Perform methods to avoid the spread of infections.
- Use appropriate hand hygiene.
- Avoid sharing clothing, hats, combs, brushes, or towels.
- Keep the child from touching or scratching the affected area by using distraction.
- Do not squeeze vesicles.
- Apply topical medications as prescribed.
- Administer oral medications as prescribed.

Arthropod bites and stings

Scorpions, black widow, and brown recluse spiders inject venom that requires immediate attention.

DATA COLLECTION

RISK FACTORS

Geographic area

EXPECTED FINDINGS

History of causative agent/exposure (29.4)

PATIENT-CENTERED CARE

NURSING CARE (29.4)

CLIENT EDUCATION

- Prevent secondary infections.
- Children at risk for or who have a history of severe reactions should wear a medical alert bracelet. Qs
- Inspect skin after possible exposure.
- Prevent bites.
  - Avoid areas of tall grass.
  - Use insect repellent.
  - Avoid contact with insects.
  - Avoid wood piles.
  - Inspect and treat pets, carpets, and furniture.
  - Avoid flowery prints and bright clothing.
  - Avoid perfumes and colognes.

29.5 Skin infestations

	MANIFESTATIONS	NURSING INTERVENTIONS
Scabies mite: Sarcoptes scabiei	Intense itching, especially at night Rash, especially between fingers, popliteal folds, and inguinal regions Thin, pencil-like marks on the skin. Mites look like black dot on end of a grayish-brown burrow **INFANTS** Widespread on the body Pimples on the trunk Blisters on the palms of the hands and soles of the feet **YOUNG CHILDREN:** Most common on head, neck, shoulders, palms, and soles **OLDER CHILDREN:** Most common on hands, wrists, genitals, and abdomen	Apply a scabicide such as 5% permethrin cream over the entire body to remain on the skin for 8 to 14 hr; repeat in 1 to 2 weeks. Treat entire family and persons that have been in contact with infected person during and 60 days after infection. Wash underwear, towels, clothing, and sleepwear in hot water. Vacuum carpets and furniture. Apply calamine lotion or cool compresses until itching subsides following treatment. Difficult cases: Can use oral ivermectin.
Pediculosis capitis (head lice): Pediculus humanus capitis	Intense itching Small, red bumps on the scalp Nits (white specks) on the hair shaft	1% permethrin shampoo. Spinosad 0.9% topical suspension for children 4 years and older. Benzyl alcohol 5% in infants 6 months and older. Remove nits with a nit comb, repeat in 7 days after shampoo treatment. Wash clothing, bedding in hot water with detergent. Place items unable to be laundered in a sealed plastic bag for 14 days. Difficult cases: use malathion 0.5%.

Skin infestations

- Scabies mite, *Sarcoptes scabiei*, is spread by direct contact with an infected person. The mite burrows into the skin and lays eggs.
- *Pediculosis capitis* (head lice), *Pediculus humanus capitis*, is spread by direct contact with an infected person, bedding, and objects (hair brush, clothing). The life span of the adult louse life is 1 month and they can live up to 48 hr without a human host. The female lays eggs at night, close to the skin surface and at the junction of the hair shaft. The nits hatch in 7 to 10 days.

DATA COLLECTION

RISK FACTORS

SCABIES: long-term care facilities, nursing facilities, and day care settings

HEAD LICE: day care and schools; overcrowded conditions; sharing of combs, brushes, or hats

EXPECTED FINDINGS

Itching (29.5)

DIAGNOSTIC TESTS

SCABIES: examination under a microscope or skin biopsy

PATIENT-CENTERED CARE

NURSING CARE (29.5)

- Reinforce teaching with the child and caregivers about the medications. Qpcc
- Monitor for infestation.
  ○ SCABIES: Pencil-like marks on skin
  ○ HEAD LICE: Adult lice are hard to see: small, grayish-tan, and no wings. Nits look like dandruff on the hair shaft and are firmly attached.
- Monitor for secondary skin infection.

CLIENT EDUCATION

- Avoid home remedies, as it can worsen infection.
- Understand correct laundering of potentially infected clothing, bedding.
- Bag items that cannot be laundered into tightly sealed bag for 14 days.
- Boil combs, brushes and hair accessories for 10 min or soak in lice-killing products for 1 hr.
- Avoid sharing of personal items.

COMPLICATIONS

Secondary infections

Examples include staphylococcus, streptococcus, *Haemophilus influenzae*

NURSING ACTIONS
- Ensure the family understands prescribed plan of care to prevent secondary infections.
- Monitor for secondary infections.
- Administer medications as prescribed for secondary infection.

CLIENT EDUCATION: Observe for manifestations of secondary infections.

Active Learning Scenario

A nurse is reinforcing teaching with a group of caregivers about preventing skin infections. Use the ATI Active Learning Template: System Disorder to complete this item.

CLIENT EDUCATION: Describe five instructions the nurse should reinforce with the caregivers.

Active Learning Scenario Key

Using the ATI Active Learning Template: System Disorder
CLIENT EDUCATION
- Use good hand hygiene.
- Avoid sharing clothing, hats, combs, brushes, and towels.
- Keep the child from touching or scratching the affected area by using distraction.
- Do not squeeze vesicles.
- Apply topical medications as prescribed.
- Administer oral medications as prescribed.

Ⓝ *NCLEX® Connection: Health Promotion and Maintenance, Health Promotion/Disease Prevention*

Application Exercises

1. A nurse is collecting data from an infant who has scabies. Which of the following findings should the nurse expect? (Select all that apply.)

   A. Presence of nits on the hair shaft

   B. Pencil-like marks on hands

   C. Blisters on the soles of the feet

   D. Small, red bumps on the scalp

   E. Pimples on the trunk

2. A nurse is reinforcing teaching with a group of parents about preventing insect bites. Which of the following information should the nurse include? (Select all that apply.)

   A. Wear perfumes when outside.

   B. Avoid areas of tall grass.

   C. Wear bright-colored clothing.

   D. Wear insect repellent.

   E. Check house pets frequently.

3. A nurse is reinforcing teaching with the guardian of a child who has pediculosis capitis. Which of the following instructions should the nurse include?

   A. Apply mayonnaise to the affected area at night.

   B. Treat all household pets.

   C. Use an over-the-counter medication containing 1% permethrin.

   D. Discard the child's stuffed animals.

4. A nurse is caring for a child who has cellulitis on the hand. Which of the following actions should the nurse take?

   A. Administer oral antibiotics to the child.

   B. Cleanse area using Burrow solution.

   C. Prepare the child for cryotherapy.

   D. Apply a topical antifungal medication.

5. A nurse is contributing to the plan of care for a child who has tinea capitis. Which of the following interventions should the nurse include? (Select all that apply.)

   A. Treat infected house pets.

   B. Use selenium sulfide shampoo.

   C. Cleanse area with Burrow solution.

   D. Administer antiviral medication.

   E. Use moist, warm compresses.

Application Exercises Key

1. A. Presence of nits on the hair shaft is a manifestation of pediculosis capitis.
   B. **CORRECT:** Pencil-like marks on hands is a manifestation of scabies.
   C. **CORRECT:** Blisters on the soles of the feet is a manifestation of scabies.
   D. Small, red bumps on the scalp are a manifestation of pediculosis capitis.
   E. **CORRECT:** Pimples on the trunk is a manifestation of scabies.

   Ⓝ *NCLEX® Connection: Physiological Adaptation, Basic Pathophysiology*

2. A. Perfumes attract insects and should be avoided.
   B. **CORRECT:** Insects live in tall grasses; these areas should be avoided.
   C. Bright-colored clothing attracts insects and should be avoided.
   D. **CORRECT:** Insect repellent should be applied to prevent insect bites.
   E. **CORRECT:** House pets should be inspected and treated for insects to prevent exposing family members.

   Ⓝ *NCLEX® Connection: Health Promotion and Maintenance, Health Promotion/Disease Prevention*

3. A. Home remedies (mayonnaise) increase the risk of infection and should be avoided.
   B. Pediculosis capitis is transmitted person-to-person; household pets are not hosts.
   C. **CORRECT:** Pediculosis capitis is treated with 1% permethrin, which can be purchased over the counter.
   D. Items that cannot be placed in the laundry can be placed in a sealed bag for 14 days to kill the lice.

   Ⓝ *NCLEX® Connection: Physiological Adaptation, Alterations in Body Systems*

4. A. **CORRECT:** Oral antibiotics are often prescribed for the treatment of cellulitis.
   B. Cleansing with Burow's solution is recommended for staphylococcal scalded skin syndrome or herpes simplex virus.
   C. Cryotherapy is recommended for human papillomavirus.
   D. Topical antifungal medications are indicated for the treatment of candidiasis or tinea corporis.

   Ⓝ *NCLEX® Connection: Physiological Adaptation, Alterations in Body Systems*

5. A. **CORRECT:** Tinea capitis can be transmitted from household pets, especially cats, to persons. Pets should be treated, if infected.
   B. **CORRECT:** Selenium sulfide shampoo is recommended for use for children who have tinea capitis.
   C. A topical antifungal medication is recommended for children who have tinea capitis.
   D. Tinea capitis is a fungal infection. Antifungal medications are administered.
   E. Moist, warm compresses are applied for bacterial skin infections and not recommended for children who have tinea capitis.

   Ⓝ *NCLEX® Connection: Physiological Adaptation, Alterations in Body Systems*

CHAPTER 30 Dermatitis and Acne

Common skin conditions of the pediatric population include contact dermatitis, atopic dermatitis, and acne.

Contact dermatitis

Contact dermatitis is an inflammatory, hypersensitive reaction of the skin. It is caused when the skin comes into contact with chemicals or other irritants (feces, urine, soaps, poison ivy, animals, metals, dyes, medications).

Diaper dermatitis can be caused by detergents, soaps, or chemicals that come in contact with the genital area. It can also be a result of *Candida albicans*.

Seborrheic dermatitis (cradle cap, blepharitis, otitis externa) has an unknown etiology but is most common in infancy and puberty.

DATA COLLECTION

RISK FACTORS

- Use of diapers
- Exposure to an irritant

EXPECTED FINDINGS

Pruritus

Depends on the cause of the irritant and the client
- **Contact dermatitis**
  - Red bumps that can form moist, weeping blisters
  - Skin warm and tender to the touch
  - Presence of oozing, drainage, or crusts
  - Skin becomes scaly, raw, or thickened
- **Diaper dermatitis**
  - Bright red rash that extends gradually
  - Fiery red and scaly areas on the scrotum and penis
  - Red or scaly areas on the labia
  - Pimples, blisters, ulcers, large bumps, or pus-filled sores
  - Smaller red patches that blend together

PATIENT-CENTERED CARE

NURSING CARE

Diaper dermatitis
- Promptly remove the soiled diaper.
- Remove urine from the perineal area with a nonirritating cleanser.
- Expose the affected area to air.
- Use superabsorbent disposable diapers to reduce skin exposure.
- Apply a skin barrier (zinc oxide, petrolatum ointment). Do not wash it off with each diaper change.

Contact dermatitis: Remove irritant, and limit further exposure.

Poisonous plant exposure
- Cleanse exposed area as soon as possible with cold running water, then shower with soap and water.
- Clothes and shoes should be cleansed in hot water with detergent.
- Apply calamine lotion, Burow's solution compresses, or natural colloidal oatmeal baths.
- Use topical corticosteroid gel.
- Oral corticosteroids for severe reactions or for irritation on the face, neck, or genitalia.

Seborrheic dermatitis
- Treat by gently scrubbing the scalp to remove scales and crusted areas. Petrolatum, vegetable oil, or mineral oil can be helpful.
- Use a fine-tooth comb to gently remove the loosened crusts from the hair.
- Shampoo daily with antiseborrheic shampoo.

MEDICATIONS

Antihistamines

Hydroxyzine or diphenhydramine
Administer in cases of allergic/medication reactions.

CLIENT EDUCATION
- Reinforce education with the child's family on the importance of the medication and administering it on schedule.
- Reinforce the sedating effect of some antihistamines and the need for guardians to monitor the child and provide for safety during use. Qs

Antibiotics

Used to treat secondary infections

CLIENT EDUCATION: Reinforce education with the child's family about the importance of finishing the medication completely, even if the child is feeling better.

Antifungal ointments

Clotrimazole
Used to treat *Candida albicans*

CLIENT EDUCATION: Educate the family on the importance of the medication and administering schedule.

CLIENT EDUCATION

- Change diapers frequently.
- Avoid bubble baths and harsh soaps.
- Wear long sleeves and pants when there is risk of possible exposure to irritants.
- Remove an offending agent as soon as exposure takes place.
- Use proper hand hygiene.

COMPLICATIONS

Bacterial infections

Caused by breaks in the skin from scratching

NURSING ACTIONS
- Monitor the area for manifestations of infection.
- Keep fingernails trimmed short.
- Cleanse the area with mild soap and water.
- Administer antipruritics and antibiotics.

CLIENT EDUCATION: Reinforce education with the family and child about avoiding offending agents. Qpcc

Atopic dermatitis

- Atopic dermatitis (AD) is a type of eczema (eczema describes a category of integumentary disorders, not a specific disorder with a determined etiology) that is characterized by pruritus and associated with a history of allergies that are of an inherited tendency (atopy).
- Classifications of atopic dermatitis are based on the child's age, how the lesions are distributed, and the appearance of the lesions.
- AD cannot be cured but can be well-controlled.

DATA COLLECTION

RISK FACTORS

- Presence of allergic condition and family history of atopy
- Previous skin disorder and exacerbation of present skin disorder
- Exposure to irritating and/or causative agents

EXPECTED FINDINGS

- Recent exposure to any irritant (medication, food, soap, contact with animals).
- Intense pruritus.
- Affected skin can appear dry and rough.
- Hypopigmentation of skin can occur in small, diffuse areas.
- Pallor surrounds the nose, mouth, and ears.
- Bluish discoloration present underneath the eyes.
- Numerous infections of the nails are present.
- Lymphadenopathy occurs, especially around affected areas.
- Manifestations of a wound infection are present (swelling, purulent drainage, pain, increased temperature, redness extending beyond the wound margin).

Infants

Onset at 2 to 6 months of age with spontaneous remission by 3 years of age

DISTRIBUTION: Generalized distribution of lesions on cheeks, scalp, trunk, hands and feet, as well as extensor surfaces of extremities

LESIONS
- Erythema
- Vesicles, papules
- Weeping, oozing, crusting, scaling

Children

Onset at 2 to 3 years of age with 90% of children having manifestations by 5 years of age; can follow infantile eczema

DISTRIBUTION: Lesions in the flexural areas (antecubital and popliteal fossae, neck), wrists, ankles, and feet with symmetric involvement

LESIONS
- Clusters
- Erythematous or flesh-colored papules
- Dry
- Lichenification
- Keratosis pilaris

Adolescents

Onset at age 12 and can continue into adulthood

DISTRIBUTION: Similar distribution to children

LESIONS
- Same as for children
- Dry, thick
- Confluent papules

PATIENT-CENTERED CARE

NURSING CARE

- Keep skin hydrated with tepid baths (with/without mild soap or emulsifying oil), then apply an emollient within 3 min of bathing. Two or three baths can be given daily with one prior to bedtime. After bathing, pat skin to dry, do not rub.
- Dress the child in cotton clothing. Avoid wool and synthetic fabrics.
- Avoid excessive heat and perspiration, which increases itching.
- Avoid irritants (bubble baths, soaps, perfumes, fabric softeners).
- Provide support to the child and family.
- Wash skin folds and genital area frequently with water.
- Assist in identifying causative agent.
- Keep child's nails short and filed smooth to eliminate sharp edges.

MEDICATIONS

Antihistamines

Hydroxyzine or diphenhydramine
CLIENT EDUCATION
- Reinforce the sedating effect of some antihistamines and the need for guardians to monitor the child during use.
- Reinforce safety of the child when using sedating antihistamines. Qs

Loratadine or fexofenadine
Oral antihistamine for antipruritic effect
NURSING ACTIONS: Administer as prescribed.
CLIENT EDUCATION: Preferred for daytime use.

Antibiotics

- Antibiotics are used to treat secondary infections.
- Reinforce education with the family about the importance of finishing the medication.

Topical corticosteroids

Topical corticosteroids can be used intermittently to reduce or control flare-ups. They can be low-, moderate-, or high-potency and are prescribed based on the degree of skin involvement (extremity versus eyelids), age of the child, and consequences from adverse effects.

Topical immunomodulators (nonsteroidal)

Tacrolimus or pimecrolimus
- Used to decrease inflammation during flare-ups
- Safe to apply to face

NURSING ACTIONS
- Use for children older than 2 years of age.
- Use at the start of an exacerbation of AD when skin turns red and starts to itch.

CLIENT EDUCATION
- Observe for manifestations of infection.
- Change diapers when wet or soiled.
- Keep nails short and trimmed.
- Place gloves or cotton socks over hands for sleeping.
- Dress young children in soft, cotton, one-piece, long-sleeve, long-pant outfits.
- Remove items that can promote itching (woolen blankets, scratchy fabrics). Use cotton items whenever possible.
- Use mild detergents to wash clothing and linens. The wash cycle can be repeated without soap.
- Avoid latex products, second-hand smoke, furry pets, dust, and molds.
- Encourage tepid baths without the use of soap. Avoid oils and powders.
- Follow specific directions regarding topical medications, soaks, and baths. Emphasize the importance of understanding the sequence of treatments to maximize the benefit of therapy and prevent complications.
- Avoid overheating the bedroom during winter months. Use a room humidifier.
- Maintain treatment to prevent flare-up.
- Follow up with the provider as directed.
- Participate in support groups.

COMPLICATIONS

Infection

Caused by breaks in the skin from scratching

NURSING ACTIONS
- Keep nails trimmed.
- Administer antipruritics.
- Monitor the area for manifestations of infection.
- Cleanse the area with mild soap and water.

CLIENT EDUCATION: Educate the family and child to avoid offending agents. Qpcc

Acne

- Acne is the most common skin condition during adolescence.
- Acne is self-limiting and not life-threatening. However, it poses a threat to self-image and self-esteem for adolescents.
- Acne involves the pilosebaceous follicles (hair follicle and sebaceous gland complex) of the face, neck, chest, and upper back.
- *Propionibacterium acnes* is the bacteria associated with inflammation in acne.

DATA COLLECTION

RISK FACTORS

- Acne has a genetic link.
- More common in males.
- Hormonal fluctuations can result in acne flares in females.
- The use of cosmetic products containing ingredients (petrolatum and lanolin) can increase acne outbreaks.
- Adolescents working at fast-food restaurants can have an increased incidence of acne due to exposure to cooking grease.
- There is a possible dietary link with acne and the intake of high glycemic index foods and dairy products.

EXPECTED FINDINGS

- Report of exacerbations and remissions.
- Lesions (comedones) are either open (blackheads) or closed (whiteheads). Both are most often found on the face, neck, back, and chest.
- *P. acnes* can lead to inflammation manifesting as papules, pustules, nodules, or cysts.

PATIENT-CENTERED CARE

NURSING CARE

- Discuss the process of acne with the child and family.
- Discuss the importance of adherence with the prescribed plan of care.

CLIENT EDUCATION

- Gently wash the face and other affected areas, avoiding scrubbing and abrasive cleaners.
- Observe for adverse effects of prescribed medications.

MEDICATIONS

Tretinoin

Interrupts abnormal keratinization that causes microcomedones

CLIENT EDUCATION

- Tretinoin can irritate the skin. Wait 20 to 30 min after washing the face before application in order to decrease skin irritation.
- Use a pea-size amount of medication and apply at night.
- Avoid sun exposure.
- Use sunscreen (SPF 15 or greater) daily to avoid sunburn.

Benzoyl peroxide

- Antibacterial agent
- Inhibits growth of *P. acnes*
- Benzoyl peroxide can bleach bed linens, towels, and clothing, but not skin.

Topical and oral antibacterial agents

Inhibits growth of *P. acnes*

CLIENT EDUCATION

- Various topical antibacterial agents (clindamycin, azelaic acid, dapsone) can be used. Monitor for allergic reactions.
- Every-other-day application decreases adverse effects (drying of the skin, burning sensations, and erythema).
- Oral antibacterial medications (tetracycline, doxycycline, erythromycin, minocycline) are indicated for severe acne that is unresponsive to topical agents.
- Avoid sun exposure due to photosensitivity.
- Use sunscreen with an SPF of 15 or greater when exposure to sun is unavoidable.

Isotretinoin

Affects factors involved in the development of acne

NURSING ACTIONS

- Isotretinoin is only prescribed by dermatologists for severe acne that is unresponsive to other therapies.
- Monitor for behavioral changes.
- Isotretinoin is teratogenic. It is contraindicated in clients of childbearing age who are not taking oral contraceptives. If sexually active, the client must agree to use two forms of effective contraception for 1 month before and during treatment, and at least 1 month following treatment.

CLIENT EDUCATION: Adverse effects include dry skin and mucous membranes, dry eyes, decreased night vision, headaches, photosensitivity, elevated cholesterol and triglycerides, depression, suicidal ideation, and violent behaviors.

Oral contraceptive pills

Decreases endogenous androgen production and bioavailability, resulting in decreased acne development

NURSING ACTIONS

- Indicated only for adolescent females.
- Therapeutic effects can take 4 to 6 months to achieve.
- Therapy is combined with a topical acne treatment.

CLIENT EDUCATION

- Reinforce that adherence to the therapeutic plan is essential to preventing acne flares.
- Encourage the child to eat a balanced, healthy diet.
- Encourage sleep, rest, and daily exercise.
- Wash the affected area gently with a mild cleanser once or twice daily, and not to pick or squeeze comedones.
- Encourage frequent shampooing.
- Encourage family support of the child and family members to assist the child in coping with body-image changes. Qpcc
- Wear protective clothing and sunscreen when outside.
- Avoid the use of tanning beds.
- Reinforce the need for follow-up and monitoring of cholesterol and triglycerides for adolescents who are taking isotretinoin.
- Reinforce the importance of using effective contraception while taking isotretinoin.

COMPLICATIONS

Infection and cellulitis

Caused by lesions of dermatitis and/or acne or breaks in the skin from scratching

NURSING ACTIONS

- Monitor the area for manifestations of infection.
- Cleanse the area with mild soap and water.
- Monitor for redness, swelling, and pain, which can indicate cellulitis.
- Check for fever.
- Examine the client's face, back, and chest for the presence of scarring.

CLIENT EDUCATION Qpcc

- Observe for manifestations of cellulitis and notify the provider if these occur.
- Scarring can be caused by loss of skin tissue due to acne formation.
- Avoid vigorous scrubbing of the skin.
- Avoid squeezing or picking at acne.
- Discuss possible treatments for scarring (chemical peels or laser therapy).

Application Exercises

1. A nurse is reinforcing teaching with the guardian of an infant who has seborrheic dermatitis of the scalp. Which of the following instructions should the nurse include?

   A. "You can use petrolatum to help soften and remove patches from your infant's scalp."

   B. "When patches are present, you should keep your infant away from others."

   C. "You should avoid washing your infant's hair while patches are present on the scalp."

   D. "When patches are present, it indicates that your infant has a systemic infection."

2. A nurse is caring for a child who has contact dermatitis due to poison ivy exposure. Which of the following actions should the nurse take? (Select all that apply.)

   A. Remove the clothing over the rash.

   B. Initiate contact isolation precautions while the rash is present.

   C. Expose the rash to a heat lamp for 15 min.

   D. Cleanse the affected areas with hydrogen peroxide solution.

   E. Apply calamine lotion to the skin.

3. A nurse is caring for an adolescent who has acne and a new prescription for isotretinoin. Which of the following laboratory findings should the nurse plan to monitor?

   A. Cholesterol and triglycerides

   B. BUN and creatinine

   C. Blood potassium

   D. Blood sodium

4. A nurse is contributing to the plan of care for an infant who has diaper dermatitis. Which of the following interventions should the nurse include? (Select all that apply.)

   A. Apply talcum powder with every diaper change.

   B. Allow the buttocks to air dry.

   C. Use commercial baby wipes to cleanse the area.

   D. Use cloth diapers until the rash is gone.

   E. Apply zinc oxide ointment to the affected area.

5. A nurse is collecting data from an infant who has eczema. Which of the following findings should the nurse expect? (Select all that apply.)

   A. Generalized distribution of lesions

   B. Papules

   C. Ecchymosis in flexural areas

   D. Crusting lesions

   E. Keratosis pilaris

Active Learning Scenario

A nurse is reinforcing teaching with the guardian of a child who has eczema. Use the ATI Active Learning Template: System Disorder to complete this item.

ALTERATION IN HEALTH (DIAGNOSIS)

CLIENT EDUCATION: Include at least five instructions the nurse should give to the guardian.

1. A. **CORRECT:** Recommend that the guardian use petrolatum, vegetable oil, or mineral oil to help soften and remove scales and crusted areas.
    B. Seborrheic dermatitis is not contagious, so it is not necessary to keep the infant away from others.
    C. Washing the infant's hair daily with an antiseborrheic shampoo can help remove scales and crusted areas and can help prevent recurrence.
    D. The cause of seborrheic dermatitis is unknown and is not associated with a systemic infection.

    Ⓝ *NCLEX® Connection: Physiological Adaptation, Alterations in Body Systems*

2. A. **CORRECT:** Removing the irritant from the skin will decrease the child's exposure. Remove the clothing over the affected area.
    B. Poison ivy is not spread by contact with the rash. Once the plant oils are removed, it cannot be transmitted to others.
    C. Avoid using a heat lamp, which can cause skin burns.
    D. Cleanse the affected area with cold running water, followed by soap and water as soon as possible following exposure.
    E. **CORRECT:** Apply calamine lotion to assist in relieving discomfort.

    Ⓝ *NCLEX® Connection: Physiological Adaptation, Alterations in Body Systems*

3. A. **CORRECT:** Adverse effects of isotretinoin include elevated cholesterol and triglycerides. Plan to monitor these laboratory values during treatment.
    B. Medications (cephalosporins and furosemide) can alter blood BUN and creatinine levels. However, they do not need to be monitored in clients taking isotretinoin.
    C. Medications (diuretics and corticosteroids) can alter blood potassium levels. However, it does not need to be monitored in clients taking isotretinoin.
    D. Medications(IV fluids and corticosteroids) can alter the blood sodium level. However, it does not need to be monitored in clients taking isotretinoin.

    Ⓝ *NCLEX® Connection: Pharmacological Therapies, Expected Actions/Outcomes*

4. A. Talcum powder can cake and cause inhalation injury. It should not be used for infants who have diaper dermatitis.
    B. **CORRECT:** Allowing the buttocks to air dry facilitates thorough drying of the skin and should be included in the plan of care.
    C. Commercial baby wipes contain chemicals that can irritate the skin. They should not be used for infants who have diaper dermatitis.
    D. Superabsorbent diapers should be used for infants who have diaper dermatitis to assist in keeping the skin dry.
    E. **CORRECT:** Zinc oxide ointment protects the skin from moisture and irritation and should be included in the plan of care.

    Ⓝ *NCLEX® Connection: Physiological Adaptation, Alterations in Body Systems*

5. A. **CORRECT:** Generalized distribution of lesions is an expected finding in infants who have eczema.
    B. **CORRECT:** Papules are an expected finding in infants who have eczema.
    C. Lesions, rather than ecchymosis, in the flexural areas are an expected finding in children 2 years of age and older.
    D. **CORRECT:** Crusting lesions are an expected finding in infants who have eczema.
    E. Keratosis pilaris is an expected finding in children 2 years of age and older.

    Ⓝ *NCLEX® Connection: Physiological Adaptation, Basic Pathophysiology*

Using the ATI Active Learning Template: System Disorder

ALTERATION IN HEALTH (DIAGNOSIS): Eczema describes a category of integumentary disorders, not a specific disorder with a determined etiology, that is characterized by pruritus and associated with a history of allergies that are of an inherited tendency (atopy).

CLIENT EDUCATION

- Clinical manifestations of infection.
- Change diapers when wet or soiled.
- Keep nails short and trimmed.
- Place gloves or cotton socks over hands for sleeping.
- Dress young children in soft, cotton, one-piece, long-sleeve, long-pant outfits.
- Remove items that can promote itching (woolen blankets, scratchy fabrics). Use cotton items whenever possible.
- Use mild detergent to wash clothing and linens. The wash cycle can be repeated without soap.
- Avoid latex products, second-hand smoke, furry pets, dust, and molds.
- Encourage tepid baths without the use of soap. Avoid oils and powders.
- Follow specific directions regarding topical medications, soaks, and baths.
- Emphasize the importance of understanding the sequence of treatments to maximize the benefit of therapy and prevent complications.
- Avoid overheating the bedroom during winter months. Use a room humidifier.
- Maintain treatment to prevent flare-ups.
- Follow up with the provider as directed.
- Participate in support groups.

Ⓝ *NCLEX® Connection: Physiological Adaptation, Alterations in Body Systems*

CHAPTER 31 *Burns*

Thermal, cold, chemical, electrical, and radioactive agents can cause burns, which result in cellular destruction of the skin layers and underlying tissue. The type and severity of the burn affects the treatment plan.

Thermal burns occur when there is exposure to flames, hot surfaces, or hot liquids. Chemical burns occur when there is exposure to a caustic agent (acid, alkali, or organic compound). Cleaning agents used in the home and industrial setting cause chemical burns.

Electrical burns occur when an electrical current passes through the body. This type of burn can result in severe damage, including loss of organ function, tissue destruction with the subsequent need for amputation of a limb, and cardiac and respiratory arrest.

HEALTH PROMOTION AND DISEASE PREVENTION

- Provide adequate supervision.
- Establish a safe play area.
- Keep hot liquids, electrical cords, and dangling objects out of reach.

DATA COLLECTION

RISK FACTORS

- Abuse, neglect, or lack of supervision
- Developmental growth of the child

EXPECTED FINDINGS

- Type of burning agent (dry heat, moist heat, chemical, electrical, ionizing radiation)
- Duration of contact
- Area of the body in which the burn occurred
- Younger children tend to have deeper injuries due to thinner skin. Children less than 2 years old have a higher mortality rate due to decreased protein stores and immature renal and immune functioning.
- Extent, depth, and severity of injury

PHYSICAL FINDINGS

Refer to chart (31.1)

EXTENT OF INJURY

Total body surface area (TBSA)

- Age-related charts determine the extent of injury to body surface, which is expressed in percentages.
- Infants' skin is thin, so injury is likely to be deeper.

31.1 Stages of burns

	FIRST-DEGREE	SECOND-DEGREE		THIRD-DEGREE	FOURTH-DEGREE
	Superficial	*Superficial partial thickness*	*Deep partial thickness*	*Full thickness*	*Deep full thickness*
	Damage to epidermis	Damage to the entire epidermis Dermal elements are intact	Damage to the entire epidermis and some parts of the dermis Sweat glands and hair follicles remain intact	Damage to the entire epidermis and dermis and possible damage to the subcutaneous tissue Nerve endings, hair follicles, and sweat glands are destroyed	Damage to all layers of the skin that extends to muscle, fascia, and bones
APPEARANCE	Pink to red in color with no blisters Blanches with pressure	Painful, moist, red in color with blisters, mild to moderate edema, and no eschar Blanches with pressure	Mottled, red to white in color, with blisters and moderate edema Blanches with pressure	Red to tan, black, brown, or waxy white in color Dry, leathery appearance No blanching	Color variable Dull and dry Charring Possible visible ligaments, bone or tendons
SENSATION/HEALING	Painful Heals within 3 to 7 days No scarring	Painful Heals in less than 21 days Variable amounts of scarring Sensitive to temperature changes, exposure to air, and light touch	Painful Sensitive to temperature changes and light touch Healing time can extend beyond 21 days Scarring is likely	As burn heals, painful sensations return and severity of pain increases Heals within weeks to months Scarring is present Autografting is required	No pain is present Heals within weeks to months Scarring is present Autografting is required Amputation possible

Severity grading system (31.2)

Classification

The severity of the injury depends on the child's age, causative agent, body area involved, and the extent and depth of the burn.

Minor: treated in outpatient setting

Moderate: treated in a hospital with expertise in burn care

Major: requires medical services of a burn center

LABORATORY TESTS

MAJOR BURNS: CBC, blood electrolytes, BUN, ABGs, random glucose levels, liver enzymes, urinalysis

PATIENT-CENTERED CARE

NURSING CARE

Minor burns

- Stop the burning process.
  - Place the child in a horizontal position and roll him in a blanket to extinguish the fire.
  - Remove clothing or jewelry that can conduct heat.
  - Apply tepid water soaks or run water over the injury. Do not use ice.
  - Flush burns caused by liquid chemicals with large amounts of water.
  - While wearing gloves, brush dry chemicals from skin before flushing with large amounts of water.
- Cover the burn with a clean cloth to prevent contamination.
- Cleanse with mild soap and tepid water (avoid excess friction).
- Removing blisters is not recommended.
- Use antimicrobial ointment.
- Apply dressing.
  - Nonadherent: fine–mesh gauze
  - Hydrocolloid: occlusive dressing
- Provide warmth.
- If necessary, child is seen in a health care facility for medical care.
- Provide analgesia.
- Check immunization status. Administer tetanus vaccine if it has been more than 5 years since last immunization.
- Instruct the family to avoid using greasy lotions or butter on burns.
- Instruct the family to monitor for manifestations of infection.

Major burns

- Maintain airway and ventilation.
- Provide humidified 100% supplemental oxygen as prescribed.
- Monitor vital signs.
- Maintain cardiac output.
- Fluid replacement is important during the first 24 hr.
  - Isotonic crystalloid solutions (lactated Ringer's) are used during the early stage of burn recovery.
  - Colloid solutions (albumin or plasma) can be used after the first 24 to 48 hr of burn recovery.
  - Maintain urine output of 0.5 to 1 mL/kg/hr if the child weighs less than 30 kg (66 lb).
  - Maintain urine output of 30 mL/hr if the child weighs more than 30 kg (66 lb).
  - Be prepared to witness administration of blood products as prescribed.
- Monitor for manifestations of septic shock, and notify the provider of findings.
  - Alterations in sensorium (confusion)
  - Increased capillary refill
  - Increased temperature
  - Mottled or cool extremities
  - Decreased bowel sounds
  - Tachycardia
  - Tachypnea
  - Decreased urine output
- Manage pain.
  - Establish ongoing method to monitor pain level and effectiveness of pain management.
  - Avoid IM or subcutaneous injections.
  - Monitor IV opioid analgesics (morphine sulfate, midazolam, and fentanyl).
  - Monitor for respiratory depression when using opioid analgesics. Ⓢ
  - Collaborate with the RN for administration of IV pain medications prior to dressing changes or procedures.
  - Use nonpharmacologic methods for pain control (guided imagery, music therapy, therapeutic touch) to enhance the effects of analgesics and promote improved pain management.
- Prevent infection.
  - Follow standard precautions when performing wound care.
  - Restrict plants and flowers in client rooms due to the risk of contact with pseudomonas.
  - Change position frequently to prevent contractures and prolonged pressure.

31.2 Severity grading system

Adopted by the American Burn Association

	MINOR	MODERATE	MAJOR
Partial-thickness burns	Less than 10% of TBSA	10% to 20% of TBSA	Greater than 20% of TBSA
Full-thickness burns	Usually outpatient Can require 1- to 2-day admission	Admission to hospital, preferably one with expertise in burn care	Admission to a burn center

From Vaccarro P., Trofino, R.: Care of the patient with minor to moderate burns. In Trofino R., editor: Nursing care of the burn-injured patient, Philadelphia, 1991, Davis.

- Limit visitors.
- Use reverse isolation if prescribed.
- Monitor for manifestations of infection, and report to the provider.
- Use client-designated equipment (blood pressure cuffs and thermometers).
- Administer tetanus toxoid if indicated.
- Administer antibiotics if infection is present.
- Provide nutritional support.
  - Increase caloric intake to meet increased metabolic demands and prevent hypoglycemia.
  - Increase protein intake to prevent tissue breakdown and promote healing.
  - Provide enteral therapy or total parenteral nutrition (TPN) if necessary due to decreased gastrointestinal motility and increased caloric needs.
  - Administer vitamins A and C to facilitate cell growth, and zinc for wound healing.
- Restore mobility.
  - Maintain correct body alignment, splint extremities, and facilitate position changes to prevent contractures.
  - Maintain active and passive range of motion.
  - Assist with ambulation as soon as the child is stable.
  - Apply pressure dressings to prevent contractures and scarring.
  - Closely monitor areas at high risk for pressure injury (heels, sacrum, back of head).
- Provide psychological support.
  - Provide developmentally appropriate support for the child.
  - Assist with coping.
  - Use family-centered approach.
  - Make referrals as needed.

MEDICATIONS

Topical agents

Silver sulfadiazine
- Use with second- and third-degree burns.
- Apply to cleansed, debrided area.
- Wear sterile gloves for application.

Mafenide acetate
- Use with second- and third-degree burns.
- Apply to cleansed, debrided area.
- Wear sterile gloves for application.

Bacitracin: Use for prevention of secondary infection.

Morphine sulfate

Analgesia

NURSING ACTIONS
- Administer via continuous IV infusion with boluses prior to procedures.
- Monitor for respiratory depression.
- Monitor pain relief.

CLIENT EDUCATION: Perform safety precautions needed with opioid administration.

Midazolam, fentanyl , propofol , and nitrous oxide

Sedation and analgesia

NURSING ACTIONS
- Determine the need for sedation.
- Assist with IV administration just prior to the start of a procedure.
- Monitor pain relief.

CLIENT EDUCATION: Follow the rights of medication administration and use correct procedures for all routes.

Nitrous oxide/oxygen mixture

Short term analgesic gas, 50%

NURSING ACTIONS
- Peak effect in 3 to 5 min and eliminated via lungs in 2 to 5 min
- Useful for relieving anxiety and increasing pain threshold during procedures

THERAPEUTIC PROCEDURES

Wound care

NURSING ACTIONS
- Premedicate as prescribed prior to wound care.
  - Administer analgesics.
  - Administer hydroxyzine or diphenhydramine for pruritus.
- Remove previous dressings.
- Examine for odors, drainage, and discharge.
- Cleanse the wound as prescribed.
- Assist with debridement.
  - Provide hydrotherapy (place client or affected extremity in a warm tub of water or use warm running water, as if to shower) to cleanse the wound. Use once or twice a day. Use mild soap or detergent to gently wash burns, and then rinse with tepid water.
  - Encourage active range of motion during hydrotherapy.
  - Monitor for indications of cold stress and hypothermia.

Skin coverings

Biologic skin coverings can be used to promote healing of large burns. Requires repeated surgical application.
- **Allograft (homograft):** Skin from human cadavers that is used for partial and full thickness burn wounds
- **Xenograft:** Obtained from animals (pigs) for partial-thickness burn wounds
- **Synthetic skin coverings:** Used for partial-thickness burn wounds
- **Artificial skin:** A biologic product that allows the dermis to regenerate, used for partial- and full-thickness burns (healing is faster)

Permanent skin coverings can be the treatment of choice for burns covering large areas of the body.
- **Autografts:** Client's skin
- **Sheet graft:** Sheet of skin used to cover the wound
- **Mesh graft:** Sheet of skin placed in a mesher so skin graft has small slits in it; allows graft to cover larger areas of burn wound
- **Cultured epithelium:** Epithelial cells cultured for use when grafting sites are limited

NURSING ACTIONS

- Maintain immobilization of the graft site.
- Elevate the extremity.
- Provide wound care to the donor site.
- Administer analgesics.
- Monitor for infection before and after skin coverings or grafts are applied.
  - Discoloration of unburned skin surrounding burn wound
  - Green color to subcutaneous fat
  - Degeneration of granulation tissue
  - Development of subeschar hemorrhage
  - Hyperventilation indicating systemic involvement of infection
  - Unstable body temperature

CLIENT EDUCATION

- The child should keep the extremity elevated.
- Report evidence of infection.

INTERPROFESSIONAL CARE

Refer to services (nutrition, child life, social support, respiratory therapy, occupational/physical therapy, individual and family counseling) as prescribed.

CLIENT EDUCATION Qᴛᴄ

- The child should continue to perform range-of-motion exercises and to work with a physical therapist to prevent contractures.
- Examine the wound for infection and perform wound care.
- Perform age-appropriate safety measures for the home (covering electrical outlets, supervising children when in the bath, keeping irons out of reach of children, reinforcing teaching about the dangers of playing with matches). Qₛ
- Avoid sun exposure between 1000 and 1400, wear protective clothing, and apply sunscreen to prevent sunburn.
- Expect delays in growth and weight for up to three years post burn injury
- Increased risk of bone remodeling.

CARE AFTER DISCHARGE

- Initiate a referral for home health services.
- Initiate a referral to occupational therapy for evaluation of the home environment and assistance to relearn how to perform ADLs.
- Initiate a referral to social services for community support services.

COMPLICATIONS

Inhalation injury

Direct thermal injury

- Occurs with burns to the face and lips. Damage occurs to the tracheobronchial tree after inhalation of heated gases and toxic chemicals produced during combustion.
- Can be delayed 24 to 48 hr.
- Findings include wheezing, increased secretions, hoarseness, wet rales in the lungs, singed nasal hairs, laryngeal edema, and carbonaceous secretions.

Carbon monoxide injury

- Occurs when incident takes place in an enclosed area.
- Findings include mucosal erythema and edema followed by sloughing of the mucosa.

NURSING ACTIONS: Maintain airway and ventilation, and provide 100% oxygen as prescribed.

Shock/systemic sepsis

NURSING ACTIONS

- Administer IV crystalloid solutions for the first 24 hr followed by colloid solutions.
- Meticulously monitor I&O.
- Monitor laboratory findings, noting indications of anemia and infection.
- Monitor vital signs.
- Check sensorium.
- Monitor capillary refill in extremities.

Pulmonary problems

Include edema, bacterial pneumonia, aspiration, embolus, and pulmonary insufficiency

NURSING ACTIONS

- Maintain airway via intubation, sometimes tracheostomy.
- Administer oxygen as prescribed.

Wound infections

NURSING ACTIONS

- Examine for discoloration, edema, odor, and drainage.
- Check for fluctuations in temperature and heart rate.
- Obtain a wound culture.
- Administer antibiotics as prescribed.
- Monitor laboratory findings, noting indications of anemia and infection.
- Maintain surgical aseptic technique with dressing changes.

Application Exercises

1. A nurse is caring for a client who has a superficial partial-thickness burn. Which of the following actions should the nurse take?

   A. Monitor IV infusion of 0.9% sodium chloride.

   B. Apply cool, wet compresses to the affected area.

   C. Clean the affected area using a soft-bristle brush.

   D. Administer morphine sulfate.

2. A nurse is collecting data from a client who has major burns and suspected septic shock. Which of the following findings should the nurse expect? (Select all that apply.)

   A. Increased body temperature

   B. Altered sensorium

   C. Decreased capillary refill time

   D. Decreased urine output

   E. Increased bowel sounds

3. A nurse is assisting with the care of a client who has a major burn and is experiencing severe pain. Which of the following actions should the nurse take?

   A. Monitor morphine sulfate IV.

   B. Monitor meperidine IM.

   C. Administer acetaminophen PO.

   D. Administer hydrocodone PO.

4. A nurse is caring for a client who has a skin graft. Which of the following findings indicate infection? (Select all that apply.)

   A. Pink color to subcutaneous fat

   B. Unstable body temperature

   C. Generation of granulation tissue

   D. Subeschar hemorrhage

   E. Change in skin color around the affected area

5. A nurse is caring for a client who has a moderate burn. Which of the following actions should the nurse take?

   A. Maintain immobilization of the affected area.

   B. Expose affected area to the air.

   C. Initiate a high-protein, high-calorie diet.

   D. Implement contact isolation.

Active Learning Scenario

A nurse is assisting with an in-service for newly licensed nurses about manifestations of burns. Which of the following information should the nurse plan to include? Use the ATI Active Learning Template: Basic Concept to complete this item.

UNDERLYING PRINCIPLES: List the depth, appearance, sensation, and healing of first-, second-, third-, and fourth-degree burns.

Application Exercises Key

1. A. Fluid replacement is indicated for clients who have sustained moderate to major burns.
    B. **CORRECT**: Applying cool, wet compresses stops the burn process.
    C. Gentle cleansing with tepid water, not a soft-bristle brush, is recommended for a superficial partial-thickness burn.
    D. Morphine sulfate for pain relief is indicated for clients who have sustained moderate to major burns.

    Ⓝ NCLEX® Connection: Physiological Adaptation, Alterations in Body Systems

2. A. **CORRECT**: Increased body temperature is a manifestation of septic shock.
    B. **CORRECT**: Altered sensorium is a manifestation of septic shock.
    C. Increased capillary refill time is a manifestation of septic shock.
    D. **CORRECT**: Decreased urine output is a manifestation of septic shock.
    E. Decreased bowel sounds are a manifestation of septic shock.

    Ⓝ NCLEX® Connection: Physiological Adaptation, Basic Pathophysiology

3. A. **CORRECT**: Opioids administered IV via continuous infusion are recommended for clients who have major burns.
    B. IM medications are contraindicated for clients who have major burns.
    C. Oral acetaminophen is recommended for clients who have minor burns.
    D. IV opioid medications are recommended for clients who have major burns.

    Ⓝ NCLEX® Connection: Pharmacological Therapies, Pharmacological Pain Management

4. A. Pink color to subcutaneous fat is a manifestation of wound healing.
    B. **CORRECT**: Unstable body temperature is a manifestation of infection.
    C. Degeneration of granulation tissues is a manifestation of infection.
    D. **CORRECT**: Subeschar hemorrhage is a manifestation of infection.
    E. **CORRECT**: A discoloration of the skin around the burn is a manifestation of infection.

    Ⓝ NCLEX® Connection: Physiological Adaptation, Unexpected Response to Therapies

5. A. Active and passive range of motion of the affected area is recommended to prevent contractures.
    B. Dressings should be applied to the burned area to prevent infection.
    C. **CORRECT**: A high-protein, high-calorie diet is initiated to meet increased metabolic demands and promote healing.
    D. Reverse isolation precautions are recommended to prevent wound infections.

    Ⓝ NCLEX® Connection: Physiological Adaptation, Alterations in Body Systems

Active Learning Scenario Key

Using the ATI Active Learning Template: Basic Concept

UNDERLYING PRINCIPLES

Superficial (first-degree)
- Damage to the epidermis
- Pink to red in color with no blisters
- Blanches with pressure
- Painful
- Heals within 3 to 7 days with no scarring

Superficial partial thickness (second-degree)
- Damage to the entire epidermis with intact dermal elements
- Moist
- Red in color with blisters
- Blanches with pressure
- Mild to moderate edema
- No eschar
- Painful
- Sensitive to temperature changes and light touch
- Heals in less than 21 days with variable scarring

Deep partial thickness (second-degree)
- Damage to the entire epidermis and some parts of the dermis
- Sweat glands and hair follicles remain intact
- Mottled
- Red to white in color with blisters
- Blanches with pressure
- Moderate edema
- Painful
- Sensitive to temperature changes and light touch
- Healing can go beyond 21 days with scarring

Full thickness (third degree)
- Damage to the entire epidermis and dermis with possible damage to the subcutaneous tissue
- Nerve endings, hair follicles, and sweat glands are destroyed
- Red to tan, black, brown, or waxy white in color
- Dry, leathery appearance
- No blanching
- As burn heals, painful sensations return and severity of pain increases
- Heals within weeks to months
- Scarring is present
- Grafting is required

Deep full thickness (fourth-degree)
- Damage to all layers of the skin that extends to the muscle, tendons, and bones.
- Color variable, dull, and dry with charring
- Possible visible ligaments, bone, or tendons
- No pain is present
- Heals within weeks to months
- Scarring is present and grafting is required
- Amputation possible

Ⓝ NCLEX® Connection: Physiological Adaptation, Basic Pathophysiology

ⓝ NCLEX® Connections

When reviewing the following chapters, keep in mind the relevant topics and tasks of the NCLEX outline, in particular:

Pharmacological Therapies

DOSAGE CALCULATIONS
Collect required data prior to medication administration.

Use clinical decision making when calculating doses.

EXPECTED ACTIONS/OUTCOMES: Apply knowledge of pathophysiology when addressing pharmacological agents.

MEDICATION ADMINISTRATION: Reinforce client teaching on client self-administration of medications.

Reduction of Risk Potential

DIAGNOSTIC TESTS: Perform diagnostic testing.

THERAPEUTIC PROCEDURES: Assist with the performance of a diagnostic or invasive procedure.

Physiological Adaptation

ALTERATIONS IN BODY SYSTEMS
Reinforce education to client regarding care and condition.

BASIC PATHOPHYSIOLOGY
Identify signs and symptoms related to an acute or chronic illness.

Apply knowledge of pathophysiology to monitoring client for alterations in body systems.

CHAPTER 32 *Diabetes Mellitus*

Diabetes mellitus is characterized by a partial or complete metabolic deficiency of insulin. Type 1 is characterized by destruction of pancreatic beta cells. Type 2 arises when the body fails to use insulin properly combined with insulin insufficiency.

Diabetes mellitus is a contributing factor for the development of cardiovascular disease, hypertension, renal failure, blindness, and stroke as individuals age.

DATA COLLECTION

RISK FACTORS

- Genetics can predispose a person to the occurrence of type 1 and type 2 diabetes mellitus.
- Toxins and viruses can predispose an individual to diabetes by destroying the beta cells, leading to type 1 diabetes mellitus.
- Obesity, physical inactivity, high triglycerides (greater than 250 mg/dL), and hypertension can lead to insulin resistance and type 2 diabetes mellitus.

EXPECTED FINDINGS

BLOOD GLUCOSE ALTERATIONS

- **Hypoglycemia:** blood glucose less than 60 mg/dL
  - Hunger, lightheadedness, and shakiness
  - Headache
  - Anxiety and irritability
  - Pallor, cool skin
  - Diaphoresis
  - Irritability
  - Normal or shallow respirations
  - Tachycardia and palpitations
  - Strange or unusual feelings
  - Decreasing level of consciousness
  - Difficulty in thinking and inability to concentrate
  - Change in emotional behavior
  - Slurred speech
  - Headache and blurred vision
  - Seizures leading to coma

- **Hyperglycemia:** blood glucose usually greater than 250 mg/dL
  - Thirst
  - Polyuria (early), oliguria (late)
  - Nausea, vomiting, abdominal pain
  - Skin that is warm, dry, and flushed with poor turgor
  - Dry mucous membranes
  - Confusion
  - Weakness
  - Lethargy
  - Weak pulse
  - Diminished reflexes
  - Rapid, deep respirations with acetone/fruity odor due to ketones (Kussmaul respirations)
  - Recurrent vaginal yeast (early indication of type 2)

LABORATORY TESTS

DIAGNOSTIC CRITERIA FOR DIABETES

- An 8-hr fasting blood glucose level of 126 mg/dL or more
- A random (casual) blood glucose of 200 mg/dL or more with manifestations of diabetes
- An oral glucose tolerance test of 200 mg/dL or more in the 2-hr sample
- HbA1C greater than 6.5%

Fasting blood glucose

CLIENT EDUCATION: Ensure that the child has fasted (no food or drink other than water) for 8 hr prior to the blood draw. Antidiabetic medications should be postponed until after the level is drawn.

Oral glucose tolerance test

CLIENT EDUCATION

- Instruct the child to consume a balanced diet for the 3 days prior to the test, then, to fast for 8 hr prior to the test. A fasting blood glucose level is drawn at the start of the test.
- The child is then instructed to consume a specified amount of glucose. Blood glucose levels are drawn at 30 and 60 min, and then at hourly intervals depending on the type of test.
- The child must be monitored for hypoglycemia throughout the procedure.

Glycosylated hemoglobin (HbA1c)

Used to evaluate diabetes management by providing an average of the child's blood glucose level over a period of about 3 months. The expected reference range is 4% to 6%, but an acceptable target for children who have diabetes can be 6.5% to 8% depending on the child's age.

DIAGNOSTIC PROCEDURES

Self-monitored blood glucose (SMBG) Qpcc

- Blood glucose monitoring is essential to management of diabetes. Measurements should be checked at a minimum before meals and at bedtime.
- Follow or ensure that the child follows the proper procedure for blood sample collection and use of a glucose meter.

CLIENT EDUCATION

- Instruct the child to check the accuracy of the strips with the control solution provided.
- Advise the child to keep a record of the SMBG that includes time, date, blood glucose level, insulin dose, food intake, and other events that can alter glucose metabolism (activity level or illness).

PATIENT-CENTERED CARE

NURSING CARE Qtc

- Monitor the following.
  - Vital signs
  - Blood glucose levels and factors affecting levels (other medications, diet, and/or activity)
  - I&O and weight
  - Skin integrity and healing status of any wounds, paying close attention to the feet and folds of the skin
  - Findings of poor glucose control (paresthesias, visual changes, recurrent infections).
  - Dietary practices
  - Exercise patterns
  - The child's proficiency at self-monitoring blood glucose
  - The child's proficiency at self-administering medication
- Follow agency policy for nail care. Some protocols allow for trimming toenails straight across with clippers and filing edges with a nail file. If clippers or scissors are contraindicated, the child should file the nails straight across.
- Reinforce teaching about personal hygiene.
- Caution the child against wearing sandals, walking barefoot, or wearing shoes without socks.
- Instruct the child to cleanse cuts with warm water and mild soap, gently dry, and apply a dry dressing. Instruct the child and parents to monitor healing and seek intervention promptly.
- Reinforce with the child the importance of having medical identification.
- Examine the child's eyes yearly.
- Emphasize the importance of regular dental and health care visits.
- Provide nutritional guidelines.
  - Read labels for nutritional value.
  - Meal planning is based on the requirements of growth and development of the child.
  - Plan meals to match the timing of food to activity, and the onset, peak and duration of antidiabetic medications. Calories and food composition should be similar each day.
  - Eat at regular intervals and do not skip meals.
  - Count grams of carbohydrates consumed.

- Recognize that 15 g of carbohydrates are equal to 1 carbohydrate exchange.
  - Avoid high-fat and high-sugar/high-carbohydrate food items.
  - Use artificial sweeteners in moderation.
- Reinforce teaching about appropriate techniques for SMBG, including obtaining blood samples, recording and responding to results, and correctly handling supplies and equipment.
- Assist with an exercise plan.
  - Children active with team sports will require a snack 30 min prior to activity.
  - Prolonged activities will require food intake every 45 to 60 min.
  - Adjustment in diet and medications can be required with changes in activities.
- Reinforce illness management guidelines.
  - Monitor blood glucose and urinary ketone levels every 3 hr.
  - Continue to take antidiabetic agents. However, dosages can differ.
  - Encourage sugar-free, noncaffeinated liquids to prevent dehydration.
  - Meet carbohydrate needs by eating soft foods if possible. If not, consume liquids that are equal to the usual carbohydrate content.
  - Rest.
  - Call the provider for the following.
    - Blood glucose greater than 240 mg/dL
    - Positive ketones in the urine
    - Disorientation or confusion
    - Rapid breathing
    - Vomiting occurs more than once
    - Liquids cannot be tolerated
- Reinforce manifestations of hypoglycemia (tremors, diaphoresis, anxiety, nervousness, chills, headache, confusion, labile, difficulty focusing, hunger, dizziness, pallor, palpations).
  - Check blood glucose levels.
  - Follow guidelines outlined by the provider or diabetes educator. Guidelines can include the following. Qs
    - Treat with 10 to 15 g simple carbohydrate (1 Tbsp sugar). Examples are 4 oz orange juice, 8 oz milk, 3 to 4 glucose tablets, or 4 oz regular soft drink.
    - For mild reactions, use milk or fruit juice.
    - Monitor blood glucose frequently.
    - After 15 min, if the blood glucose level does not increase by 15 mg/dL, consume more carbohydrates.
    - Follow with complex carbohydrate.
    - If the child is unconscious or unable to swallow, administer glucagon SC or IM and notify the provider. Administer simple carbohydrate as soon as tolerated. Watch for vomiting, and take precautions against aspiration.
- Reinforce manifestations of hyperglycemia (lethargy, confusion, thirst, nausea, vomiting, abdominal pain, manifestations of dehydration, rapid respirations, fruity breath).
  - Encourage oral fluid intake.
  - Administer insulin as prescribed.
  - Test urine for ketones, and report if findings they remain high.
  - Consult the provider if manifestations persist or progress.

32.1 Rate of onset, peak, and duration of action by insulin type

	TYPE	ONSET	PEAK	DURATION
Rapid-acting	Insulin lispro	15 min	30 to 90 min	3 to 6 hr
Short-acting	Regular insulin	30 min to 1 hr	1 to 5 hr	6 to 10 hr
Intermediate-acting	NPH insulin	1 to 2 hr	6 to 14 hr	16 to 24 hr
Long-acting	Insulin glargine U-100	70 min	None	18 to 24 hr

MEDICATIONS

- Insulin is used to manage type 1 diabetes.
- The rate of onset, peak, and duration of action varies for each different type of insulin. (32.1)

Insulin pumps
- Delivers a programmed amount of insulin on a consistent basis.
- Boluses can be administered before meals.

Insulin injections
- Self-administered injections two or more times per day
- Mixing insulin: usually rapid- and intermediate-acting

NURSING ACTIONS
- Do not mix insulin glargine with other insulin due to incompatibility.
- Observe the child and/or parent drawing up and administering the insulin injection, and reinforce instructions as indicated.
- Observe the child and/or parent using the insulin pump and reinforce instructions as indicated.

CLIENT EDUCATION
Perform self-administration of insulin.
- Rotate injection sites (prevents lipohypertrophy) within one anatomic site four or six injections before switching to another anatomic site (prevents day-to-day changes in absorption rates).
- Inject at a 90° angle. (Use pinch technique if skin is thin.) Aspiration for blood is not necessary.
- When mixing a rapid- or short-acting insulin with a longer-acting insulin, draw up the shorter-acting insulin into the syringe first and then the longer-acting insulin (this reduces the risk of introducing the longer-acting insulin into the vial of the shorter-acting insulin).

INTERPROFESSIONAL CARE

- Refer the child and family to a diabetes nurse educator for comprehensive education in diabetes management.
- Referrals often include pediatric endocrinologist, nutritionist, and exercise physiologist.
- School teachers, school nurses, guidance counselors, and coaches should also be involved.

COMPLICATIONS

Diabetic ketoacidosis (DKA)

- DKA is an acute, life-threatening condition characterized by hyperglycemia (greater than 330 mg/dL), glycosuria, and acidosis (pH 7.30 and bicarbonate 15 mmol/L), resulting in the breakdown of body fat for energy and an accumulation of ketones from the blood, urine, and lungs. The onset is rapid, and the mortality rate is high.
- Causes of DKA include insufficient insulin, acute stress, and poor management of acute illness.

NURSING ACTIONS
- Assist with admitting the child to an intensive care unit.
  - Place the child on a cardiac monitor.
  - Obtain venous access for administration of fluids, electrolytes, and insulin.
- Monitor subjective and objective data for DKA.
  - Ketone levels in the blood and urine
  - Blood glucose levels
  - Labs: glucose, electrolytes, BUN, ABG, CBC
  - Fruity scent to the breath
  - Mental confusion
  - Dyspnea
  - Nausea and vomiting
  - Dehydration
  - Weight loss
  - Electrolyte imbalances
  - Untreated: Coma, which can progress to death
- Provide rapid isotonic fluid (0.9% sodium chloride) replacement to maintain perfusion to vital organs. Large quantities are often required to replace losses. Monitor for evidence of fluid volume excess and cerebral edema.
- When blood glucose levels approach 250 mg/dL, add glucose to IV fluids in order to maintain 120 to 240 mg/dL blood glucose levels. Administer regular insulin continuously through an IV infusion at 0.1 unit/kg/hr.
- Monitor glucose levels hourly, or more frequently if required.
- Monitor blood potassium levels. Potassium levels will initially be elevated. With insulin therapy, potassium will shift into cells and the child will need to be monitored for hypokalemia. Provide potassium replacement therapy in IV fluids as indicated by laboratory values. Make sure urinary output is adequate before administering potassium.

- Assist with administration of sodium bicarbonate by slow IV infusion for severe acidosis (pH less than 7.0). Monitor potassium levels because a correction of acidosis that occurs too quickly can lead to hypokalemia. Monitor closely for changes in level of consciousness.
- Administer oxygen to children who are cyanotic and whose arterial oxygen level is less than 80%.

CLIENT EDUCATION: Reinforce instructions to manage diabetes. $\mathcal{Q}_{PCC}$

Long-term complications

- Kidney disease
- Eye disease
- Neurologic complications

Active Learning Scenario

A nurse is reinforcing teaching with the guardian of a school-age child who has type 1 diabetes mellitus. Use the ATI Active Learning Template: System Disorder to complete this item.

ALTERATION IN HEALTH (DIAGNOSIS)

MEDICATIONS: List the types of insulin used for children who have type 1 diabetes mellitus.

NURSING CARE: Describe eight interventions.

CLIENT EDUCATION: Describe three client outcomes.

Application Exercises

1. A nurse is reinforcing teaching about sick-day management with a parent of a child who has type 1 diabetes mellitus. Which of the following instructions should the nurse include? (Select all that apply.)

   A. Monitor blood glucose levels every 3 hr.

   B. Discontinue taking insulin until feeling better.

   C. Drink 8 oz of fruit juice every hour.

   D. Test urine for ketones.

   E. Call the provider if blood glucose is greater than 240 mg/dL.

2. A nurse is reinforcing teaching with a child who has type 1 diabetes mellitus about self-care. Which of the following statements by the child indicates understanding of the teaching?

   A. "I should skip breakfast when I am not hungry."

   B. "I should increase my insulin with exercise."

   C. "I should drink a glass of milk when I am feeling irritable."

   D. "I should draw up the NPH insulin into the syringe before the regular insulin."

3. A nurse is collecting data from a child who has type 1 diabetes mellitus. Which of the following manifestations indicate of diabetic ketoacidosis? (Select all that apply.)

   A. Blood glucose 58 mg/dL

   B. Weight gain

   C. Dehydration

   D. Mental confusion

   E. Fruity breath

4. A nurse is reinforcing teaching with a school-age child who has diabetes mellitus about insulin administration. Which of the following instructions should the nurse include?

   A. "You should inject the needle at a 30-degree angle."

   B. "You should combine your glargine and regular insulin in the same syringe."

   C. "You should aspirate for blood before injecting the insulin."

   D. "You should give four to six injections in one area before switching sites."

5. A nurse is reinforcing teaching with an adolescent who has diabetes mellitus about manifestations of hypoglycemia. Which of the following findings should the nurse include? (Select all that apply.)

   A. Increased urination

   B. Hunger

   C. Poor skin turgor

   D. Irritability

   E. Sweating and pallor

   F. Kussmaul respirations

Application Exercises Key

1. A. **CORRECT:** A child who is experiencing illness can have waning blood glucose levels. Frequent monitoring of blood glucose levels is done to identify hyperglycemic or hypoglycemic episodes.
   B. A child who is experiencing illness should continue taking insulin during to prevent hyperglycemic episodes.
   C. A child who is experiencing illness should drink fluids without sugars.
   D. **CORRECT:** A child who is experiencing an illness should test their urine for ketones to assist in early detection of ketoacidosis.
   E. **CORRECT:** A child who is experiencing illness should notify the provider of blood glucose levels greater than 240 mg/dL to obtain further instructions in caring for the hyperglycemia.

   Ⓝ *NCLEX® Connection: Physiological Adaptation, Alterations in Body Systems*

2. A. A child who has diabetes should eat three meals per day with snacks and avoid skipping meals to prevent hypoglycemic episodes.
   B. The insulin requirements of a child who has type 1 diabetes will decrease with exercise. Increasing the amount of insulin with exercise could precipitate a hypoglycemic episode.
   C. **CORRECT:** An early manifestation of hypoglycemia is irritability. Drinking a glass of milk, which is approximately 15 g of carbohydrates, indicates understanding of the teaching.
   D. Regular insulin should be drawn up into the syringe prior to drawing up NPH to avoid altering the regular insulin.

   Ⓝ *NCLEX® Connection: Physiological Adaptation, Alterations in Body Systems*

3. A. Diabetic ketoacidosis is classified as a blood glucose level greater than 300 mg/dL.
   B. Children who have diabetic ketoacidosis display weight loss.
   C. **CORRECT:** Children who have diabetic ketoacidosis experience osmotic diuresis because of the electrolyte shift.
   D. **CORRECT:** Children who have diabetic ketoacidosis experience mental confusion because of the electrolyte shift.
   E. **CORRECT:** Children who have diabetic ketoacidosis experience fruity breath because of the body's attempt to eliminate ketones.

   Ⓝ *NCLEX® Connection: Physiological Adaptation, Medical Emergencies*

4. A. Instruct the child to inject the needle at a 90° angle.
   B. Instruct the child to not mix glargine with any other insulin due to incompatibility.
   C. Instruct the child that it is not necessary to aspirate for blood prior to administering insulin.
   D. **CORRECT:** Instruct the child to administer four to six injections about 2.5 cm (1 in) apart before switching to another site.

   Ⓝ *NCLEX® Connection: Pharmacological Therapies, Medication Administration*

5. A. An increase in urination is a manifestation of hyperglycemia.
   B. **CORRECT:** Hunger is a manifestation of hypoglycemia because of the increased adrenergic nervous system activity.
   C. Monitor for poor skin turgor due to dehydration as a manifestation of hyperglycemia.
   D. **CORRECT:** Irritability is a manifestation of hypoglycemia because of the depleted glucose in the CNS.
   E. **CORRECT:** Sweating and pallor are manifestations of hypoglycemia because of the increased adrenergic nervous system activity.
   F. Kussmaul respirations are a manifestation of hyperglycemia.

   Ⓝ *NCLEX® Connection: Reduction of Risk Potential, Alterations in Body Systems*

Active Learning Scenario Key

Using the ATI Active Learning Template: System Disorder

ALTERATION IN HEALTH (DIAGNOSIS): Diabetes mellitus is characterized by a partial or complete metabolic deficiency of insulin.

MEDICATIONS
- Insulin lispro: Rapid-acting
- Regular insulin: Short-acting
- NPH insulin: Intermediate-acting
- Insulin glargine U-100: Long-acting

NURSING CARE
- Monitor for manifestations of hyperglycemia and hypoglycemia.
- Provide nail care according to policy.
- Reinforce teaching about wound care.
- Provide nutritional guidelines.
- Encourage yearly eye exams.
- Encourage dental and medical follow-up.
- Instruct self-monitoring of blood glucose.
- Reinforce teaching about guidelines to follow when sick.
- Reinforce teaching about medications.

CLIENT EDUCATION
- The child will have blood glucose levels within the prescribed range.
- The child will maintain a glycosylated hemoglobin within the target range.
- The child and/or family will be able to administer insulin.
- The child and/or family will be able to monitor for complications and intervene as necessary.
- The child and/or family will maintain adequate dietary intake to support growth and development.

Ⓝ *NCLEX® Connection: Physiological Adaptation, Alterations in Body Systems*

UNIT 2   SYSTEM DISORDERS

SECTION: ENDOCRINE DISORDERS

CHAPTER 33   *Growth Hormone Deficiency*

Human growth hormone (GH), somatotropin, is a naturally-occurring substance that is secreted by the pituitary gland. GH is important for normal growth, development, and cellular metabolism. A deficiency in GH prevents somatic growth throughout the body.

Other hormones that work with GH to control metabolic processes include adrenocorticotropic hormone (ACTH), thyroid stimulating hormone (TSH), and the gonadotropins: follicle-stimulating hormone and luteinizing hormone.

Hypopituitarism is the diminished or deficient secretion of pituitary hormones (primarily GH). Consequences of the condition depend on the degree of the deficiency.

DATA COLLECTION

RISK FACTORS

- Structural factors (tumors, trauma, structural defects, surgery)
- Heredity disorders
- Other pituitary hormone deficiencies (deficiencies of TSH or ACTH)
- Most often, GH deficiencies are idiopathic

EXPECTED FINDINGS

PHYSICAL FINDINGS
- Short stature but proportional height and weight
- Delayed epiphyseal closure
- Increased insulin sensitivity
- Delayed dentition
- Underdeveloped jaw
- Delayed sexual development
- Linear growth velocity consistently less than –1 standard deviation (SD) for age, or an absolute height of less than –2 SD

LABORATORY TESTS

Plasma insulin–like growth factor–1 (IGF–1) and IGF binding protein–3 (IGFBP–3) levels

Further evaluation is indicated if the values are one standard deviation below the expected mean for age.

NURSING ACTIONS
- Collect the specified amount of blood for the test.
- Explain the laboratory procedure to the family and child.

CLIENT EDUCATION: The child should fast the night before the test. Qpcc

DIAGNOSTIC PROCEDURES

GH stimulation

GH stimulation testing is generally done for children who have a low level of IGF-1 and IGFBP-3, and short stature.

NURSING ACTIONS
- Draw baseline blood sample between 0600 and 0800.
- Administer medication that triggers the release of GH (arginine or GH–releasing hormone).
- Obtain blood sample every 30 min for a 3-hr period following medication administration

CLIENT EDUCATION
- Nothing to eat or drink 10 to 12 hr before the test.
- Limit physical activity 10 to 12 hr before the test.

Radiologic evaluations

- Determine skeletal maturity by comparing epiphyseal centers to age-appropriate published standards.
- A general skeletal survey is done in children under 3 years of age; older children should have radiographs of the hands and wrists. This will provide information about growth as well as epiphyseal function.
- A series of skull films can detect structural abnormalities (small sella turcica).

NURSING ACTIONS: Assist in positioning the child.

Computed tomographic scanning, magnetic resonance imaging

Used to identify tumors or other brain lesions

NURSING ACTIONS: Monitor the child during the procedure.

CLIENT EDUCATION: Provide emotional support. Qpcc

Evaluation of the growth curve

NURSING ACTIONS
- Accurately obtain and plot height and weight measurements on a recommended growth chart.
- Determine height velocity or height over time.
- Determine height-to-weight relationship.
- Project target height in context of genetic potential.

PATIENT-CENTERED CARE

NURSING CARE

- The child's height and weight are measured and marked on a growth chart as part of every visit to the provider.
  - The height of a child is more affected than weight. Bone age usually matches height age.
  - Measure children who are younger than 3 years of age at least every 6 months and children older than 3 years of age every year.
- Monitor effectiveness of GH replacement. GH is supplied by recombinant DNA technology.
- Assist with administration of other hormone replacements (thyroid hormone) if prescribed.
- Provide support to the child and family regarding psychosocial concerns (altered body image, depression). Reassure the child and family that there are no cognitive delays or deficits.
- Stress the importance of maintaining realistic expectations based on the child's age and abilities.

MEDICATIONS

Somatropin

Used as a human growth hormone that is a replacement for deficiency and growth failure

NURSING ACTIONS
- Administer the medication via subcutaneous injections into the abdomen, thigh, or buttock.
- Use cautiously in children who are receiving insulin.
- Rotate injection sites to prevent tissue atrophy.

INTERPROFESSIONAL CARE

- Consult with an endocrinologist.
- Recommend psychological counseling to help the child and family cope during this period of time.

CLIENT EDUCATION

- There should not be any significant adverse effects when GH replacement therapy is used in appropriate doses for GH deficiency.
- GH will assist with muscle growth and help improve self-esteem.
- Understand home administration of medication by subcutaneous injection. Qpcc
- Instruct the child and guardians that GH should be administered 6 to 7 days a week.
- Reinforce teaching with the guardians on the need for compliance with injections.
- Encourage the child and family to seek evaluation during early adulthood to determine the need for continued replacement therapy.
- Child, family, and health care team make the decision to stop treatment together. Expected growth is 5 cm/year; therefore, if growth is not equal to or greater than 2.5 cm/year, treatment is discontinued.

COMPLICATIONS

GH deficiency without hormone replacement can result in disruption of vertical growth, delayed epiphyseal closure, retarded bone age, delayed sexual development, and premature aging later in life.

Application Exercises

1. A nurse is caring for a child who has short stature. Which of the following diagnostic tests should the nurse expect to confirm a growth hormone (GH) deficiency? (Select all that apply.)

   A. CT scan of the head

   B. Skeletal x-rays

   C. GH stimulation test

   D. Blood IGF-1

   E. DNA testing

2. A nurse is reinforcing teaching with the guardian of a child who has a growth hormone deficiency. Which of the following complications of untreated growth hormone deficiency should the nurse include? (Select all that apply.)

   A. Delayed sexual development

   B. Premature aging

   C. Advanced bone age

   D. Short stature

   E. Increased epiphyseal closure

3. A parent of a school-age child who has GH deficiency asks the nurse how long the child will need to take injections for growth delay. Which of the following responses should the nurse make?

   A. "Injections are usually continued until age 10 for girls and age 12 for boys."

   B. "Injections continue until your child reaches the fifth percentile on the growth chart."

   C. "Injections might be stopped once your child grows less than 1 inch/year."

   D. "The injections will need to be administered throughout your child's entire life."

4. A nurse is collecting data from a child who has short stature. Which of the following findings would indicate a growth hormone deficiency?

   A. Proportional height to weight

   B. Height proportionally greater than weight

   C. Oversized jaw

   D. Early-onset puberty

Active Learning Scenario

A nurse is contributing to the plan of care for a child who is to undergo a growth hormone (GH) stimulation test. What interventions should the nurse include? Use the ATI Active Learning Template: Nursing Skill to complete this item.

NURSING INTERVENTIONS: Include two preprocedure nursing actions and three intraprocedure actions.

Application Exercises Key

1. A. **CORRECT:** A CT scan of the head is conducted to determine whether there is a structural component to the short stature.
   B. **CORRECT:** Skeletal x-rays are conducted to determine the development of the bones.
   C. **CORRECT:** A GH stimulation test is conducted to confirm diagnosis of GH deficiency.
   D. **CORRECT:** A blood IGF-1 is obtained as a preliminary test to determine GH deficiency.
   E. DNA testing is not a diagnostic test to determine GH deficiency.

   Ⓝ *NCLEX® Connection: Reduction of Risk Potential, Diagnostic Tests*

2. A. **CORRECT:** A complication of untreated growth hormone deficiency includes delayed sexual development.
   B. **CORRECT:** A complication of untreated growth hormone deficiency includes premature aging.
   C. A complication of untreated growth hormone deficiency includes retarded bone age.
   D. **CORRECT:** A complication of untreated growth hormone deficiency includes short stature.
   E. A complication of untreated growth hormone deficiency includes delayed epiphyseal closure.

   Ⓝ *NCLEX® Connection: Physiological Adaptation, Alterations in Body Systems*

3. A. Standards for stopping therapy include a bone age of more than 14 years for females or more than 16 years for males.
   B. While the child's growth is tracked on growth charts, stopping treatment is not based on percentile markings.
   C. **CORRECT:** Treatment usually stops when the child grows less than 1 inch per year and has reached required bone maturity.
   D. Injections are stopped once sufficient growth is obtained, which will be variable among clients.

   Ⓝ *NCLEX® Connection: Pharmacological Therapies, Expected Actions/Outcomes*

4. A. **CORRECT:** Children who have growth hormone deficiency present with short stature with proportional height and weight.
   B. Height greater than weight is unexpected.
   C. An underdeveloped jaw is an expected finding.
   D. Delayed sexual development is an expected finding.

   Ⓝ *NCLEX® Connection: Physiological Adaptation, Basic Pathophysiology*

Active Learning Scenario Key

Using the ATI Active Learning Template: Nursing Skill

NURSING INTERVENTIONS

Preprocedure
- Ensure child has nothing to eat or drink 10 to 12 hr prior to procedure.
- Limit child's activity 10 to 12 hr prior to procedure.

Intraprocedure
- Draw baseline blood sample between 0600 and 0800.
- Administer medication that triggers the release of GH (arginine or GH-releasing hormone).
- Obtain blood sample every 30 min during a 3-hr period following medication administration.

Ⓝ *NCLEX® Connection: Reduction of Risk Potential, Diagnostic Tests*

ⓝ NCLEX® Connections

When reviewing the following chapters, keep in mind the relevant topics and tasks of the NCLEX outline, in particular:

Safety and Infection Control

STANDARD PRECAUTIONS/TRANSMISSION-BASED PRECAUTIONS/SURGICAL ASEPSIS
Identify communicable diseases and modes of transmission.

Identify client knowledge of infection control procedures.

Apply principles of infection control.

Health Promotion and Maintenance

HEALTH PROMOTION/DISEASE PREVENTION
Identify clients in need of immunizations.

Identify precautions and contraindications to immunizations.

Assist client in disease prevention activities.

HIGH RISK BEHAVIORS: Reinforce client teaching
related to client high risk behavior.

Basic Care and Comfort

NON-PHARMACOLOGICAL COMFORT INTERVENTIONS:
Provide non–pharmacological measures for pain relief.

Pharmacological Therapies

MEDICATION ADMINISTRATION: Administer a
subcutaneous, intradermal, or intramuscular medication.

Reduction of Risk Potential

THERAPEUTIC PROCEDURES: Reinforce client
teaching on treatments and procedures.

Physiological Adaptation

ALTERATIONS IN BODY SYSTEMS: Reinforce
education to client regarding care and condition.

BASIC PATHOPHYSIOLOGY

Identify signs and symptoms related to an acute or chronic illness.

Consider general principles of client disease process when
providing care (injury and repair, immunity, cellular structure).

Apply knowledge of pathophysiology to monitoring
client for alterations in body systems.

UNIT 2 SYSTEM DISORDERS
  SECTION: IMMUNE AND INFECTIOUS DISORDERS

CHAPTER 34 *Immunizations*

Administration of a vaccine stimulates the immune system to produce antibodies against a specific disease. Vaccines contain the infectious organism, but it is either killed or weakened to prevent causing the disease. Antibodies disappear after they destroy the infection/antigen, but memory cells are formed to protect from future exposures to that same infection. This builds immunity against that antigen to protect against future exposure.

The Advisory Committee on Immunization Practices (ACIP) makes recommendations and creates guidelines regarding immunizations. Children who are born preterm should receive the dose of each vaccine according to the immunization schedule. The most up-to-date information can be found at the Centers for Disease Control and Prevention website.

CHILDHOOD IMMUNIZATIONS

For children who have missed scheduled immunizations, use the "catch-up" schedule located on the CDC website. (34.1)

PURPOSE

- Decrease or eliminate certain infectious diseases in society.
- Prevent infectious diseases and their complications.

34.1 Childhood immunizations

MINIMUM AGE	NUMBER OF DOSES	SCHEDULE	CONSIDERATIONS
Hepatitis B (HepB)			
Birth	Three	Birth 1 to 2 months 6 to 18 months	Minimum of 4 weeks between doses one and two. Minimum of 8 weeks between doses two and three. Final dose no earlier than age of 24 weeks of age and at least 16 weeks after first dose. Should be withheld for infants born prematurely and weighing less than 2,000 g if the mother is negative for hepatitis B.
Rotavirus (RV)			
6 weeks	Two (RV1) or Three (RV5)	2 and 4 months (Rotarix [RV1]) or 2, 4, and 6 months (RotaTeq [RV5])	Maximum age for the first dose is 24 weeks, 6 days. Maximum age for the last dose is 8 months, 0 days. Series should not be initiated for children 15 weeks, 0 days or older.
Diphtheria, tetanus, and acellular pertussis (DTaP)			
6 weeks	Five	2 months 4 months 6 months 15 to 18 months 4 to 6 years	Minimum of 6 months between doses three and four. Dose four can be given as early as 12 months of age Dose five dose is not needed if dose four was given at 4 years of age or older.
Tetanus, diphtheria, and acellular pertussis (Tdap); tetanus and diphtheria (Td)			
11 years	One (Tdap) Every 10 years (Td)	11 to 12 years then Booster every 10 years (Td)	Administer one dose to adolescents who are pregnant (with each pregnancy) regardless of timing of previous Td or Tdap vaccine (between 27 and 36 weeks of gestation). Booster with Td every 10 years after administration of Tdap. Administer Tdap or Td according to recommendations for wounds other than clean, minor if 5 years or longer since previous dose of tetanus toxoid.

34.1 Childhood immunizations (continued)

MINIMUM AGE	NUMBER OF DOSES	SCHEDULE	CONSIDERATIONS
Haemophilus influenzae type b (Hib)			
6 weeks (all except Hiberix) 12 months (Hiberix)	Four (ActHIB, MenHibrix, or Pentacel) or Three (PedvaxHib or COMVAX)	2 months 4 months 6 months (only if four-dose series) 12 to 15 months (booster dose with any Hib-containing vaccine)	Administer Hiberix as a booster dose at 12 months to 4 years of age only if a prior dose of Hib was received. Only 1 dose is recommended for children who are 15 months of age or older, and not immunized.
Pneumococcal conjugate (PCV13)			
6 weeks	Four	2 months 4 months 6 months 12 to 15 months	Administer a one-time dose of PCV13 to children who are 24 to 59 months of age and received age-appropriate dosing with PCV7. Follow current recommendations for dual vaccination series with PCV13 and PPSV23 for children who have high-risk conditions.
Inactivated poliovirus (IPV)			
6 weeks	Four	2 months 4 months 6 to 18 months 4 to 6 years	Final dose should be administered on or after the age of 4 years and at least 6 months from the previous dose.
Inactivated influenza vaccine (IIV)			
6 months	Yearly	Yearly	Must be 2 years or older to receive live, attenuated influenza vaccine (LAIV). Children who have medical conditions that predispose them to influenza should not receive LAIV. Administer starting with availability, usually in early fall. Administration recommendations can change yearly because the vaccine is created with different influenza strains each year.
Measles, mumps, rubella (MMR)			
12 months	Two	12 to 15 months 4 to 6 years	Administer one dose to infants age 6 to 11 months if traveling internationally. However, a two-dose series is still recommended starting at 12 to 15 months. Dose two of the series can be given prior to the age of 4 years if it has been at least 4 weeks since the first dose.
Varicella (VAR)			
12 months	Two	12 to 15 months 4 to 6 years	Dose two of the series can be given prior to the age of 4 years if it has been at least 3 months since the first dose.
Hepatitis A (HepA)			
12 months	Two	12 to 23 months 6 to 18 months following	Administer the final dose 6 to 18 months after the first. Two-dose series is recommended for anyone over the age of 2 years who needs immunity to hepatitis A virus.
Meningococcal conjugate (MenACWY)			
2 months (MenACWY-CRM) 9 months (MenACWY-D)	One	11 to 12 years 16 years (booster)	Follow recommendations for earlier administration to children who have high-risk conditions or who travel to areas with hyperendemic or epidemic rates of meningococcal disease.
Meningococcal (MenB)			
10 years	Two or three dose series	16 to 18 years	Maximum age 23 years. Administer 2 doses of Bexsero at least 1 month apart. Trumenba is given in 2 doses at least 6 months apart; clients who have certain risk factors should receive 3 doses of Trumenba at 0, 1 to 2 months, and 6 months time spacing.
Human papillomavirus (HPV)			
9 years	Two or three dose series	11 to 12 years 6 to 12 months following	9v-HPV is vaccine approved through 45 years of age. If first dose after the 16th birthday, give the second dose at least 4 weeks later, and the third dose at least 12 weeks after the second (at least 6 months after the first).

34.2 Immunization considerations

ADVERSE EFFECTS	CONTRAINDICATIONS	PRECAUTIONS
DTaP		
Mild • Redness, swelling, and tenderness at the injection site • Poor appetite • Vomiting • Low fever • Behavioral changes (drowsiness, irritability, anorexia) **Moderate** • Inconsolable crying for 3 hr or more • Fever 40.6° C (105° F) or higher • Seizures (with or without fever) • Shock-like state Severe: Acute encephalopathy (rare)	Occurrence of encephalopathy within 7 days following prior doses of the vaccine	Occurrence of Guillain-Barré syndrome within 6 weeks of prior dose of tetanus toxoid Progressive neurologic disorders; uncontrolled seizures Fever 40.6° C (105° F) or higher within 48 hr of prior dose Shock-like state within 48 hr of prior dose Seizures within 3 days of prior dose Inconsolable crying for 3 hr or more within 48 hr of prior dose
Hib		
Redness, swelling, warmth, and tenderness at the injection site Fever greater than 37.8° C (101° F), vomiting, diarrhea, and crying	Age younger than 6 weeks	
RV		
Irritability Mild, temporary diarrhea or vomiting Intussusception	History of intussusception Severe combined immunodeficiency (SCID), which is a rare disorder that is inherited	Chronic gastrointestinal disease Spina bifida Bladder exstrophy Immunocompromised (other than SCID)
MMR		
Mild: Local reactions (rash; fever; swollen glands in cheeks and/or neck) **Moderate** • Pain at the site of the injection • Joint pain and stiffness lasting for days to weeks • Febrile seizure • Low platelet count **Severe** • Transient thrombocytopenia • Deafness • Long-term seizures • Brain damage	Pregnancy Immunodeficiency	History of thrombocytopenia or thrombocytopenic purpura Anaphylactic reaction to eggs, gelatin, or neomycin Transfusion with blood product containing antibodies within the prior 3 months Simultaneous tuberculin skin testing
VAR		
Mild • Tenderness and swelling at injection site • Fever • Rash (mild) possible for up to 1 month after vaccination **Moderate:** Seizures **Severe** • Pneumonia • Low blood count (extremely rare) • Severe brain reactions (extremely rare)	Pregnancy Anaphylactic reaction to gelatin or neomycin	Transfusion with blood product containing antibodies within the prior 3 to 11 months Treatment with antiviral medication within 24 hr prior to immunization (avoid taking antivirals for 14 days following immunization) Treatment with immunosuppressants (corticosteroids) for 2 weeks or longer Cancer Aspirin or products containing aspirin
PCV13		
Swelling, redness and tenderness at site of injection Fever Irritability Drowsiness Anorexia Headache Chills	Anaphylactic reaction to any vaccine containing diphtheria toxoid; yeast	

ADVERSE EFFECTS	CONTRAINDICATIONS	PRECAUTIONS
HepA		
Tenderness at the injection site Headache Anorexia Malaise Low grade fever	Severe allergy to latex	Pregnancy
HepB		
Tenderness at the injection site Temperature of 37.7° C (99.9° F) or higher	Anaphylactic allergy to yeast	Infant weight less than 2 kg (4 lb, 6.4 oz)
IIV		
Mild: • Swelling, redness and tenderness at the injection site • Hoarseness • Fever • Malaise • Headache • Cough • Aches Severe: • Increased risk for Guillain-Barré syndrome • Increased risk of seizures in young children receiving PCV13 and/or DTaP simultaneously		Occurrence of Guillain-Barré syndrome within 6 weeks of prior influenza vaccine Moderate or severe acute illness
LAIV		
Vomiting, diarrhea Cough Fever Headache Myalgia Nasal congestion, runny nose Wheezing Sore throat	Age less than 2 years Pregnancy	Occurrence of Guillain-Barré syndrome within 6 weeks of prior influenza vaccine History of asthma for greater than 5 years Treatment with antiviral medication within 48 hr prior to immunization (avoid taking antivirals for 14 days following immunization) Certain chronic conditions ACIP recommends the option of the LAIV to clients regardless of the severity of egg allergy. Clients who have a history of an egg allergy, other than a hive-only reaction, should receive the immunization where a provider is present and emergency equipment is available. (At the time of publication these recommendations are awaiting approval by the CDC. Please refer to CDC's website for the current approval status.)
MenACWY		
Redness and tenderness at the injection site Fever Joint pain		
MenB		
Injection site pain Headache Fatigue Muscle pain	Prior hypersensitivity Bexsero: latex allergy (prefilled syringes contain latex)	Use Bexsero in pregnancy only if clearly indicated; add client to pregnancy registry. Trumenba safety is not established for children under 10 years of age.
HPV9		
Redness, swelling and tenderness at the injection site Mild to moderate fever Headache Fainting (shortly after receiving the vaccine)	Severe allergy to yeast	Pregnancy
IPV		
Tenderness at the injection site	Anaphylactic reaction to neomycin, streptomycin or polymyxin B	Pregnancy

COMPLICATIONS, CONTRAINDICATIONS, AND PRECAUTIONS

- A severe allergic reaction (anaphylaxis) can occur in response to any vaccine and is a contraindication for receiving further doses of that vaccine or other vaccines containing that substance. Q EBP
- Moderate or severe illnesses with or without fever are precautions to receiving immunizations.
- The common cold and other minor illnesses are not contraindications to immunizations.
- Severe febrile illness is a contraindication to all immunizations.
- Do not administer live virus vaccines (varicella or MMR) to a child who is severely immunocompromised, pregnant, or has received treatment that provide acquired passive immunity (blood products) within 3 months.
- Precautions to immunizations require providers to analyze data and weigh the risks that come with immunizing or not immunizing. (34.2)

NURSING ADMINISTRATION

- Assist with obtaining consent from the child's legal guardian prior to administration.
- Prior to administration, provide vaccine information sheets (VIS) and review the content with legal guardians and older children. Include the publication date of each VIS given in documentation.
- Reassure guardians that there is no association of autism with the MMR vaccine.
- Give IM immunizations in the vastus lateralis or ventrogluteal muscle in infants and young children, and into the deltoid muscle for older children and adolescents.
- Give subcutaneous injections in the outer aspect of the upper arm or anterolateral thigh.
- Select needle size based on the route, site, age, and amount of medication. Adequate needle length reduces the incidence of swelling and tenderness at the injection site. Q PCC
- Use strategies to minimize discomfort.
  - Provide distraction.
  - Apply a topical anesthetic prior to injection.
  - Give infants a concentrated oral sucrose solution 2 min prior to, during, and 3 min after immunization administration.
  - Use non-nutritive sucking (pacifiers) during procedure.
- Have emergency medications and equipment on standby in case the child experiences an allergic response (anaphylaxis [rare]).

- Encourage caregivers to use comforting measures during and after the procedure (applying cool compresses to injection site, gentle movement of involved extremity).
- Provide praise afterward.
- Apply a colorful bandage, if appropriate.
- Document the administration of the vaccine.
  - Date, route, and site of immunization
  - Type, manufacturer, lot number, and expiration date of the vaccine
  - Evidence of informed consent from the legal guardian
  - Name, address and title of administering nurse
- Encourage guardians to maintain up-to-date immunizations for the child.
- Instruct guardians to avoid administering aspirin to the child to treat fever or local reaction following administration of a live virus vaccine due to the risk of developing Reye syndrome.
- Instruct the family to observe for complications and notify the provider if adverse effects occur.
- Report any adverse reactions to the Vaccine Adverse Event Reporting System (VAERS).

NURSING EVALUATION OF MEDICATION EFFECTIVENESS

Depending on therapeutic intent, effectiveness can be evidenced by the following.
- Improvement of local reaction to immunization with absence of pain, fever, and swelling at the site of injection
- Development of immunity

Active Learning Scenario

A nurse is preparing to administer LAIV, 9v-HPV, and MenACWY to a 12-year-old client. Use the ATI Active Learning Template: Medication to complete this item.

COMPLICATIONS: Include adverse effects for each vaccine.

Application Exercises

1. A nurse is preparing to administer immunizations to a 4-month-old infant. Which of the following actions should the nurse take to provide atraumatic care?

   A. Administer 81 mg of aspirin.

   B. Use the Z-track method when injecting.

   C. Ask the guardians to leave the room during the injection.

   D. Provide sucrose solution on the pacifier.

2. A nurse is planning to administer recommended immunizations to a 2-month-old infant. Which of the following vaccines should the nurse plan to give? (Select all that apply.)

   A. Rotavirus (RV)

   B. Diphtheria, tetanus, and acellular pertussis (DTaP)

   C. *Haemophilus influenzae* type b (Hib)

   D. Hepatitis A (HepA)

   E. Pneumococcal conjugate (PCV13)

   F. Inactivated poliovirus (IPV)

3. A nurse is planning to administer recommended immunizations to a 4-year-old child. Which of the following vaccines should the nurse plan to give? (Select all that apply.)

   A. Inactivated poliovirus (IPV)

   B. *Haemophilus influenzae* type b (Hib)

   C. Measles, mumps, rubella (MMR)

   D. Varicella (VAR)

   E. Hepatitis B (HepB)

   F. Diphtheria, tetanus, and acellular pertussis (DTaP)

4. A nurse is preparing to administer the varicella vaccine to an adolescent. Which of the following questions should the nurse ask to determine whether there is a contraindication to administering the vaccine?

   A. "Do you have an allergy to eggs?"

   B. "Have you ever had encephalopathy following immunizations?"

   C. "Are you currently taking corticosteroid medication?"

   D. "Have you ever had an anaphylactic reaction to yeast?"

5. A nurse is caring for a 15-month-old child in a clinic. Which of the following actions should the nurse take? (See the chart for additional client information.)

   ### IMMUNIZATION RECORD

   HepB: 1 month, 2 months, 12 months

   Rotavirus: 2 months, 4 months, 6 months

   DTaP: 2 months, 4 months, 6 months

   Hib: 2 months, 4 months, 12 months

   IPV: 2 months, 4 months, 6 months

   MMR: 12 months

   Varicella: 12 months

   HepA: 12 months

   ### NURSES NOTES

   Temperature: 37.8° C (100.1° F)

   Sore throat

   Family history of seizures

   A. Administer DTaP vaccine.

   B. Administer rotavirus vaccine.

   C. Hold immunizations until fever subsides.

   D. Administer hepatitis A vaccine.

Application Exercises Key

1. A. Administering aspirin to the infant can increase his risk for developing Reye syndrome.
   B. Using the Z-track method is not recommended with immunizations.
   C. Separating the guardians from the infant can produce anxiety in the infant.
   D. **CORRECT:** Allowing an infant to suck on a pacifier with sucrose solution can decrease pain with immunizations and is an appropriate action for the nurse to take in providing atraumatic care.

   Ⓝ *NCLEX® Connection: Basic Care and Comfort, Non-Pharmacological Comfort Interventions*

2. A. **CORRECT:** RV is given as a two-or three-dose series starting at 2 months of age.
   B. **CORRECT:** DTaP is given as a five-dose series starting at 2 months of age.
   C. **CORRECT:** Hib is given as a three-or four-dose series starting at 2 months of age.
   D. HepA is given as a two-dose series starting at 12 months of age.
   E. **CORRECT:** PCV13 is given as a four-dose series starting at 2 months of age.
   F. **CORRECT:** IPV is given as a four-dose series starting at 2 months of age.

   Ⓝ *NCLEX® Connection: Health Promotion and Maintenance, Health Promotion/Disease Prevention*

3. A. **CORRECT:** Four doses of IPV are given during childhood with a dose given at 4 years of age.
   B. The series of Hib vaccines is complete by the age of 15 months.
   C. **CORRECT:** Two doses of MMR are given during childhood with a dose given at 4 years of age.
   D. **CORRECT:** Two doses of VAR are given during childhood with a dose given at 4 years of age.
   E. The series of HepB vaccines is complete by the age of 18 months.
   F. **CORRECT:** Five doses of DTaP are given during childhood with a dose given at 4 years of age.

   Ⓝ *NCLEX® Connection: Health Promotion and Maintenance, Health Promotion/Disease Prevention*

4. A. The varicella vaccine is contraindicated for clients who have an allergy to gelatin or neomycin.
   B. DTaP vaccine is contraindicated for clients who have a history of encephalopathy within 7 days following prior doses of the vaccine.
   C. **CORRECT:** Varicella vaccine is contraindicated for clients who have been taking corticosteroids or other medications that affect the immune system for 2 weeks or longer.
   D. HepB vaccine is contraindicated for clients who have had an anaphylactic reaction to yeast.

   Ⓝ *NCLEX® Connection: Health Promotion and Maintenance, Health Promotion/Disease Prevention*

5. A. **CORRECT:** Five diphtheria, tetanus, and acellular pertussis immunizations are given during childhood, with one at 15 months of age.
   B. This child completed the three-dose rotavirus vaccine series at age 6 months.
   C. Temperature of 37.8° C (100.1° F) is not a contraindication to administering immunizations.
   D. Two hepatitis A immunizations are given during childhood, with the second one 6 to 18 months after the first.

   Ⓝ *NCLEX® Connection: Health Promotion and Maintenance, Health Promotion/Disease Prevention*

Active Learning Scenario Key

Using the ATI Active Learning Template: Medication

COMPLICATIONS

LAIV
- Allergic reaction
- Vomiting and/or diarrhea
- Cough
- Fever
- Headache
- Myalgia
- Nasal congestion/runny nose

9v-HPV
- Redness, swelling and tenderness at the injection site
- Mild to moderate fever
- Headache
- Fatigue
- Fainting (shortly after receiving the vaccine)

MenACWY
- Allergic reaction
- Redness and tenderness at the injection site
- Fever

Ⓝ *NCLEX® Connection: Health Promotion and Maintenance, Health Promotion/Disease Prevention*

UNIT 2   SYSTEM DISORDERS

SECTION: IMMUNE AND INFECTIOUS DISORDERS

CHAPTER 35 *Communicable Diseases*

Communicable diseases are spread through airborne, droplet, or direct contact transmission. Most communicable diseases can be prevented with immunizations.

Antibiotics and antitoxins reduce serious complications. Primary prevention refers to immunizations. Secondary prevention controls the spread of the disease to others.

See immunization recommendations at the CDC website.

HEALTH PROMOTION AND DISEASE PREVENTION

Conjunctivitis

SPREAD: Direct contact (viral and bacterial)

INCUBATION: Depends on the infection

COMMUNICABILITY
- Viral: Appears secondary to a viral infection; starts in one eye and then spreads to the other, clears on its own in 7 to 14 days.
- Bacterial: Caused by certain bacteria, clears with topical antibiotics
- Allergic: Occurs in people who have other allergic conditions; clears with allergy medications.

Epstein-Barr virus (EBV)/mononucleosis

SPREAD: Saliva

INCUBATION: 30 to 50 days

COMMUNICABILITY
- Healthy people can carry EBV in saliva, transmitting the virus for a lifetime.
- People who have mononucleosis can transmit for weeks.

Erythema infectiosum (fifth disease)/parvovirus B19

SPREAD
- Droplet
- Blood

INCUBATION: 4 to 14 days, sometimes up to 21 days

COMMUNICABILITY: Onset of manifestations before rash appears

Mumps/paramyxovirus (35.1)

SPREAD
- Direct contact
- Droplet

INCUBATION: 14 to 21 days

COMMUNICABILITY: Immediately before and after swelling begins

Pertussis (whooping cough)/Bordetella pertussis

SPREAD
- Direct contact
- Droplet
- Indirect contact with freshly contaminated articles

INCUBATION: 6 to 20 days, usually 7 to 10 days

COMMUNICABILITY: Greatest during catarrhal stage before onset of paroxysmal stage

Rubella (German measles)/rubella virus

SPREAD
- Direct contact
- Droplet

INCUBATION: 14 to 21 days

COMMUNICABILITY: 7 days before to 5 days after the rash appears

Rubeola (measles)/rubeola virus

SPREAD
- Direct contact
- Droplet (airborne)

INCUBATION: 10 to 20 days

COMMUNICABILITY: 4 days before to 5 days after the rash appears

Varicella (chickenpox)/ varicella-zoster virus

SPREAD
- Direct contact
- Droplet (airborne)
- Contaminated objects

INCUBATION: 2 to 3 weeks, usually 14 to 16 days

COMMUNICABILITY: 1 to 2 days before lesions appear and until all the lesions have formed crusts

DATA COLLECTION

RISK FACTORS

- History of communicable disease
- Immunocompromised status
- Crowded living conditions
- Poor sanitation
- Poor nutrition
- Poor oxygenation and impaired circulation
- Chronic illness
- Recent exposure to a known case of a communicable disease
- Not immunized or up-to-date on immunizations
- Prodromal manifestations

EXPECTED FINDINGS

Conjunctivitis

- Pink or red color in the sclera of the eyes
- Swelling of the conjunctiva
- Excessive tearing
- Yellow-green, purulent discharge from the eyes (bacterial)
- Watery eye discharge (viral)
- Crusting of the eyelids in the morning (bacterial)

Fifth disease (Erythema infectiosum)

BEFORE RASH (SEVERAL DAYS): Fever, runny nose, headache

RASH (7 DAYS TO SEVERAL WEEKS)
- Red rash on face (slapped cheek) which disappears around day 1 to 4
- Maculopapular red spots symmetrically distributed on upper and lower extremities progressing proximal to distal surfaces through 1 week
- Secondary itchy rash that can appear on rest of body, especially on the soles of the feet

Measles (rubeola)

3 TO 4 DAYS PRIOR TO RASH
- Mild to moderate fever
- Conjunctivitis
- Fatigue
- Cough, runny nose, red eyes, sore throat

RASH
- Koplik spots (tiny white spots) appear in mouth 2 days before rash
- Red or reddish-brown rash beginning on the face spreading downward
- Spike in fever with rash

Epstein-Barr virus (EBV)/mononucleosis

- Fever
- Lethargy
- Sore throat
- Swollen lymph glands
- Loss of appetite
- Headache
- Increased WBC
- Atypical lymphocytes
- Splenomegaly
- Hepatic involvement

Mumps

- Painful, swollen parotid glands
- Fever and muscle aches
- Headache
- Earache made worse by chewing
- Fatigue and loss of appetite

Pertussis (whooping cough)

- Common cold manifestations: runny nose, congestion, sneezing, mild fever, mild cough (catarrhal stage)
- Severe coughing starts in 1 to 2 weeks (paroxysmal stage)
  - Coughing fits
  - Violent and rapid coughing
  - Loud "whooping" sound upon inspiration

Rubella (German measles)

- Low-grade fever and sore throat
- Headache
- Malaise
- Cough
- Lymphadenopathy
- Red rash that starts on the face and spreads to the rest of the body, lasting 2 to 3 days

Varicella (chickenpox)

MANIFESTATIONS 1 TO 2 DAYS PRIOR TO RASH
- Fever
- Fatigue
- Loss of appetite
- Headache

RASH
- Macules start in center of trunk, spreading to the face and proximal extremities.
- Progresses from macules, to papules, to vesicles, and crust formation follows.
- Scabs appear in approximately 1 week.

LABORATORY TESTS

- CBC
- Electrolyte panels
- Mono spot blood test for infectious mononucleosis

PATIENT-CENTERED CARE

NURSING CARE Qᴛᴄ

SYMPTOMATIC TREATMENT
- Administer an antipyretic for fever. Do not administer aspirin, due to the risk of Reye syndrome.
- Administer an antipruritic for severe itching.
- Administer analgesics for pain.
- Provide fluids and nutritious foods of the child's preference. Qᴘᴄᴄ
- Provide quiet diversional activities.
- Promote adequate rest with naps if necessary.
- Keep lights dim if the child develops photophobia.
- Keep the child out of the sun.
- Notify the child's school or day care center of the child's infection. Obtain a plan from the school so that the child can continue working on schoolwork at home.
- Notify the health department of communicable diseases.

SKIN CARE

- Provide calamine lotion for topical relief.
- Keep the skin clean and dry to prevent secondary infection.
- Keep the child cool, but prevent chilling.
- Dress the child in lightweight, loose clothing.
- Give baths in tepid water.
- Keep the child's fingernails clean and short.
- Apply mittens if the child scratches.
- Reinforce good oral hygiene. A sore throat can be managed with analgesics, lozenges, and saline rinses.
- Change linens daily.

ISOLATION PRECAUTIONS

- **Airborne/Contact:** Varicella, Measles
- **Droplet**
  ○ Fifth disease
  ○ Mumps
  ○ Pertussis
  ○ Rubella
- **Standard**
  ○ Conjunctivitis
  ○ Mononucleosis

MEDICATIONS

Antihistamine

Diphenhydramine hydrochloride and hydroxyzine used to control pruritus

NURSING ACTIONS

- Monitor the reaction to the medication, because some children can become hyperalert with the administration of a medication from this group.
- Monitor for drowsiness.
- Educate the family about safety precautions. Qs

Antibiotic or antiviral therapy

- Acyclovir for high-risk clients who have varicella
- Antibiotics for pertussis
- Antibiotic eye drops for bacterial conjunctivitis

NSAIDs or acetaminophen

Decreases fever

NURSING ACTIONS

- Be alert for allergies.
- Reinforce to guardians the proper dosing for acetaminophen. Qpcc

CLIENT EDUCATION Qpcc

- Good hand hygiene prevents the spread of infection.
- Adhere to the antibiotic or antiviral therapy.
- Cover the nose and mouth when coughing or sneezing.
- Wash bed linens daily in mild detergent.
- If immunocompromised, seek prompt medical care if manifestations develop.
- Adolescents can participate in decision-making.

COMPLICATIONS

Fifth disease: Self-limited arthritis and arthralgia (more common in adult females)

Mononucleosis: Ruptured spleen

Mumps: Orchitis, encephalitis, meningitis, oophoritis, mastitis, deafness, myocarditis, arthritis, hepatitis

Pertussis
- Infants and children: pneumonia, seizures, apnea, encephalopathy, death, ear infections, hemorrhage, weight loss, hernias
- Teens and adults: weight loss, loss of bladder control, syncope, rib fractures, pneumonia

Rubella
- Complications generally rare with this communicable disease
- Birth defects (deafness; heart defects; mental, liver, and spleen damage) in fetus of clients infected during pregnancy

Rubeola: Ear infections, pneumonia, encephalitis, death, laryngitis

Varicella: Pneumonia, bleeding problems, bacterial infection of the skin, encephalitis

Active Learning Scenario

A nurse is contributing to the plan of care for a group of clients who have communicable diseases. Use the ATI Active Learning Template: Basic Concept to complete this item.

RELATED CONTENT: List the communicable diseases that require more than standard isolation precautions during hospitalization.

NURSING INTERVENTIONS: Identify the type of isolation precaution to be implemented with the communicable disease identified above.

Active Learning Scenario Key

Using the ATI Active Learning Template: Basic Concept
RELATED CONTENT
- Varicella
- Rubella
- Fifth disease
- Pertussis
- Mumps

NURSING INTERVENTIONS
- Airborne/contact: Varicella
- Droplet: Rubella, fifth disease, pertussis, mumps

Ⓝ *NCLEX® Connection: Safety and Infection Control, Standard Precautions/Transmission-Based Precautions Surgical Asepsis*

Application Exercises

1. A nurse is reinforcing teaching with a group of family members about complications of communicable diseases. Which of the following communicable diseases can lead to pneumonia? (Select all that apply.)

   A. Rubella (German measles)

   B. Rubeola (measles)

   C. Pertussis (whooping cough)

   D. Varicella (chickenpox)

   E. Mumps

2. A nurse is caring for a client who has rubeola. The nurse should monitor for which of the following complications? (Select all that apply.)

   A. Otitis media

   B. Constipation

   C. Laryngitis

   D. Arthralgia

   E. Syncope

3. A nurse is collecting data from a client who has pertussis. Which of the following findings should the nurse expect? (Select all that apply.)

   A. Runny nose

   B. Mild fever

   C. Cough with whooping sound

   D. Swollen salivary glands

   E. Red rash

4. A nurse is reinforcing teaching with a group of family members about communicable diseases. The nurse should include that which of the following is the best method to prevent a communicable disease?

   A. Hand washing

   B. Avoiding persons who have active disease

   C. Covering your cough

   D. Obtaining immunizations

Application Exercises Key

1. A. Complications of rubella include birth defects (deafness; heart defects; mental, liver, and spleen damage) in the fetus of a client infected during pregnancy.
   B. **CORRECT:** Complications of rubeola include ear infections, pneumonia, diarrhea, encephalitis, and death.
   C. **CORRECT:** Complications of pertussis include pneumonia, convulsions, apnea, encephalopathy, and death in infants and children; and weight loss, loss of bladder control, syncope, and rib fractures in teens and adults.
   D. **CORRECT:** Complications of varicella include dehydration, pneumonia, bleeding problems, bacterial infection of the skin, sepsis, toxic shock syndrome, bone or joint infections, and death.
   E. Complications of mumps include orchitis, encephalitis, meningitis, oophoritis, mastitis, and deafness.

   Ⓝ *NCLEX® Connection: Safety and Infection Control, Standard Precautions/Transmission–Based Precautions Surgical Asepsis*

2. A. **CORRECT:** Otitis media is a complication of rubeola.
   B. Constipation is not a complication of rubeola.
   C. **CORRECT:** Laryngitis is a complication of rubeola.
   D. Arthralgia is a complication of fifth disease and mumps.
   E. Syncope is a complication of pertussis.

   Ⓝ *NCLEX® Connection: Physiological Adaptation, Basic Pathophysiology*

3. A. **CORRECT:** A client who has pertussis has coldlike manifestations, including runny nose, congestion, and mild fever.
   B. **CORRECT:** A client who has pertussis has coldlike manifestations, including runny nose, congestion, and mild fever.
   C. **CORRECT:** A client who has pertussis will experience coughing fits and a whooping sound.
   D. A client who has mumps will have enlarged lymph nodes.
   E. A client who has measles will have a red rash.

   Ⓝ *NCLEX® Connection: Physiological Adaptation, Basic Pathophysiology*

4. A. Hand washing will decrease the spread of infection. However, this is not the best method to prevent communicable disease.
   B. Avoiding people who have active disease will decrease the spread of infection. However, this is not the best method to prevent communicable disease.
   C. Covering coughs will decrease the spread of infection. However, this is not the best method to prevent communicable disease.
   D. **CORRECT:** Obtaining immunizations has decreased the rate of communicable diseases and is the best method to prevent further spread of illness.

   Ⓝ *NCLEX® Connection: Safety and Infection Control, Standard Precautions/Transmission–Based Precautions/Surgical Asepsis*

CHAPTER 36 *Acute Otitis Media*

Acute otitis media (AOM) is an infection of the structures of the middle ear. Otitis media with effusion (OME) is a collection of fluid in the middle ear but no infection.

Repeated infections can cause impaired hearing and speech. Many infections clear spontaneously in a few days. The majority of incidences are related to Eustachian tube malfunction.

DATA COLLECTION

RISK FACTORS

- Eustachian tubes in children are shorter and more horizontal than those of adults. Otitis media is most common in the first 24 months of life and again when children enter school (ages 5 to 6). Otitis media occurs infrequently after age 7.
- Otitis media is usually triggered by a bacterial infection (*Streptococcus pneumoniae, Haemophilus influenzae, Moraxella catarrhalis*), a viral infection (respiratory syncytial virus or influenza), allergies, or enlarged adenoids.
- There is a lower incidence of otitis media in infants who are breastfed possibly due to the presence of immunoglobulin A (IgA) in breasts and the semi-vertical feeding position of breastfed babies. Q_{EBP}
- Incidence is higher in the winter and spring months.
- Exposure to large numbers of children (day care).
- Exposure to secondhand smoke.
- Cleft lip and/or cleft palate.
- Noncompliance with childhood immunizations.
- Down syndrome.

EXPECTED FINDINGS

- Recent history of upper respiratory infection
- Acute onset of changes in behavior
- Frequent crying, irritability, and fussiness
- Inconsolability
- Tugging at ear
- Turning head from side to side
- Reports of ear pain, loss of appetite, nausea, and vomiting
- Fever

PHYSICAL FINDINGS
- **AOM**
  - Rubbing or pulling on ear
  - Crying
  - Lethargy
  - Bulging yellow or red tympanic membrane
  - Purulent material in middle ear or drainage from external canal
  - Decreased or no tympanic movement with pneumatic otoscopy
  - Lymphadenopathy of the neck and head
  - Temperature: can be as high as 40° C (104° F)
  - Hearing difficulties and speech delays if otitis media becomes a chronic condition
- **OME**
  - Feeling of fullness in the ear
  - Orange discoloration of the tympanic membrane with decreased movement
  - Vague findings including rhinitis, cough, and diarrhea
  - Transient hearing loss and balance disturbances

DIAGNOSTIC PROCEDURES

Pneumatic otoscope

A pneumatic otoscope is used to visualize the tympanic membrane and middle ear structures. The otoscope also evaluates tympanic membrane movement.

NURSING ACTIONS: Gently assist with pulling the pinna down and back to visualize the tympanic membrane of a child younger than 3 years old. For a child older than 3 years, gently assist with pulling the pinna up and back.

PATIENT-CENTERED CARE

NURSING CARE

- Provide comfort measures.
  - Administer pain medication as needed.
  - Provide diversional activities.
- Place child in an upright position.
- Management of fevers.

MEDICATIONS

Acetaminophen or ibuprofen

Used to provide analgesia and reduce fever

Antibiotics

- Amoxicillin, amoxicillin–clavulanate, or azithromycin PO (10 to 14 days)
- Ceftriaxone IM (once)

NURSING ACTIONS
- Antibiotics are recommended for children over 6 months of age who have severe manifestations (increased pain or temperature above 39° C [102.2° F]) for more than 2 days, or for children 6 to 23 months with bilateral AOM and no manifestations.
- In other cases, antibiotic therapy can be withheld. If the child does not improve or worsens within 48 to 72 hours, antibiotics are started at that time.
- Administer in high doses orally, usually 80 to 90 mg/kg/day in two divided doses.

- The usual course of oral treatment is 10 days in children younger than 6 years of age. The course can be shorter for older children.
- IM is used for resistant organisms or for client-specific reasons (difficulty taking oral medications, inability to complete the oral course).

CLIENT EDUCATION
- The child should complete the total course of antibiotic treatment.
- Observe for manifestations of allergy to the antibiotic (rash or difficulty breathing).

Topical anesthetics

Benzocaine or lidocaine drops can help relieve pain.

THERAPEUTIC PROCEDURES

Myringotomy and placement of tympanoplasty tubes can be indicated for a child who has multiple episodes of otitis media. This procedure can be performed by laser treatment.
- This procedure is performed in an outpatient setting with the administration of general anesthesia. It is usually completed in 15 min.
- A small incision is made in the tympanic membrane, and tiny plastic or metal tubes are placed into the eardrum to equalize pressure and minimize effusion.
- Recovery takes place in a PACU, and discharge usually occurs within 1 hr.
- Postoperative pain is not common and, if present, will be mild.
- The tubes usually come out spontaneously (in 8 to 18 months).

CLIENT EDUCATION
- Limit the child's activities for a few days following surgery.
- Notify the provider when tubes come out. This usually does not require replacement of tubes.
- Avoid getting water into the child's ears while the tubes are in place. The effectiveness of earplugs is not conclusive. Advise the guardians to follow the health care provider's instructions.

CLIENT EDUCATION
- Use comfort measures.
- Feed the child in an upright position when bottle- or breastfeeding.
- If drainage is present, clean the external ear with sterile cotton swabs. Apply antibiotic ointment.
- Avoid exposure of child to risk factors if possible (secondhand smoke, individuals with viral/bacterial respiratory infections).
- Seek medical care at initial manifestations of infections (change in behavior, tugging on ear).
- Maintain up-to-date immunizations.

COMPLICATIONS

Hearing loss and/or speech delays

NURSING ACTIONS
- Monitor for deficits.
- Request a referral for audiology testing if needed.

CLIENT EDUCATION: Speech therapy can be necessary.

Application Exercises

1. A nurse is caring for a toddler who has acute otitis media. Which of the following is the priority action for the nurse to take?

   A. Provide emotional support to the family.

   B. Reinforce teaching with the family on care of the child.

   C. Provide a diversional activity for the toddler.

   D. Administer analgesics to the toddler.

2. A nurse is caring for an infant who has manifestations of acute otitis media (AOM). The nurse should identify that which of the following factors places the infant at risk for otitis media? (Select all that apply.)

   A. Breastfeeds without formula supplementation

   B. Attends day care 4 days per week

   C. Immunizations are up to date

   D. History of a cleft palate repair

   E. Parents smoke cigarettes outside

3. A nurse is caring for a toddler who has had rhinitis, cough, and diarrhea for 2 days. The tympanic membrane has an orange discoloration and decreased movement. Which of the following statements should the nurse make?

   A. "Your child has an ear infection that requires antibiotics."

   B. "Your child could experience transient hearing loss."

   C. "Your child will need to be on a decongestant until this clears."

   D. "Your child will need to have a myringotomy."

4. A nurse is caring for a toddler who has had three ear infections in the past 5 months. The nurse should identify that this places the toddler at risk for developing which of the following long-term complications?

   A. Balance difficulties

   B. Rash

   C. Speech delays

   D. Mastoiditis

5. A nurse is collecting data from an infant who has acute otitis media. Which of the following findings should the nurse expect? (Select all that apply.)

   A. Decreased pain in the supine position

   B. Rolling head side to side

   C. Loss of appetite

   D. Increased sensitivity to sound

   E. Crying

Active Learning Scenario

A nurse is caring for an infant who has acute otitis media for the first time. Use the ATI Active Learning Template: System Disorder to complete this item.

ALTERATION IN HEALTH (DIAGNOSIS)

NURSING CARE: Describe two interventions.

MEDICATIONS: List two.

CLIENT EDUCATION: Describe two teaching points.

COMPLICATIONS: Identify one.

Application Exercises Key

1. A. Providing emotional support to the family will promote psychological well-being. However, it is not the priority action.
   B. Reinforcing teaching with the family on the care of the child will promote recovery from illness. However, it is not the priority action.
   C. Providing a diversional activity for the toddler will help provide normalcy during care. However, it is not the priority action.
   D. **CORRECT:** The priority action when using Maslow's hierarchy of needs is to meet the toddler's physiological need first. Administering analgesics to alleviate or decrease physical pain is the priority action for the nurse to take.

   Ⓝ *NCLEX® Connection: Coordinated Care, Establishing Priorities*

2. A. Breastfeeding helps to protect against AOM because breast milk contains secretory immunoglobulin A.
   B. **CORRECT:** Infants who attend day care have an increased risk of OM because of the exposure to multiple people.
   C. The pneumococcal conjugate vaccine decreases the incidence of OM.
   D. **CORRECT:** Infants born with cleft palate are more prone to AOM because micro-organisms can easily enter the Eustachian tubes.
   E. **CORRECT:** Exposure to secondhand smoke increases an infant's risk for AOM.

   Ⓝ *NCLEX® Connection: Health Promotion and Maintenance, Health Promotion/Disease Prevention*

3. A. Rhinitis, cough, diarrhea, and an orange discoloration of the tympanic membrane are findings of otitis media with effusion (OME). Therefore, antibiotics are not recommended.
   B. **CORRECT:** Transient hearing loss is a complication of OME.
   C. Decongestants are not recommended for OME.
   D. Myringotomy is recommended for clients who have chronic OME.

   Ⓝ *NCLEX® Connection: Physiological Adaptation, Unexpected Response to Therapies*

4. A. Balance difficulties can be present with otitis media. However, it is not a long-term complication.
   B. Although rash can indicate antibiotic sensitivity, it is not a long-term complication of otitis media.
   C. **CORRECT:** Speech delay is a common complication of otitis media.
   D. Mastoiditis can be a result of otitis media. However, it is not a long-term complication.

   Ⓝ *NCLEX® Connection: Physiological Adaptation, Basic Pathophysiology*

5. A. Infants who have acute otitis media will have an increase in pain in the supine position from the fluid and pressure in the ear.
   B. **CORRECT:** Infants who have acute otitis media will roll their head side to side because of the pain and pressure in the ear.
   C. **CORRECT:** Infants who have acute otitis media will exhibit a loss of appetite due to the pain and pressure in the ear.
   D. Infants who have acute otitis media have a decreased sensitivity to sound from the fluid and pressure in the ear.
   E. **CORRECT:** Infants who have acute otitis media will exhibit crying and irritability from the pain.

   Ⓝ *NCLEX® Connection: Physiological Adaptation, Basic Pathophysiology*

Active Learning Scenario Key

Using the ATI Active Learning Template: System Disorder

ALTERATION IN HEALTH (DIAGNOSIS): Acute otitis media is an infection of the structures of the middle ear with rapid manifestations of infection.

NURSING CARE
- Comfort care with pain medications and distraction.
- Management of fevers.
- Place child in an upright position.

MEDICATIONS
- Amoxicillin, amoxicillin-clavulanate or azithromycin PO or ceftriaxone IM
- Acetaminophen or ibuprofen for pain and fever
- Benzocaine

CLIENT EDUCATION
- Inform the guardians about comfort measures.
- Encourage the guardians to feed the child in an upright position when bottle or breastfeeding.
- If drainage is present, clean the external ear with sterile cotton swabs. Apply antibiotic ointment.
- Remind guardians to avoid risk factors (secondhand smoke, exposure to individuals with viral/bacterial respiratory infections).
- Stress the importance of seeking medical care at the onset of findings of infections (change in child's behavior, tugging on ear).
- Encourage the guardians to keep the child's immunizations up to date.

POTENTIAL COMPLICATION: Hearing loss and/or speech delays

Ⓝ *NCLEX® Connection: Physiological Adaptation, Basic Pathophysiology*

CHAPTER 37 *HIV/AIDS*

HIV infection is a viral infection in which the virus primarily infects a specific subset of T-lymphocytes, the CD4 T cells, causing immune dysfunction. The virus impairs or destroys cells of the immune system and progressively destroys the body's ability to fight off infections. This leads to organ dysfunction and a variety of opportunistic illnesses in a weakened host.

DATA COLLECTION

RISK FACTORS

- Infants can become infected perinatally or by ingesting breast milk from an HIV infected woman perinatally or by breast milk.
- Exposure to blood products or body fluids that contain the HIV virus
- Sexual assault survivor
- Risky behaviors (unprotected sexual activity and IV substance use)
- Sexually transmitted infections
- Lack of awareness of risk factors and modes of transmission

EXPECTED FINDINGS

37.1 HIV infection stages

	LESS THAN 12 MONTHS (CELLS/µL*)	1 TO 5 YEARS (CELLS/µL)	6 YEARS AND OLDER (CELLS/µL)
Stage 1	1,500 or more	1,000 or more	500 or more
Stage 2	750 to 1,499	500 to 999	200 to 499
Stage 3	Less than 750	Less than 500	Less than 200

*CD4+ T-lymphocyte count
Source: CDC.gov

HIV clinical classification

To read more about HIV, go to the website of the Centers for Disease Control and Prevention.

Category N: Asymptomatic
No manifestations are present, considered to be the result of HIV infection, or the child has only one of the conditions listed in the mildly symptomatic category (A).

Category A: Mildly symptomatic
Children have two or more of the following mildly symptomatic manifestations, but none of the conditions listed in the moderately or severely symptomatic categories (B or C).
- Lymphadenopathy
- Hepatomegaly
- Splenomegaly
- Recurrent upper respiratory infections, sinusitis, or otitis media
- Oral candidiasis
- Parotitis

Category B: Moderately symptomatic
Children have more serious manifestations, including:
- Anemia
- Bacterial meningitis, pneumonia, or sepsis (single episode)
- Oropharyngeal candidiasis
- Cytomegalovirus infection
- Cardiomyopathy
- Herpes zoster
- Herpes simplex virus (HSV), bronchitis, pneumonitis, or esophagitis
- Hepatitis
- Lymphoid interstitial pneumonia (LIP) or pulmonary lymphoid hyperplasia complex
- Leiomyosarcoma
- Toxoplasmosis

Category C: Severely symptomatic
Children who have the following conditions are considered severely symptomatic.
- Multiple serious bacterial infections (meningitis, bone or joint, abscesses of internal organ or body cavity, septicemia, mycobacterial pneumonia)
- Esophageal or pulmonary candidiasis, (bronchi, trachea, lungs)
- Cytomegalovirus disease (greater than 1 month of age with site other than liver, spleen, or lymph nodes)
- HSV stomatitis, bronchitis, pneumonitis, or esophagitis lasting longer than 1 month
- Kaposi's sarcoma
- Tuberculosis
- Encephalopathy with developmental delays
- Extrapulmonary cryptococcosis
- Cryptosporidiosis
- Disseminated histoplasmosis
- Pneumocystis carinii pneumonia
- Encephalopathy
- Septicemia
- Wasting syndrome
- Lymphoma

HIV infection: 13 to 20 years

Refer to **ADULT MEDICAL SURGICAL REVIEW MODULE, CHAPTER 76: HIV/AIDS**.

DIAGNOSTIC PROCEDURES

LABORATORY CRITERIA FOR DIAGNOSIS

- 18 months or older: Positive result from HIV enzyme-linked immunosorbent assay (ELISA) and Western blot immunoassay.
- Infants less than 18 months of age and were born to infected mothers: Positive result from polymerase chain reaction and virus culture.

CLASSIFICATION: Children are classified by the following criteria.

- **N:** No manifestations
  - N1 = no evidence of suppression
  - N2 = evidence of moderate suppression
  - N3 = severe suppression
- **A:** Mild manifestations
  - A1 = no evidence of suppression
  - A2 = evidence of moderate suppression
  - A3 = severe suppression
- **B:** Moderate manifestations
  - B1 = no evidence of suppression
  - B2 = evidence of moderate suppression
  - B3 = severe suppression
- **C:** Severe manifestations
  - C1 = no evidence of suppression
  - C2 = evidence of moderate suppression
  - C3 = severe suppression

PATIENT-CENTERED CARE

NURSING CARE

- Encourage a balanced diet that is high in calories and protein. Obtain the child's preferred food and beverages. Give nutritional supplements.
- Administer total parental nutrition if prescribed.
- Provide good oral care, and report abnormalities for treatment.
- Keep the child's skin clean and dry.
- Provide nonpharmacological methods of pain relief.
- Determine pain level, and provide adequate pain management. Use of medications can include nonsteroidal anti-inflammatory drugs (NSAIDs), acetaminophen, opioids, muscle relaxants, and/ or a eutectic mixture of local anesthetics (lidocaine and prilocaine topical ointment) for numerous diagnostic procedures.
- Prevent infection. Qs
  - Use standard precautions.
  - Encourage deep breathing and coughing.
  - Maintain good hand hygiene.
  - Reinforce teaching with the child and guardians to avoid individuals who have colds/infections/viruses.
  - Encourage immunizations (pneumococcal vaccine and yearly seasonal influenza vaccine).
  - Monitor for indications of opportunistic infections.

- Administer medications as prescribed for opportunistic infections.
- Provide psychosocial support to client and family and assist them in disclosing the diagnosis.
- Reinforce teaching with the child and parents about transmission of the virus (high-risk behaviors).
- Identify stressors affecting the family, and make appropriate referrals (school/community response to child, finances, access to health care).
- Discuss with adolescents the various routes of HIV transmission (sexual transmission, IV substance use).

MEDICATIONS

Antiretroviral medications

Antiretroviral medications are given at various stages of the HIV cycle to inhibit reproduction of the virus, therefore slowing progression of the HIV disease process.

- Combinations of antiretroviral medications are prescribed to decrease the client's development of medication resistance.
- Antiretroviral medication therapy is lifelong.

Nucleoside reverse transcriptase inhibitors: Zidovudine, didanosine, stavudine, lamivudine, and abacavir suppress the synthesis of viral DNA.

Non-nucleoside reverse transcriptase inhibitors: Delavirdine, efavirenz, and nevirapine bind to the viral DNA, causing direct inhibition.

Protease inhibitors: Indinavir, ritonavir, nelfinavir, amprenavir, saquinavir, and lopinavir inhibit an enzyme needed for the virus to replicate.

NURSING ACTIONS: Monitor laboratory results (CBC, WBC, liver function tests). Antiretroviral medications can increase alanine aminotransferase, aspartate aminotransferase, bilirubin, mean corpuscular volume, high-density lipoproteins, total cholesterol, and triglycerides.

CLIENT EDUCATION
- Observe for adverse effects of the medications and perform ways to decrease the severity of the adverse effects.
- Take the medication on a regular schedule and do not miss doses.

Antibiotics

Trimethoprim-sulfamethoxazole
Administer to all infants who are born to infected mothers until HIV infection is excluded. QEBP

IV gamma globulin

To prevent recurrent or serious bacterial infections

INTERPROFESSIONAL CARE

- Social services can help with access to health care and medication acquisition.
- Dietitian can assist with nutritional support and promote good nutrition.

CLIENT EDUCATION

- This illness is chronic and there is a need for lifelong medication administration.
- Notify the provider for manifestations requiring medical care, including headache, fever, lethargy, warmth, tenderness, redness at joints, and neck stiffness.
- Perform safe practice when using needles/syringes and administering medications.
- Discuss with adolescents the various routes of HIV transmission, including sexual transmission and IV substance use. Ensure the adolescent understands safe sex practices.

COMPLICATIONS

Failure to thrive

NURSING ACTIONS

- Obtain a baseline height and weight, and continue to monitor.
- Promote optimal nutrition. This can require the administration of total parenteral nutrition.
- Observe growth and development characteristics. Monitor for delays.
- Provide opportunities for normal development (age-appropriate toys, playing with children of the same age).

CLIENT EDUCATION: Consume recommended nutrition to meet nutritional needs.

Pneumocystis carinii pneumonia

NURSING ACTIONS

- Monitor respiratory status, which includes respiratory rate and effort, oxygen saturation, and breath sounds.
- Administer appropriate antibiotics.
- Administer an antipyretic and/or analgesics.
- Provide adequate hydration and maintain fluid and electrolyte balance.
- Use postural drainage and chest physiotherapy to mobilize and remove fluid from the lungs.
- Promote adequate rest.
- Reinforce teaching with the child and guardians about the infectious process and how to prevent infection.
- Reinforce teaching with the child and guardians about the importance of medication and the need to maintain the medication regimen.

Application Exercises

1. A nurse is reinforcing teaching with the guardian of a child who has HIV. Which of the following information should the nurse include? (Select all that apply.)
   - A. Obtain yearly influenza vaccination.
   - B. Monitor a fever for 24 hr before seeking medical care.
   - C. Avoid individuals who have colds.
   - D. Provide nutritional supplements.
   - E. Administer aspirin for pain.

2. A nurse is caring for a child who has AIDS. Which of the following isolation precautions should the nurse initiate?
   - A. Contact
   - B. Airborne
   - C. Droplet
   - D. Standard

3. A nurse is assisting with the admission of a child who has HIV. The nurse should identify which of the following findings as an indication that the child is in the mildly symptomatic category of the infection? (Select all that apply.)
   - A. Herpes zoster
   - B. Anemia
   - C. Oral candidiasis
   - D. Hepatomegaly
   - E. Lymphadenopathy

4. A nurse in a community center is reinforcing teaching with a group of adolescents about HIV/AIDS. Which of the following statements should the nurse include in the teaching?
   - A. "You can contract HIV through casual kissing."
   - B. "HIV is transmitted through IV substance use."
   - C. "HIV is now curable if caught in the early stages."
   - D. "Medications inhibit transmission of the HIV virus."

5. A nurse is caring for a child who has severely symptomatic HIV. Which of the following findings should the nurse expect? (Select all that apply.)
   - A. Kaposi's sarcoma
   - B. Hepatitis
   - C. Wasting syndrome
   - D. Pulmonary candidiasis
   - E. Cardiomyopathy

Application Exercises Key

1. A. **CORRECT:** Obtaining a yearly influenza vaccination is recommended to protect the child from opportunistic infections.
   B. The child who has HIV should receive prompt medical care for a fever, as this is an indication of an infection.
   C. **CORRECT:** Avoiding individuals who have colds will assist in protecting the child from opportunistic infections.
   D. **CORRECT:** Nutritional supplements are recommended to promote improved nutrition of the child who has HIV.
   E. Acetaminophen, NSAIDs, or opioids should be administered to a child who has pain.

   Ⓝ *NCLEX® Connection: Physiological Adaptation, Alterations in Body Systems*

2. A. Contact isolation precautions are used to protect transmission of disease that is skin-to-skin or direct contact.
   B. Airborne isolation precautions are used to protect transmission of disease that is small-particle droplets.
   C. Droplet isolation precautions are used to protect transmission of disease that is large-particle droplets.
   D. **CORRECT:** Standard isolation precautions are used to protect transmission of disease that is bloodborne or present in a body fluid.

   Ⓝ *NCLEX® Connection: Safety and Infection Control, Standard Precautions/Transmission–Based Precautions/Surgical Asepsis*

3. A. Herpes zoster is a manifestation of a child who is moderately symptomatic.
   B. Anemia is a manifestation of a child who is moderately symptomatic.
   C. **CORRECT:** Oral candidiasis is a manifestation of a child who is mildly symptomatic.
   D. **CORRECT:** Hepatomegaly is a manifestation of a child who is mildly symptomatic.
   E. **CORRECT:** Lymphadenopathy is a manifestation of a child who is mildly symptomatic.

   Ⓝ *NCLEX® Connection: Physiological Adaptation, Basic Pathophysiology*

4. A. HIV is transmitted via blood, semen, vaginal secretions, and breast milk. There is no evidence that casual contact (kissing) spreads the virus.
   B. **CORRECT:** HIV is transmitted via blood, semen, vaginal secretions, and breast milk. IV substance use is a potential mode of transmission.
   C. Antiretroviral therapy slows the progression of HIV but does not cure the disease.
   D. Medications suppress the progression of the virus but do not prevent transmission from one individual to another.

   Ⓝ *NCLEX® Connection: Health Promotion and Maintenance, Community Resources*

5. A. **CORRECT:** Kaposi's sarcoma is a manifestation of a child who is severely symptomatic.
   B. Hepatitis is a manifestation of a child who is moderately symptomatic.
   C. **CORRECT:** Wasting syndrome is a manifestation of a child who is severely symptomatic.
   D. **CORRECT:** Pulmonary candidiasis is a manifestation of a child who is severely symptomatic.
   E. Cardiomyopathy is a manifestation of a child who is moderately symptomatic.

   Ⓝ *NCLEX® Connection: Physiological Adaptation, Basic Pathophysiology*

Active Learning Scenario

A nurse is reinforcing teaching with the guardian of a child who has AIDS. Use the ATI Active Learning Template: System Disorder to complete this item.

COMPLICATIONS: List two complications of AIDS and include four nursing actions for each.

Active Learning Scenario Key

Using the ATI Active Learning Template: System Disorder
COMPLICATIONS

Failure to thrive
- Obtain a baseline height and weight, and continue to monitor.
- Promote optimal nutrition. This can require the administration of total parenteral nutrition.
- Observe growth and development characteristics. Monitor for delays.
- Provide opportunities for normal development (age-appropriate toys, playing with children of the same age).
- Reinforce teaching with the child and guardians about appropriate nutrition and how to meet nutritional needs.

Pneumocystis carinii pneumonia (PCP)
- Monitor respiratory status, which includes respiratory rate and effort, oxygen saturation, and breath sounds.
- Administer appropriate antibiotics.
- Administer an antipyretic and/or analgesics.
- Provide adequate hydration, and maintain fluid and electrolyte balance.
- Use postural drainage and chest physiotherapy to mobilize and remove fluid from the lungs.
- Promote adequate rest.
- Reinforce teaching with the child and guardians about the infectious process and how to prevent infection.
- Reinforce teaching with the child and guardians about the importance of medication and the need to maintain the medication regimen.

Ⓝ *NCLEX® Connection: Physiological Adaptation, Alterations in Body Systems*

N NCLEX® Connections

When reviewing the following chapters, keep in mind the relevant topics and tasks of the NCLEX outline, in particular:

Basic Care and Comfort

NUTRITION AND ORAL HYDRATION: Monitor impact of disease/illness on client nutritional status.

Physiological Adaptation

ALTERATIONS IN BODY SYSTEMS: Reinforce education to client regarding care and condition.

BASIC PATHOPHYSIOLOGY
Identify signs and symptoms related to an acute or chronic illness.

Consider general principles of client disease process when providing care.

UNEXPECTED RESPONSE TO THERAPIES: Intervene in response to client unexpected negative response to therapy.

CHAPTER 38 *Pediatric Cancers*

Working with a child who has cancer requires caring and competency. The nurse should provide individualized care and support to the child and the child's family. Pediatric cancers have a low rate of incidence compared to cancer in adults. However, some neoplasms occur predominantly in children. Types of pediatric cancers include organ neoplasms, blood neoplasms, and bone and soft tissue cancers.

For more information, see ADULT MEDICAL SURGICAL REVIEW MODULE, CHAPTER 79: GENERAL PRINCIPLES OF CANCER. Refer to ADULT MEDICAL SURGICAL REVIEW MODULE, CHAPTER 82: CANCER DISORDERS for organ neoplasms that both adults and children can acquire (lymphoma, brain tumor, liver and testicular cancer).

Organ neoplasms

- Wilms' tumor (nephroblastoma) is a malignancy that occurs in the kidneys or abdomen. The tumor is usually unilateral, with 10% of cases affecting both kidneys. Diagnosis typically occurs before age 5, with most cases diagnosed between 2 and 3 years of age. Metastasis is rare.
- Neuroblastoma is a malignancy that occurs in the adrenal gland, sympathetic chain of the retroperitoneal area, head, neck, pelvis, or chest. It is usually manifested during the toddler years, with 95% of cases prior to age 10. Median age at diagnosis is 22 months. It is more common in males than females. Half of all cases have metastasized before diagnosis.
- Treatment varies by child and can be any combination of surgery, chemotherapy, and radiation.

DATA COLLECTION

RISK FACTORS

There are no known risk factors for Wilms' tumor or neuroblastoma. Q͟EBP

EXPECTED FINDINGS

Wilms' tumor

- Mass is usually found by guardians during routine bathing or dressing of their child
- Painless, firm, nontender unilateral abdominal swelling or mass
- Fatigue, malaise, weight loss
- Fever
- Hematuria
- Hypertension
- Manifestations of metastasis include dyspnea, cough, shortness of breath, and chest pain

Neuroblastoma

- Manifestations depend upon the location and stage of disease.
- Manifestations of metastasis include an ill appearance, periorbital ecchymoses, proptosis, bone pain, weight loss, and irritability.

LABORATORY TESTS

Wilms' tumor

- BUN, creatinine
- CBC
- Urinalysis

Neuroblastoma

- CBC and coagulation studies
- Urine catecholamines (vanillylmandelic acid, homovanillic acid, dopamine, and norepinephrine)

DIAGNOSTIC PROCEDURES

NURSING ACTIONS
- Determine if the child has allergies to dye or shellfish.
- Reinforce education of the guardian and child prior to procedure on expectations.
- Assist the child to remain still during the procedure.
- Reinforce instructions with the child to drink oral contrast if prescribed.
- Assist with sedation of the child if prescribed.
- Provide emotional support. Q͟PCC

Wilms' tumor

- Abdominal ultrasonography
- Abdominal and chest computed tomography (CT) scan
- Inferior venacavogram (rule out involvement with the vena cava)
- Bone marrow aspiration (rule out metastasis)

Neuroblastoma

- Skeletal survey
- Skull, neck, chest, abdominal, and bone CT scans
- Bone marrow aspiration (rule out metastasis)
- Metaiodobenzylguanidine scan (determine bone, bone marrow, and soft tissue involvement)
- Biopsy of tumor

PATIENT-CENTERED CARE

NURSING CARE

- If any abdominal tumor is suspected, do not palpate the abdomen.
- Use extreme caution when handling or bathing the client to prevent trauma to the tumor site. Qs
- Monitor the child's and family's coping and support.
- Check for developmental delays related to illness.
- Monitor physical growth (height and weight).
- Reinforce education and support to the child and family regarding diagnostic testing, treatment plan, ongoing therapy, and prognosis.
- Monitor for findings of infection.
- Administer antibiotics as prescribed for infection.
- Keep the child's skin clean and dry.
- Provide oral hygiene.
- Provide age-appropriate diversional activities.
- Provide support to the child and family.
  - Avoid false reassurance.
  - Listen to the child's concerns.
  - Allow time for the child and family to discuss feelings regarding grief and loss.

THERAPEUTIC PROCEDURES

Treatment for Wilms' tumor

- Varies according to the stage and histology of the tumor
- Surgical removal of the tumor and kidney soon after diagnosis
- Preoperative chemotherapy or radiation if both kidneys are involved to decrease the size of the tumors and potentially preserve one kidney
- Postoperative radiation and/or chemotherapy for children who have large tumors, metastasis, recurrence, and residual disease

Treatment for neuroblastoma

- Varies according to the tumor stage
- Surgical removal of the tumor
- Chemotherapy and/or radiation for metastasis and residual disease

Chemotherapy

The child can have a long-term central venous access device or peripherally inserted central catheter in place.

NURSING ACTIONS

- Provide an antiemetic prior to administration of chemotherapy.
- Allow the child several food choices, including their favorite foods.
- Observe the mouth for mucosal ulcerations.
- Offer cool fluids to prevent dehydration and soothe sore mucous membranes.

CLIENT EDUCATION Qpcc

- Monitor for adverse effects of chemotherapy (mouth sores, loss of appetite, nausea and vomiting, hair loss, diarrhea or constipation, increased risk of infection, easy bruising or bleeding, and fatigue).
- Receive immunizations and follow-up appointments.
- Perform good infection control practices.

ADVERSE EFFECTS OF CHEMOTHERAPY

Monitor for adverse effects of chemotherapy and provide interventions to prevent and minimize manifestations.

Skin breakdown
- Inspect skin daily.
- Examine rectal mucosa for fissures.
- Avoid rectal temperatures.
- Provide sitz baths as needed.
- Reposition frequently.
- Use a pressure reduction system.

Constipation
- Encourage a diet high in fiber.
- Administer stool softeners and laxatives as needed.
- Encourage fluids.

Foot drop
- Use a footboard in bed.
- Wear high-top shoes.
- Causes weakness and numbness of extremities.
- Assist with ambulation.

Pain
- Collect data for pain.
- Administer analgesics as prescribed.
- Assist with determining the effectiveness of pain interventions.
- For jaw pain, provide a soft or liquid diet.

Loss of appetite
- Monitor fluid intake and hydration status.
- Weigh the child daily.
- Monitor electrolyte values.
- Provide small, frequent, well-balanced meals.
- Encourage high protein and caloric foods and supplements.
- Involve the child in meal planning.
- Administer enteral nutrition if needed.
- Ensure that chemotherapy is administered early in the day.
- If nausea or vomiting is present, administer antiemetics prior to or after therapy (ondansetron).

Hemorrhage cystitis
- Encourage fluids.
- Encourage frequent voiding.
- Ensure that chemotherapy is administered early in the morning to promote adequate fluid intake and voiding.
- Administer mesna to provide protection to the bladder.

Bone marrow depression: From chemotherapy resulting in anemia, neutropenia, and/or thrombocytopenia

- Monitor vital signs and report them to the health care provider. Report a temperature greater than 37.8° C (100° F).
- Monitor for findings of infection (lung congestion; redness, swelling and pain around IV sites) and lesions in the mouth. Monitor the wound site and immunization status.
- Administer antimicrobial, antiviral, and antifungal medications as prescribed.
- Protect the child from sources of possible infection.
- Use good hand hygiene.
- Encourage the child and family to use good hand hygiene.
- Encourage the child to avoid crowds while undergoing chemotherapy.
- Screen visitors and staff for manifestations of infection.
- Reinforce with the child to avoid fresh fruits and vegetables.
- Avoid invasive procedures (injections, rectal temperatures, catheters). Apply pressure to puncture sites for 5 min.
- Monitor for indications of bleeding.
- Avoid aspirin and NSAIDs.
- Administer filgrastim, a granulocyte colony-stimulating factor that stimulates WBC production, subcutaneously daily.
- Monitor the child for headache, fever, and mild to moderate bone pain.
- Administer epoetin alfa subcutaneously two to three times per week as prescribed to stimulate RBC formation.
- Monitor blood pressure.
- Administer oprelvekin subcutaneously daily as prescribed to stimulate platelet formation.
- Encourage the use of a soft toothbrush.
- Use gentle handling and positioning to protect from injury.
- Organize care to provide for rest. Schedule rest periods.
- CLIENT EDUCATION ◯PCC
  - Perform infection control procedures at home.
  - Provide support.

Anorexia, nausea, vomiting: Adverse effects of chemotherapy and radiation therapy

- Avoid strong odors. Provide a pleasant atmosphere for meals.
- Avoid offering the child's favorite foods during chemotherapy because they can develop an aversion to these foods.
- Suggest and assist in selecting foods/fluids.
- Provide small, frequent meals.
- Administer antiemetics as prescribed, usually before meals.

Alteration in bowel elimination: Diarrhea is a result of radiation to the abdominal area. Some chemotherapeutic agents can cause constipation. If mobility and nutrition decrease, the child is more likely to develop constipation.

- Provide meticulous skin care.
- Provide a nutritious diet.
- Determine if certain foods or drinks (high-fiber, lactose-rich) worsen the child's condition.
- Monitor I&O and daily weight.

Mucositis and dry mouth

- Provide a soft toothbrush and/or swabs.
- Lubricate the child's lips.
- Give soft, nonacidic foods. A pureed or liquid diet can be required.
- Provide analgesics.
- Avoid hydrogen peroxide and lemon glycerin swabs due to mucosal drying and irritation on eroded tissue.
- CLIENT EDUCATION ◯PCC
  - Visit a dentist before therapy.
  - Use chlorhexidine mouth wash or salt rinses using ½ tsp table salt mixed with 1 tsp baking soda and 1 quart water.

Alopecia: Occurs with chemotherapy and radiation of the head and/or neck

- Monitor the child's feelings.
- Discuss cutting long hair short.
- Suggest wearing a disposable surgical cap for hair collection during heavy loss periods.
- Use gentle shampoos. Gently brush the child's hair.
- Avoid blow dryers and curling irons.
- Suggest wearing a cotton hat or scarf.
- CLIENT EDUCATION ◯PCC
  - Discuss the use of a wig, turbans, or hats.
  - Avoid blow dryers and curling irons.
  - Perform scalp hygiene.
  - Hair grows back in 3 to 6 months.

Radiation

- Radiation is dose-calculated and usually delivered in divided treatments over several weeks.
- Radiation affects rapidly growing cells in the body. Therefore, cells that normally have a fast turnover can be affected in addition to cancer cells.

NURSING ACTIONS

- Take care when radiation is in use. Wear lead aprons.
- Reinforce education with the child and family about the procedure, and provide support.

CLIENT EDUCATION ◯PCC

- Do not wash off marks on skin that outline the targeted areas.
- Wash the marked areas with lukewarm water, use hands instead of a washcloth, pat dry, and take care not to remove the markings. Avoid using hot or cold water.
- Avoid use of soaps, creams, lotions, and powders unless they are prescribed.
- Wear loose cotton clothing.
- Keep the areas protected from the sun by wearing a hat and long-sleeved shirts.
- Seek medical care for blisters, weeping, and red/tender skin.

Surgical interventions

Tumor debulking

PREOPERATIVE NURSING ACTIONS
- Avoid palpation of Wilms' tumor.
- Reinforce preoperative teaching to the child and family that includes length of surgery, where the child will recover, and what equipment will be in place (nasogastric tube, IV line, indwelling urinary catheter).

POSTOPERATIVE NURSING ACTIONS
- Monitor gastrointestinal activity (bowel sounds, bowel movements, distention, nausea, vomiting).
- Provide pain relief.
- Monitor vital signs and observe for any findings of infection.
- Encourage pulmonary hygiene.

INTERPROFESSIONAL CARE

- Social services can assist with access to medications and durable medical equipment if needed.
- A dietitian can be consulted for development of a diet plan.

COMPLICATIONS

- Metastasis
- Kidney failure
- Pancytopenia

Blood neoplasms

- Leukemia is the term for a group of malignancies that affect the bone marrow and lymphatic system. Peak onset in children is between ages 2 and 5 years. Leukemia is classified by the type of WBCs that becomes neoplastic and is commonly divided into two groups: acute lymphoid leukemia (ALL) and acute myelogenous or nonlymphoid leukemia (AML/ANLL). ALL is the most common childhood malignancy. Morphology, cytogenetic, chromosome and immunologic marker testing is used to further classify leukemia so that the most effective treatment is prescribed.
- Leukemia causes an increase in the production of immature WBCs (leukoblasts) with neoplastic characteristics, which leads to infiltration of organs and tissues.
- Bone marrow infiltration causes crowding of cells that would normally produce RBCs, platelets, and mature WBCs. Deficient RBCs cause anemia. Deficient mature WBCs (neutropenia) increase the risk for infection. Deficient platelets (thrombocytopenia) cause bleeding and bruising.
- Infiltration of spleen, liver, and lymph nodes leads to tissue fibrosis. Infiltration of the CNS causes increased intracranial pressure. Other tissues can also be infiltrated (testes, prostate, ovaries, gastrointestinal tract, kidneys, and lungs).

DATA COLLECTION

RISK FACTORS

- Leukemia is the most common cancer of childhood
- Male sex
- Non-Hispanic white or Hispanic clients
- Family history of leukemia
- Children who have trisomy 21 (Down syndrome)

EXPECTED FINDINGS

History and data collection findings can reveal vague reports (anorexia, headache, fatigue).

PHYSICAL FINDINGS
- EARLY MANIFESTATIONS
  - Low-grade fever
  - Pallor
  - Increased bruising and petechiae
  - Listlessness
  - Enlarged liver, lymph nodes, and joints
  - Abdominal, leg, and joint pain
  - Constipation
  - Headache
  - Vomiting and anorexia
  - Unsteady gait
- LATE MANIFESTATIONS
  - Pain
  - Hematuria
  - Ulcerations in the mouth
  - Enlarged kidneys and testicles
  - Manifestations of increased intracranial pressure

LABORATORY TESTS

Complete blood count
- Anemia (low blood count)
- Thrombocytopenia (low platelets)
- Neutropenia (low neutrophils)
- Leukemic blasts (immature WBCs)
- Blood smear (immature WBC)

DIAGNOSTIC PROCEDURES

Bone marrow aspiration or biopsy analysis

The most definitive diagnostic procedure. If leukemia is present, the specimen will show prolific quantities of immature leukemic blast cells and protein markers indicating a specific type of leukemia.

NURSING ACTIONS
- Assist the provider with the procedure.
- Topical anesthetic (a eutectic mixture of local anesthetic cream) can be applied over the biopsy area 45 min to 1 hr prior to the procedure.
- Conscious sedation is induced using a general anesthetic (propofol).
- Positioning depends on the access site to be used (posterior or anterior iliac crest is most common; tibia can be used in infants because it is easier to access and hold the infant).

POSTPROCEDURE

- Apply pressure to the site, then apply a pressure dressing.
- Monitor vital signs frequently.
- Monitor for manifestations of bleeding and infection for 24 hr.

CLIENT EDUCATION: Understand proper procedure and postprocedure care.

Cerebrospinal fluid (CSF) analysis

CSF, obtained by lumbar puncture, is analyzed to determine CNS involvement.

NURSING ACTIONS

- Assist the provider with the sterile procedure.
- A topical anesthetic cream can be applied over the biopsy area 1 hr prior to the procedure.
- Place the child in the side-lying position with the head flexed and knees drawn up toward the chest with their back arched, and assist in maintaining the position. Distraction can be required.
- Position the newborn upright with their head flexed forward.
- The child can be sedated.
- The provider will clean the skin and inject a local anesthetic.
- The provider will take pressure readings and collect three to five sterile test tubes of CSF.
- Pressure and an elastic or adhesive bandage will be applied to the puncture site after the needle is removed.
- Label specimens appropriately, and deliver them to the laboratory.
- Monitor the site for bleeding, hematoma, or infection.
- Monitor for manifestations of increased intracranial pressure (ICP) (increased blood pressure, decreased respirations, or changes in LOC).

CLIENT EDUCATION: Remain in bed for 4 to 8 hr in a flat position to prevent leakage and a resulting spinal headache. This might not be possible for an infant, toddler, or preschooler.

Liver and kidney function studies

Used for baseline functioning before chemotherapy and also during therapy to monitor effectiveness.

CLIENT EDUCATION: Understand the length of time to receive results.

PATIENT-CENTERED CARE

NURSING CARE

- Provide emotional support to the child and family.
- Encourage peer contact if appropriate.
- Check for pain using an age-appropriate pain scale.
- Use pharmacological and nonpharmacological interventions to provide around-the-clock pain management.

MEDICATIONS

Chemotherapy

- The agents to be used depend on the type of leukemia, age, and whether leukemic cells are found in the cerebrospinal fluid.
- Common agents include vincristine, doxorubicin.
- The agent must be administered by an RN through a central line or port.
- Corticosteroids can be used as treatment for certain cancers and to minimize adverse effects of treatment.
- Goal of therapy is complete remission with less than 5% of blast cells present.
- Intrathecal methotrexate can be administered prophylactically to prevent CNS complications.

Chemotherapy is administered in different phases to treat leukemia.

- **Induction/remission therapy:** To achieve complete remission or less than 5% of leukemic cells in the bone marrow
- **Intensification therapy (consolidation):** To destroy any remaining leukemic cells followed by a delayed intensification to prevent any resistant leukemic cells from emerging
- **Maintenance therapy:** To sustain the remission phase. Also requires frequent monitoring of CBC.

NURSING ACTIONS

- Control nausea and vomiting with antiemetics prior to treatment. Can be combined with dexamethasone.
- Monitor adverse effects of treatment (myelosuppression).
- Monitor for complications or adverse effects of chemotherapy.

CLIENT EDUCATION

- The use of a steroid treatment can cause moon face and changes in skin and mood.
- Observe for manifestations of infection, skin breakdown, and nutritional deficiency.
- Notify treatment team immediately if the child develops a fever.
- Maintain good hygiene.
- Avoid individuals who have infectious diseases.
- Administer medications and provide nutritional support at home.
- Understand proper use of vascular access devices.
- Understand bleeding precautions and the management of active bleeding.

THERAPEUTIC PROCEDURES

Hematopoietic stem cell transplant (HCST)

HCST can be indicated for children who have AML during the first remission and for children who have ALL after a second remission.

Allogeneic transplant: The blood-forming stem cells generally are donated by another person.

NURSING ACTIONS

- Implement protective isolation. Qs
  - Private, positive-pressure room
  - At least 12 air exchanges/hr
  - HEPA filtration for incoming air
  - Respirator mask, gloves, and gowns
  - No dried or fresh flowers, and no potted plants

CLIENT EDUCATION: The child is at an increased risk for infection and bleeding until transfused stem cells grow.

Radiation therapy

Refer to the information provided in the neoplasm section regarding nursing actions and client education for radiation therapy.

INTERPROFESSIONAL CARE

Assist with providing information regarding support services for the child and family.

COMPLICATIONS

Infection

Infection can be a complication of myelosuppression.

NURSING ACTIONS

- Provide the child with a private room. The room should be designed to allow for adequate air flow to reduce airborne pathogens.
- Restrict visitors and health personnel who have active illnesses.
- Adhere to strict hand hygiene.
- Monitor for potential sites of infections (oral ulcer, open cut), and monitor temperature.
- Administer antibiotics as prescribed after source of infection identified through chest radiographs; blood, stool, urine, and nasopharyngeal cultures.
- Encourage adequate protein and caloric intake.
- Monitor absolute neutrophil count (ANC).
- Use aseptic technique for all procedures.

CLIENT EDUCATION

- Understand infection control practices.
- Observe for manifestations of infection and call the provider if necessary.
- Avoid live vaccines while the immune system is depressed.

Hemorrhage

Bleeding (thrombocytopenia) can be a complication of myelosuppression.

NURSING ACTIONS

- Monitor for findings of bleeding: petechiae, ecchymoses, hematuria, bleeding gums, hematemesis, tarry stools.
- Avoid unnecessary skin punctures, and use surgical aseptic technique when performed. Apply pressure for 5 min to stop bleeding.
- Treat a nosebleed with cold and pressure.
- Administer platelet concentrates or platelet rich plasma as prescribed.
- Avoid obtaining temperatures rectally.
- No aspirin products.

CLIENT EDUCATION Qpcc

- Understand the importance of and how to perform meticulous oral care to prevent gingival bleeding. Use a soft toothbrush, and avoid astringent mouthwashes.
- Take measures to control epistaxis (gentle pressure, packing the nostrils).
- Avoid activities that can lead to injury or bleeding.

Kidney impairment

- Increased uric acid can obstruct renal tubules causing decreased excretion of chemotherapeutic agents.
- Administer allopurinol as prescribed to decrease uric acid production

Testicular invasion

Testicular involvement can occur.

Anemia

Anemia can be a complication of myelosuppression.

NURSING ACTIONS
- Administer blood transfusions as prescribed.
- Allow for frequent rest periods.
- Administer oxygen therapy.
- Administer IV fluid replacement.

CLIENT EDUCATION: Be aware of foods high in iron. Qpcc

Bone and soft tissue cancers

- Malignant tumors in bone can originate from all tissues involved in bone growth, including osteoid matrix, blood vessels, and cartilage.
  - Osteosarcoma usually occurs in the metaphysis of long bones, most often in the femur. Treatment frequently includes amputation or limb salvage procedure of the affected extremity as well as chemotherapy.
  - Ewing's sarcoma (a primitive neuroectodermal tumor) occurs in the shafts of long bones and of trunk bones. Treatment includes surgical biopsy, intensive radiation therapy to tumor site, and chemotherapy, but not amputation. Prognosis depends on how quickly the disease is diagnosed and whether metastasis has occurred.
- Soft tissue malignancies arise from undifferentiated cells in the soft tissues (muscles, tendons), in connective or fibrous tissue, or in blood or lymph vessels. These malignancies can begin in any area of the body.
  - Rhabdomyosarcoma originates in skeletal muscle in any part of the body, but it most commonly occurs in the head and neck, with the orbit of the eye frequently affected. Treatment consists of surgical biopsy, local radiation therapy, and chemotherapy, rather than radical surgical procedures.
- Children who undergo irradiation for malignancies in or near the pelvic area can experience sterilization and secondary cancers.

Bone tumors

DATA COLLECTION

RISK FACTORS

- Osteosarcoma peaks at age 15 during growth spurts and is more common in boys than girls.
- Ewing's sarcoma occurs prior to 30 years of age and is more common in Caucasian clients.

EXPECTED FINDINGS

- Nonspecific bone pain that is often mistaken for an injury or growing pains
- Temporary relief of pain when extremity is flexed
- Weakness, swelling, decreased movement, or limping
- Palpable lymph nodes near the tumor
- Anemia, generalized infection, or unexplained weight loss
- Inability to hold a heavy object

LABORATORY TESTS

CBC and other common tests can help rule out infection, iron deficiency anemia, and other possible causes of findings.

DIAGNOSTIC PROCEDURES

- X-rays, computed tomography (CT) scans, or magnetic resonance imaging (MRI) of the primary site
- Bone marrow biopsy
- CT of the chest and bone scans to evaluate metastasis

PATIENT-CENTERED CARE

NURSING CARE

- Use developmentally appropriate language when explaining the diagnosis and treatment.
- Allow the child time, usually several days, to prepare emotionally for surgery and chemotherapy.
- Avoid overwhelming the child with information.
- Provide emotional support for the child and family.
- Explain the possibility of sterilization to adolescents and caregivers, if indicated.

MEDICATIONS

Chemotherapy

Osteosarcoma
- Various agents used singly or in combination before and/or after surgery
- High-dose methotrexate with citrovorum factor rescue, doxorubicin, cisplatin, ifosfamide, and etoposide

Ewing's sarcoma: Vincristine, doxorubicin, and cyclophosphamide alternating with ifosfamide and etoposide

NURSING ACTIONS
- Control nausea and vomiting with antiemetics prior to treatment.
- Manage adverse effects of treatment.

CLIENT EDUCATION
- Observe for manifestations of infection, skin breakdown, and nutritional deficiency.
- Maintain good hygiene.
- Understand proper use of vascular access devices.
- Take bleeding precautions and properly manage active bleeding.

THERAPEUTIC PROCEDURES

Localized radiation therapy can be used in combination with chemotherapy and surgery.

NURSING ACTIONS
- Assist the child with positioning.
- Monitor for adverse effects.

CLIENT EDUCATION: Adhere to the course of therapy.

Surgical interventions

Surgical biopsy
- Tumor is biopsied under anesthesia to determine presence and/or tissue type of cancer.
- NURSING ACTIONS
  - Provide routine preoperative and postoperative care.
  - Provide for adequate pain relief.
  - Monitor wound for manifestations of infection.
  - Actions vary with extent and area of surgery, but nursing actions should include preprocedure and postprocedure evaluations, including vital signs, medication for pain, and wound care as necessary.
- CLIENT EDUCATION: Educate the child and family regarding postprocedure care.

Limb salvage procedure for bone cancers
- Includes a course of chemotherapy to shrink the tumor and then total bone and joint replacement after the tumor and affected bone are removed.
- NURSING ACTIONS
  - Assist with managing adverse effects.
  - Provide routine postoperative care.
  - Provide for adequate pain relief.
- CLIENT EDUCATION
  - Understand proper postoperative care.
  - Understand possible effects of preoperative chemotherapy (hair loss).

Limb amputation for bone cancer
- The child can receive chemotherapy both preoperatively and postoperatively.
- NURSING ACTIONS
  - Provide routine preoperative and postoperative care.
  - Provide emotional support.
  - Monitor for the presence of phantom limb pain postoperatively, and medicate appropriately.
  - Work with the child and family to plan for issues (appropriate clothing to wear with prosthesis).

- **CLIENT EDUCATION**
  - Assist with preparing the child for fitting of a temporary prosthesis, which can occur immediately after surgery. ○PCC
  - Cooperate with postoperative physical therapy.
  - Role-play issues that the child will need to deal with after discharge (talking to strangers who ask about the prosthesis).
  - The child's emotions (anger) are normal grief reactions after amputation, chemotherapy, and other treatments.

INTERPROFESSIONAL CARE

- Older children and adolescents can benefit from attending a support group for children who have cancer and/or have had amputations.
- Initiate a referral for mental health counseling to assist the child to resume normal activities.
- Initiate appropriate referrals to assist the child to resume normal activities (school attendance, physical activities).
- Initiate physical and occupational therapy referrals to start while in the hospital and to continue after discharge.

CLIENT EDUCATION

Follow up with the provider and community resources as instructed.

COMPLICATIONS

Skin desquamation

Either dry or moist, with permanent hyperpigmentation and possible damage to underlying structures

Myelosuppression

Elimination of normal blood cells along with cancer cells is a risk with treatment by most chemotherapeutic agents. This can cause infection (reduced leukocytes), hemorrhage (reduced thrombocytes), and anemia (reduced red blood cells).

NURSING ACTIONS

- Review laboratory data and monitor for manifestations of complications.
  - Infection: elevated WBC and fever
  - Hemorrhage: blood in urine or stool, bruising, and petechiae
  - Anemia: fatigue and decreased hemoglobin/hematocrit
- Prevent infection.
  - Provide a private room when hospitalized.
  - Restrict staff/visitors that have infections.
  - Promote frequent hand hygiene by staff/visitors.
  - Avoid all live-virus vaccines during periods of immunosuppression.
  - Ensure that household members are up-to-date on immunizations.
  - Use a strict aseptic technique for all invasive procedures.

- Provide a diet adequate in proteins and calories.
- Prevent hemorrhage or injury from bleeding.
- Use gentle technique when providing mouth care.
- Clean the perineal area carefully to prevent trauma, and avoid obtaining temperatures rectally.
- Assist with administering platelets as prescribed.
- Prevent anemia or injury from anemia.
  - Provide rest periods as needed.
  - Infuse packed red blood cells as prescribed.

CLIENT EDUCATION: Perform strategies to prevent injury from infection, hemorrhage, or bleeding and report complications as soon as possible.

Rhabdomyosarcoma

Most common soft tissue malignancy in children

DATA COLLECTION

RISK FACTORS

Rhabdomyosarcoma occurs in children of all ages (but more commonly in children younger than 5 years of age) and is more common among Caucasians.

EXPECTED FINDINGS

- Can cause pain in local areas related to compression by the tumor (sore throat can occur with tumor of the nasopharynx)
- Possible absence of pain in some parts of the body (in the retroperitoneal area) until the tumor begins to obstruct organs

BASED ON AFFECTED AREA
- **CNS:** headaches, diplopia, vomiting
- **Orbit:** unilateral proptosis, ecchymosis of conjunctiva, strabismus
- **Nasopharynx:** stuffy nose, pain, nasal obstruction, epistaxis, palpable neck nodes, visible mass (late)
- **Paranasal sinuses:** nasal obstruction, pain, discharge, sinusitis, swelling
- **Middle ear:** chronic otitis media, pain, sanguinopurulent discharge, facial paralysis
- **Retroperitoneal area:** usually no findings, abdominal mass, pain, intestinal or genitourinary obstruction
- **Perineum:** visible superficial mass, bowel or bladder obstruction
- **Extremity:** pain, palpable fixed mass, lymph node enlargement

DIAGNOSTIC PROCEDURES

- CT scans or MRI of the primary site
- Biopsy of tumor is possible
- CT of the chest, bone scans, bone marrow biopsy, and lumbar puncture to evaluate metastasis

PATIENT-CENTERED CARE

NURSING CARE

- Use developmentally appropriate language when explaining the diagnosis and treatment.
- Allow the child time, usually several days, to prepare emotionally for surgery and chemotherapy.
- Avoid overwhelming the child with information.
- Provide emotional support for the parents and child.

MEDICATIONS

Chemotherapy

Vincristine, actinomycin D, cyclophosphamide, ifosfamide, topotecan, irinotecan, and doxorubicin for about 1 year

THERAPEUTIC PROCEDURES

Localized radiation therapy

Radiation therapy can be used in combination with chemotherapy and surgery.

Surgical interventions

Surgical biopsy
Tumor is biopsied under anesthesia to determine presence and/or tissue type of cancer.

COMPLICATIONS

- Skin desquamation
- Myelosuppression

Active Learning Scenario

A nurse is reinforcing teaching with the guardian of a child who has bone cancer and is receiving chemotherapy about myelosuppression. Use the ATI Active Learning Template: Basic Concept to complete this item.

NURSING CARE: Describe two actions related to each of the following areas.

- Determining laboratory data to monitor for complications
- Preventing infection
- Preventing hemorrhage or injury from bleeding
- Preventing anemia or injury from anemia

Application Exercises

1. A nurse is assisting with the care for a toddler who has a Wilms' tumor. Which of the following actions should the nurse take?

   A. Palpate the child's abdomen to identify the size of the tumor.

   B. Assist with preparing the child for surgery.

   C. Reinforce teaching with the guardians about dialysis.

   D. Obtain a 24-hr urine specimen from the child.

2. A nurse is collecting data from a child who has leukemia. Which of the following are early manifestations of leukemia? (Select all that apply.)

   A. Hematuria

   B. Anorexia

   C. Petechiae

   D. Ulcerations in the mouth

   E. Unsteady gait

3. A nurse is assisting with the care for a child who has thrombocytopenia following chemotherapy. Which of the following actions should the nurse take? (Select all that apply.)

   A. Monitor for manifestations of bleeding.

   B. Administer routine immunizations.

   C. Obtain rectal temperatures.

   D. Avoid peripheral venipunctures.

   E. Limit visitors.

4. A nurse is assisting with the care for a child who has oral mucositis. Which of the following actions should the nurse take? (Select all that apply.)

   A. Swab the mucosa with lemon glycerin swabs.

   B. Apply viscous lidocaine.

   C. Offer soft foods.

   D. Use a soft, disposable toothbrush for oral care.

   E. Encourage gargling with a warm saline mouthwash.

5. A nurse is collecting data from a child who has rhabdomyosarcoma of the nasopharynx. Which of the following are manifestations of rhabdomyosarcoma? (Select all that apply.)

   A. Enlarged neck lymph nodes

   B. Pain

   C. Vomiting

   D. Epistaxis

   E. Diplopia

Application Exercises Key

1. A. Pressure applied to the abdomen could rupture the encapsulated tumor.
   B. **CORRECT:** Removal of the tumor occurs within 24 to 48 hr of admission. Preparation for surgery should be included in the plan of care.
   C. Wilms' tumor is usually unilateral.
   D. A urine specimen is usually obtained for diagnostic evaluation of Wilms' tumor.

   Ⓝ NCLEX® Connection: Physiological Adaptation, Alterations in Body Systems

2. A. Hematuria is a late manifestation of leukemia.
   B. **CORRECT:** Anorexia is an early manifestation of leukemia.
   C. **CORRECT:** Petechiae is an early manifestation of leukemia.
   D. Ulcerations in the mouth are a late manifestation of leukemia.
   E. **CORRECT:** Unsteady gait is an early manifestation of leukemia.

   Ⓝ NCLEX® Connection: Physiological Adaptation, Basic Pathophysiology

3. A. **CORRECT:** The child who has thrombocytopenia is at risk for hemorrhage. Monitoring for findings of bleeding is an appropriate action to take.
   B. The child who has thrombocytopenia is at risk for bleeding, and skin punctures should be avoided. Administering routine immunizations is not an appropriate action to take.
   C. The child who has thrombocytopenia is at risk for bleeding, and obtaining a rectal temperature could cause tissue injury.
   D. **CORRECT:** The child who has thrombocytopenia is at risk for bleeding. Avoiding venipunctures is an appropriate action to take.
   E. The child who has thrombocytopenia is at risk for bleeding. Limiting visitors protects the child from infection and is not an appropriate action to prevent bleeding.

   Ⓝ NCLEX® Connection: Physiological Adaptation, Unexpected Response to Therapies

4. A. Lemon glycerin swabs can cause tooth decay and erosion of the tissues.
   B. Viscous lidocaine can depress the gag reflex and cause aspiration.
   C. **CORRECT:** Offering soft foods decreases the amount of chewing needed and possible irritation.
   D. **CORRECT:** A soft toothbrush allows for adequate cleaning of the mouth and decreases irritation.
   E. **CORRECT:** A warm saline mouthwash is effective in soothing mucositis.

   Ⓝ NCLEX® Connection: Physiological Adaptation, Alterations in Body Systems

5. A. **CORRECT:** Palpable neck lymph nodes are a manifestation of rhabdomyosarcoma of the nasopharynx.
   B. **CORRECT:** Pain is a manifestation of rhabdomyosarcoma of the nasopharynx.
   C. Vomiting is a manifestation of rhabdomyosarcoma of the central nervous system.
   D. **CORRECT:** Epistaxis is a manifestation of rhabdomyosarcoma of the nasopharynx.
   E. Diplopia is a manifestation of rhabdomyosarcoma of the central nervous system.

   Ⓝ NCLEX® Connection: Physiological Adaptation, Basic Pathophysiology

Active Learning Scenario Key

Using the ATI Active Learning Template: Basic Concept

NURSING CARE

- Review laboratory data to monitor for complications
  - Infection: elevated WBC and fever
  - Hemorrhage: blood in urine or stool, bruising, and petechiae
  - Anemia: fatigue and decreased hemoglobin/hematocrit
- Preventing infection
  - Provide a private room when hospitalized.
  - Restrict staff/visitors who have infections.
  - Promote frequent hand hygiene by staff/visitors.
  - Avoid all live-virus vaccines during periods of immunosuppression.
  - Ensure that household members are up-to-date on immunizations.
  - Provide a diet adequate in proteins and calories.
- Preventing hemorrhage or injury from bleeding
  - Use a strict aseptic technique for all invasive procedures.
  - Use gentle technique when providing mouth care.
  - Clean the perineal area carefully to prevent trauma, and avoid obtaining temperatures rectally.
  - Assist with administering platelets as prescribed.
- Preventing anemia or injury from anemia
  - Provide rest periods as needed.
  - Assist with infusing packed red blood cells as prescribed.

Ⓝ NCLEX® Connection: Reduction of Risk Potential, Therapeutic Procedures

When reviewing the following chapters, keep in mind the relevant topics and tasks of the NCLEX outline, in particular:

Psychosocial Integrity

ABUSE/NEGLECT
Identify signs and symptoms of physical, psychological, or financial abuse in the client.

Provide safe environment for abused/neglected client.

Physiological Adaptation

ALTERATIONS IN BODY SYSTEMS: Reinforce education to client regarding care and condition.

BASIC PATHOPHYSIOLOGY: Identify signs and symptoms related to an acute or chronic illness.

MEDICAL EMERGENCIES: Notify primary health care provider about client unexpected response/emergency situation.

UNIT 3 OTHER SPECIFIC NEEDS

CHAPTER 39 *Complications of Infants*

It is essential for a nurse to immediately identify complications of newborns and infants, notify the charge nurse and provider, and implement recommended interventions. Providing ongoing emotional support for an infant's parents or guardians is also imperative to contribute to the plan of care.

Complications include phenylketonuria (PKU), meningocele, necrotizing enterocolitis (NEC), respiratory distress syndrome (RDS), congenital hypothyroidism, substance-exposed infants, hyperbilirubinemia, chromosomal abnormalities, neonatal seizures, complications of premature infants, newborn sepsis, and plagiocephaly.

Phenylketonuria

- PKU is an inherited metabolic disorder in which the newborn lacks the enzyme phenylalanine hydroxylase. This enzyme converts phenylalanine, an essential amino acid, into tyrosine. The lack of this enzyme leads to the accumulation of phenylalanine in the newborn's bloodstream and tissues, which causes cognitive impairment.
- The key to prevention of PKU in newborns is identification of clients in their reproductive years who have the disorder. These clients must adhere to strict dietary guidelines from 3 months before conception throughout pregnancy. Failure to follow strict dietary guidelines during pregnancy can result in fetal microcephaly, cognitive impairment, and heart defects. Clients who have PKU will have their phenylalanine levels monitored one to two times per week throughout pregnancy.
- All newborns are screened for PKU by blood spot analysis after the newborn has ingested a source of protein and usually within the first 2 days of birth. Immediate identification and providing a diet with low phenylalanine significantly decreases the occurrence of cognitive impairment.

DATA COLLECTION

RISK FACTORS

PKU is inherited as an autosomal recessive trait. Female clients who have PKU or who have had a child who has PKU can undergo genetic testing to determine the risk of PKU in future children.

EXPECTED FINDINGS

- Growth failure
- Frequent vomiting
- Irritability
- Musty odor to urine
- Microcephaly
- Heart defects
- Blue eyes, very fair skin, light blonde hair

LABORATORY TESTS

Newborn metabolic screen: Blood spot analysis performed within 2 days of birth after the newborn has ingested a source of protein.
- Expected reference range of phenylalanine in newborns is 0.5 to 1 mg/dL.
- Some states require a repeat newborn metabolic screen when the newborn is 1 to 2 weeks of age.

Guthrie test: Confirms diagnosis when blood spot analysis is positive.

PATIENT-CENTERED CARE

NURSING CARE

Nursing care focuses on dietary intake.
- Initiate dietary restrictions as soon as PKU is diagnosed, or within 7 to 10 days of birth.
- Place the newborn on a formula low in phenylalanine.
  - Intake should be 20 to 30 mg of phenylalanine per kilogram of body weight per day.
  - Monitor phenylalanine level.
  - Goal is a phenylalanine level between 2 and 8 mg/dL.
- Monitor phenylalanine levels in newborns who are breastfeeding. Breast milk contains phenylalanine, so breastfeeding exclusively might not be possible.
- Monitor the newborn for findings of PKU.
- Provide guardians with education and support.
  - Consult with a registered dietitian.
  - Provide referrals to support groups.

COMPLICATIONS

- Cognitive impairment (can be mild to severe)
- Hyperactivity with erratic behavior
- Bizarre behavior (excessive fright reactions)
- Head banging
- Arm biting
- Disorientation
- Spasticity or catatonic-like positions
- Seizures

Meningocele/ Myelomeningocele

Meningocele and myelomeningocele are neural tube defects (NTD) that are present at birth and affect the CNS and spine. These defects occur when the neural tube fails to close during the third to fourth week of embryonic development. These defects are also classified as spina bifida.

Meningocele is the protrusion of a sac-like cyst that contains meninges and spinal fluid.

Myelomeningocele is the protrusion of a sac-like cyst that contains meninges, spinal fluid, and a portion of the spinal cord and nerves.

DATA COLLECTION

RISK FACTORS

- Use of medications or illicit substances during pregnancy
- Malnutrition during pregnancy
- Insufficient intake of folic acid during pregnancy
- Exposure to radiation or chemicals during pregnancy
- Prepregnancy obesity, diabetes mellitus, hyperthermia, or low levels of vitamin B12
- Previous birth of neonate who has a neural tube defect

EXPECTED FINDINGS

- Protrusion of a sac-like cyst midline of the spine. Cysts are most commonly found in the lumbar or lumbosacral area.
- Sensory and/or neuromotor dysfunction
  - Type and severity of dysfunction dependent on location of defect
  - Observe lower extremities for movement and response to stimuli
- Constant dribbling of urine and loss of feces possible
- Potential limb deformities

DIAGNOSTIC TESTS

MATERNAL TESTING DURING PREGNANCY
- Elevated alpha-fetoprotein levels in maternal blood
- Chorionic villi sampling
- Amniocentesis
- Ultrasound

NEWBORN TESTING
- MRI
- Ultrasound
- CT scan
- Neurologic evaluation

PATIENT-CENTERED CARE

NURSING CARE
- Monitor for infant-parent attachment.
- Examine the cyst.
- Perform routine newborn examinations.

- Monitor neurologic status.
- Obtain accurate measurements of output.
- Monitor fontanels and head circumference.

THERAPEUTIC PROCEDURES

Closure of the meningocele/myelomeningocele sac

Done as soon as possible to prevent complications due to injury or infection

PREOPERATIVE NURSING ACTIONS
- Assist with preparing the family for the newborn's surgery (within 24 to 72 hr after birth).
- Protect the sac from injury.
- Place the infant in a radiant warmer, without clothing.
- Apply a sterile, moist non-adhering dressing with 0.9% sodium chloride on the cyst, re-wetting as needed to prevent drying.
- Inspect the cyst closely for leakage of fluid or manifestations of irritation.
- Monitor for manifestations of infection (fever, irritability, and lethargy).
- Administer IV antibiotics as prescribed.
- Avoid measuring temperatures rectally.
- Avoid putting pressure on the sac.

POSTOPERATIVE NURSING ACTIONS
- Monitor vital signs.
- Monitor I&O.
- Monitor weight.
- Monitor for manifestations of infection.
- Provide pain management as prescribed.
- Monitor for leakage of CSF.
- Maintain prone position until other positions are prescribed.
- Resume oral feedings.
- Provide range of motion (ROM) to extremities.
- Monitor fontanels for bulging.
- Measure head circumference.

CLIENT EDUCATION
- Reinforce education with the guardians about postoperative home care.
- Depending on degree of the newborn's disability, instruct the guardians to perform ROM techniques.

ONGOING CARE
- Monitor skin integrity, head circumference, and bowel and bladder functioning.
- Check for allergies (latex).
- Evaluate cognitive and motor development.
- Monitor for infections.
- Address concerns with body image.
- Offer support to family.
- Assist the client with independence throughout lifespan.
- Assist the family with obtaining medical equipment/services.

INTERPROFESSIONAL CARE

Neurosurgery, neurology, urology, orthopedics, physical therapy, occupational therapy, and social services can be consulted.

COMPLICATIONS

Skin pressure injury

Caused by prolonged pressure on one area

NURSING ACTIONS
- Monitor skin for breakdown.
- Reposition frequently to prevent pressure on bony prominences.
- Monitor skin under splints and braces.

CLIENT EDUCATION: Reinforce teaching with the guardians on how to monitor skin integrity.

Latex allergy

The infant can have a high risk of allergy to latex. Allergy responses range from urticaria to wheezing, which can progress to anaphylaxis.

NURSING ACTIONS
- Assist with testing for allergy.
- Reduce exposure to latex.

CLIENT EDUCATION
- Avoid exposing the infant to latex.
- Be aware of household items that can contain latex (disposable diapers, cleaning gloves, water toys).
- Observe for manifestations of an allergic reaction and report them to the provider.
- Understand proper use of epinephrine.

Increased intracranial pressure

Caused by shunt malformation or hydrocephalus

MANIFESTATIONS: High-pitched cry, lethargy, vomiting, bulging fontanels and/or widening cranial suture lines, increased head circumference

NURSING ACTIONS
- Anticipate surgery for shunt or shunt revision.
- Use gentle movements when performing ROM exercises.
- Minimize environmental stressors (noise, lights, frequent visitors).
- Monitor and manage pain.

CLIENT EDUCATION: Observe for manifestations of shunt malfunction and hydrocephalus and report them to the provider.

Bladder issues

Urinary diversion can be performed to manage bladder dysfunction (either spasticity or flaccidity).

NURSING ACTIONS
- Monitor for manifestations of bladder dysfunction.
- Monitor for manifestations of bladder infection.
- Monitor for bleeding.
- Assist with preparing the newborn and family for surgery if necessary.
- Reinforce teaching with the guardians on how to care for the stoma (vesicostomy) if applicable.

Orthopedic issues

Corrections of associated potential problems (clubfoot, scoliosis, and other malformations of the feet and legs)

NURSING ACTIONS
- Monitor for manifestations of infection.
- Administer pain medications.
- Assist with preparing the newborn and family for surgery if needed.
- Provide cast care if cast is present.
- Monitor for neurologic deficits.

CLIENT EDUCATION
- Observe for manifestations of infection.
- Understand proper cast and splint care.

Necrotizing enterocolitis

NEC is an inflammatory disease of the gastrointestinal mucosa caused by ischemia or hypoxia. Ischemia results in death of mucosal cells leading to necrotic patches that interfere with digestion.

DATA COLLECTION

RISK FACTORS

- Prematurity
- Respiratory distress syndrome
- Polycythemia
- Exchange transfusion
- Intrauterine growth restriction
- Shock
- Asphyxia
- Receiving enteral feedings
- Pre-existing infection
- GI vascular compromise
- Immature GI host defense

EXPECTED FINDINGS

- Abdominal distention
- Gastric residuals
- Bloody stools
- Periods of apnea begin or worsen
- Hypotension
- Lethargy
- Poor feeding
- Decreased urinary output

LABORATORY TESTS

- CBC with differential
- ABGs
- Coagulation studies
- Blood cultures
- Electrolytes

DIAGNOSTIC PROCEDURES

Abdominal x-rays
- Sausage-shaped dilation of intestine
- Marked distention of intestine
- Characteristic "soapsuds" appearance of the intestinal wall due to air infiltration
- Free air in abdominal cavity if perforation has occurred

PATIENT-CENTERED CARE

NURSING CARE

- Treatment begins with prevention. Withhold feedings for 24 to 48 hr from newborns who suffered birth asphyxia.
- Initiate feeding with breast milk, which has a protective effect against the development of NEC.
- Anticipate discontinuation of all feedings at first manifestation of NEC.
- Handle the abdomen carefully to prevent intestinal perforation.
- Measure abdominal girth just above the umbilicus every 4 to 8 hr.
- Assist with serial abdominal x-rays every 4 to 6 hr.
- Monitor vital signs.
- Assist with preparing the newborn and family for surgical intervention, if indicated.
  - Removal of necrotized portion of bowel.
  - Temporary colostomy is a possibility.
  - Facilitate bonding.

COMPLICATIONS

- Short-bowel syndrome (disorder of absorption)
- Colonic stricture with possible obstruction
- Fat malabsorption
- Failure to thrive

Respiratory distress syndrome

RDS occurs as a result of surfactant deficiency in the lungs and is characterized by poor gas exchange and ventilatory failure.
- Surfactant is a phospholipid that assists in alveoli expansion. Surfactant keeps alveoli from collapsing and allows gas exchange to occur.
- Atelectasis (collapsing of a portion of lung) increases the work of breathing. As a result, respiratory acidosis and hypoxemia can develop.
- Complications from RDS are related to oxygen therapy and mechanical ventilation.
  - Pneumothorax
  - Pneumomediastinum
  - Retinopathy of prematurity
  - Bronchopulmonary dysplasia
  - Infection
  - Intraventricular hemorrhage

DATA COLLECTION

RISK FACTORS

- Preterm gestation
- Perinatal asphyxia (meconium staining, cord prolapse, nuchal cord)
- Maternal diabetes mellitus
- Premature rupture of membranes
- Maternal use of barbiturates or narcotics close to birth
- Cesarean section birth
- Multifetal pregnancy
- Cold stress
- Sepsis
- Airway obstruction
- Hypoglycemia

EXPECTED FINDINGS

- Tachypnea (respiratory rate greater than 60/min)
- Nasal flaring
- Expiratory grunting
- Retractions
- Labored breathing with prolonged expiration
- Fine crackles on auscultation
- Cyanosis
- Unresponsiveness, flaccidity, and apnea with decreased breath sounds (manifestations of worsened RDS)

LABORATORY TESTS

- Culture and sensitivity of the blood, urine, and cerebrospinal fluid
- Blood glucose

DIAGNOSTIC PROCEDURES

- ABGs reveal hypercapnia (excess of carbon dioxide in the blood) and respiratory or mixed acidosis.
- Chest x-ray

PATIENT-CENTERED CARE

NURSING CARE

- Suction the newborn's mouth, trachea, and nose as needed.
- Maintain thermoregulation.
- Provide mouth and skin care.
- Maintain adequate oxygenation, prevent lactic acidosis, and avoid the toxic effects of oxygen.
- Decrease environmental stimuli.

MEDICATIONS

Beractant, poractant alfa, calfactant

CLASSIFICATION: Lung surfactant

INTENDED EFFECT: It is prescribed for newborns who are premature and have RDS. It restores surfactant and improves respiratory compliance.

NURSING ACTIONS

- Monitor ABGs, respiratory rhythm, and rate and color before and after administration of agent.
- Provide suction to the newborn prior to administration of the medication.
- Monitor endotracheal tube placement.
- Avoid suctioning of the endotracheal tube for 1 hr after administration of the medication.

Congenital hypothyroidism

Congenital hypothyroidism occurs due to an absent or nonfunctioning thyroid gland in a newborn. Thyroid hypofunction can be caused by maternal iodine deficiency or maternal antithyroid medications during pregnancy.

- Findings might not appear until 3 months of age in a formula-fed infant and 6 months of age in a breastfed infant.
- Early diagnosis is crucial due to severe progressive physical and cognitive dysfunction that will occur if left untreated.

DATA COLLECTION

RISK FACTORS

- Female sex
- Low birth weight or birth weight greater than 4.5 kg (4,500 g)
- Maternal low iodine levels during pregnancy

EXPECTED FINDINGS

PHYSICAL FINDINGS
- Sleeping excessively
- Enlarged tongue
- Respiratory difficulty
- Poor sucking
- Cool, dry skin on extremities
- Jaundice
- Subnormal temperature, respiratory rate and pulse
- Short, thick neck
- Hypotonia with decreased deep tendon reflexes
- Abdominal distention and constipation

LABORATORY TESTS

- Newborn metabolic screen: blood spot analysis performed within 2 days of birth
- T3, T4 and TSH levels
- Blood lipid levels

DIAGNOSTIC PROCEDURES

- X-rays to evaluate bone growth
- Ultrasound of thyroid

PATIENT-CENTERED CARE

NURSING CARE

- Monitor vital signs and weight.
- Monitor respiratory status.
- Observe for feeding difficulties.
- Treatment is administration of synthetic thyroid hormone (sodium levothyroxine).
  - Administer medication as prescribed.
  - Medication must be taken indefinitely.
- Administer supplemental vitamin D to support rapid bone growth.
- Monitor thyroid levels (T3, T4 and TSH).

CLIENT EDUCATION: Understand the importance of proper medication administration.

Substance-exposed infants

Maternal substance use during pregnancy consists of any use of alcohol or drugs. Intrauterine drug exposure can cause anomalies, neurobehavioral changes, and evidence of withdrawal in the neonate. These changes depend on the specific drug or combination of drugs used, dosage, route of administration, metabolism and excretion by the mother and her fetus, timing of exposure, and length of exposure.

- Substance withdrawal in the newborn occurs when the mother uses drugs that have addictive properties during pregnancy. This includes illicit substances, heroin, opiates, alcohol, tobacco, methadone, and prescription medications.
- Fetal alcohol spectrum disorder (FASD), formerly referred to as fetal alcohol syndrome (FAS), results from exposure of the fetus to the chronic or periodic intake of alcohol during pregnancy. FASD is an umbrella term used to describe the range of clinical effects. FAS refers specifically to children who exhibit a triad of characteristic facial features, growth restriction, and neurodevelopmental deficits and a confirmed history of maternal alcohol consumption.
- Newborns who have FAS are at risk for specific congenital physical defects, along with long-term complications.
  - Feeding problems
  - Central nervous system dysfunction (learning disabilities, low IQ, seizures)
  - Behavioral difficulties (hyperactivity [ADHD])
  - Language abnormalities
  - Delayed growth and development
  - Poor maternal-newborn bonding

DATA COLLECTION

RISK FACTORS

- Maternal use of substances prior to knowing they are pregnant
- Maternal substance use and addiction

EXPECTED FINDINGS

PHYSICAL FINDINGS

Monitor the neonate for abstinence syndrome (withdrawal) and increased wakefulness using the neonatal abstinence scoring system that evaluates and scores the following.

- CNS: increased wakefulness, a high-pitched, shrill cry, incessant crying, irritability, tremors, hyperactive with an increased Moro reflex, increased deep-tendon reflexes, increased muscle tone, abrasions and/or excoriations on the face and knees, and convulsions
- Metabolic, vasomotor, and respiratory: nasal congestion with flaring, frequent yawning, skin mottling, tachypnea greater than 60/min, sweating, and temperature greater than 37.2° C (99° F) or temperature greater than 38.3° C (101° F)
- Gastrointestinal: poor feeding, regurgitation (projectile vomiting), diarrhea, and excessive, uncoordinated, and constant sucking

Heroin withdrawal

Neonatal abstinence syndrome: Low birth weight and small for gestational age (SGA), decreased Moro reflexes (rather than increased), jittery, hyperactive, and hypothermia or hyperthermia. The infant has a shrill persistent cry.

Methadone withdrawal

Neonatal abstinence syndrome: Increased incidence of seizures, sleep pattern disturbances, higher birth weights, and higher risk of sudden infant death syndrome (SIDS)

Cocaine exposure

- Infant can appear normal or exhibit neurologic problems at birth. Newborn can exhibit neurobehavioral depression or excitability.
- High-pitched cry, abnormal sleep patterns, excessive sucking, hypertonicity, tremors, irritability, inability to console, and poor tolerance to changes in routine.

Marijuana exposure

Associated with a decrease in newborn birth weight and length, fetal growth

Methamphetamine withdrawal

Small head circumference, SGA, agitation, vomiting, rapid respiratory rate, bradycardia or tachycardia, jitteriness, sleep pattern disturbances, emotional disturbances, and delayed growth and development

Fetal alcohol syndrome

- Craniofacial features include microcephaly, small eyes with epicanthal folds, and short palpebral fissures, thin upper lip, flat midface, and indistinct philtrum
- Lack of stranger anxiety and appropriate judgment skills
- Many vital organ anomalies (limb defect and heart defects, including ventricular septal defects)
- Prenatal and postnatal growth restriction
- Developmental delays and neurologic abnormalities
- IQ deficit
- Diminished fine motor skills
- Attention deficit disorder

Tobacco exposure

Prematurity, low birth weight, increased risk for SIDS, increased risk for bronchitis, pneumonia, and developmental delays

LABORATORY TESTS

Blood tests should be done to differentiate between neonatal drug withdrawal and central nervous system irritability.

- CBC
- Blood glucose
- Calcium
- Electrolytes
- Drug screen of urine or meconium to reveal the agent used by the mother
- Hair analysis

DIAGNOSTIC PROCEDURES

Chest x-ray for FAS to rule out congenital heart defects

PATIENT-CENTERED CARE

NURSING CARE

Nursing care for maternal substance use and neonatal effects or withdrawal include the following in addition to normal newborn care.

- Assist with a neonatal abstinence scoring system evaluation, as prescribed.
- Elicit reflexes.
- Monitor the ability to feed and digest intake.
- Monitor fluids and electrolytes, skin turgor, mucous membranes, fontanels, and I&O.
- Observe the newborn's behavior.

MEDICATIONS

Phenobarbital

CLASSIFICATION: Anticonvulsant

INTENDED EFFECT: It is prescribed to decrease CNS irritability and control seizures for newborns who are susceptible to seizures.

NURSING ACTIONS

- Monitor IV site frequently.
- Check for any medication incompatibilities.
- Decrease environmental stimuli.
- Initiate cluster care for newborns to minimize stimulation.
- Swaddle the newborn to reduce self-stimulation and protect the skin from abrasions.
- Monitor and maintain fluids and electrolytes.
- Administer frequent, small feedings of high-calorie formula. The newborn can require gavage feedings.
- Elevate the newborn's head during and following feedings, and burp the newborn to reduce vomiting and aspiration. Qs
- Try various types of nipples to compensate for a poor suck reflex.

- Have suction available to reduce the risk for aspiration.
- For newborns who are addicted to cocaine, avoid eye contact. Use vertical rocking and a pacifier.
- Consult lactation services to evaluate whether breastfeeding is desired or contraindicated to avoid passing narcotics in breast milk. Methadone is not contraindicated during breastfeeding.
- Prevent infection.
- Initiate a consult with child protective services.
- Morphine and clonidine can be administered to decrease central nervous system irritability.

CLIENT EDUCATION

- Refer the mother to a drug and/or alcohol treatment center.
- Discuss the importance of SIDS prevention activities due to the increased rate in newborns of mothers who used methadone.

Hyperbilirubinemia

Hyperbilirubinemia is an elevation of blood bilirubin levels resulting in jaundice. Jaundice normally appears in the head (especially the sclera and mucous membranes), and then progresses down the thorax, abdomen, and extremities.

Jaundice can be either physiologic or pathologic
- Physiologic jaundice is considered benign (resulting from normal newborn physiology of increased bilirubin production due to the shortened lifespan and breakdown of fetal RBCs and liver immaturity). The newborn with physiological jaundice has no other manifestations and shows evidence of jaundice after 24 hr of age.
- Hemolytic disease of the newborn (HDN), or pathologic jaundice, is a result of an underlying disease. HDN appears before 24 hr of age. In the term newborn, normal unconjugated bilirubin levels are 0.2 to 1.4 mg/dL. Levels must exceed 5 mg/dL before jaundice is observed. HDN is usually caused by a blood group incompatibility or isoimmunization.

Kernicterus (bilirubin encephalopathy): When certain pathologic conditions exist in addition to increased bilirubin levels, the newborn has an increased permeability of the blood-brain barrier to unconjugated bilirubin. The newborn has the potential for irreversible brain damage. It is a neurologic syndrome caused by bilirubin depositing in brain cells. Survivors can experience neurologic damage, cerebral palsy, seizures and display cognitive impairment, ADHD, delayed or abnormal motor movement, behavioral disorders, perceptual problems, or sensorineural hearing loss.

DATA COLLECTION

RISK FACTORS

Pathologic hyperbilirubinemia
- Blood bilirubin level in the high-risk zone on the hour-specific nomogram
- Rh or ABO incompatibility with positive direct Coombs test
- Cephalohematoma or significant bruising
- Appearance of jaundice within 24 hr of birth
- Ineffective, difficult breastfeeding
- Gestational age 35 to 36 weeks
- Sibling who has jaundice
- Hereditary hemolytic disease
- East Asian or Asian-American race

EXPECTED FINDINGS

- Yellowish tint to skin, sclera, and mucous membranes and nails.
- To verify jaundice, press the newborn's skin on the cheek or abdomen lightly with one finger. Release pressure and observe the skin color for yellowish tint as the skin is blanched.
- Note the time of jaundice onset to distinguish between physiologic and pathologic jaundice.
- Determine the underlying cause by reviewing the maternal prenatal, family, and newborn history.
- Hypoxia, hypothermia, hypoglycemia, and metabolic acidosis can increase the risk of brain damage despite lower blood levels of bilirubin.

FINDINGS OF KERNICTERUS
- Very yellowish skin
- Lethargy
- Hypotonic
- Poor feeding
- Decreased activity
- High-pitched cry
- Temperature instability

LABORATORY TESTS

- An elevated blood bilirubin level can occur (direct and indirect bilirubin). Monitor bilirubin level until it returns to normal. Use of hour-specific blood bilirubin levels to predict newborns at risk for hyperbilirubinemia is the gold standard for monitoring newborns greater than 35 weeks gestation. Q EBP
- Monitor maternal and newborn blood type to determine whether there is a presence of ABO incompatibility. This occurs if the newborn has blood type A or B, and the mother is type O.
- Review Hgb and Hct.
- A direct Coombs test reveals the presence of antibody-coated (sensitized) Rh-positive RBCs in the newborn.
- Check electrolyte levels for dehydration from phototherapy.

DIAGNOSTIC PROCEDURES

Transcutaneous bilirubin level is a noninvasive method to measure a newborn's bilirubin level.

THERAPEUTIC PROCEDURES

Phototherapy is the primary treatment for hyperbilirubinemia. It is prescribed if a newborn's blood bilirubin is in the high-risk zone on the hour-specific blood bilirubin nomogram.

PATIENT-CENTERED CARE

NURSING CARE

- Observe the skin and mucous membranes for jaundice.
- Monitor vital signs with careful attention to temperature.
- Set up phototherapy if prescribed.
  - Maintain an eye mask over the newborn's eyes for protection of corneas and retinas.
  - Keep the newborn undressed with the exception of a diaper.
  - Avoid applying lotions or ointments to the skin because they absorb heat and can cause burns.
  - Remove the newborn from phototherapy every 4 hr, and unmask the newborn's eyes, checking for inflammation or injury.
  - Reposition the newborn every 2 hr to expose all body surfaces to the phototherapy lights and prevent pressure sores.
  - Check the lamp energy with a photometer per facility protocol.
  - Turn off the phototherapy lights before drawing blood for testing.
- Observe for effects of phototherapy.
  - Bronze discoloration: not a serious complication
  - Maculopapular skin rash: not a serious complication
  - Development of pressure areas
  - Dehydration (poor skin turgor, dry mucous membranes, decreased urinary output)
  - Elevated temperature
- Encourage the guardians to hold and interact with the newborn when phototherapy lights are off.
- Monitor elimination and daily weights for evidence of dehydration.
- Check the newborn's axillary temperature every 4 hr during phototherapy because temperature can become elevated.
- Feed the newborn early and frequently, every 3 to 4 hr. This will promote bilirubin excretion in the stools.
- Encourage continued breastfeeding of the newborn. Supplementation with donor breast milk or formula may be prescribed.

CLIENT EDUCATION: Observe for the rebound effect; bilirubin initially rises after treatment is discontinued but resolves without additional intervention.

Newborn sepsis

Infection can be contracted by the newborn before, during, or after delivery. Newborns are more susceptible to micro-organisms due to their limited immunity and inability to localize infection. The infection can spread rapidly into the bloodstream.

Newborn sepsis is the presence of micro-organisms or their toxins in the blood or tissues of the newborn during the first month after birth. Manifestations of sepsis are subtle and can resemble other diseases. The nurse often notices them during routine care of the newborn.

Organisms frequently responsible for newborn infections include Staphylococcus aureus, S. epidermidis, Escherichia coli, Haemophilus influenzae, group beta-hemolytic streptococcus, Klebsiella, and Pseudomonas.

Prevention of infection and newborn sepsis starts perinatally with maternal screening for infections, prophylactic interventions, and the use of sterile and aseptic techniques during delivery. Prophylactic antibiotic treatment of the eyes of all newborns and appropriate umbilical cord care also help to prevent newborn infection and sepsis.

DATA COLLECTION

RISK FACTORS

- Nosocomial exposure in the NICU
- Premature birth
- Prolonged rupture of membranes
- Maternal infection (cytomegalovirus, herpes, hepatitis, and human immunodeficiency virus)
- Invasive procedures (IV lines and ET tubes)
- TPN
- Congenital anomalies
- Diminished immune response

EXPECTED FINDINGS

- Temperature instability (hypothermia common)
- Suspicious drainage (eyes, umbilical stump)
- Poor feeding pattern (weak suck, decreased intake)
- Vomiting and diarrhea
- Poor weight gain
- Abdominal distention
- Large residual if feeding by gavage
- Apnea, retractions, grunting, cyanosis, and nasal flaring
- Decreased oxygen saturation
- Color changes (pallor, jaundice, and petechiae)
- Tachycardia or bradycardia
- Tachypnea or apnea
- Low blood pressure
- Irritability and seizure activity
- Poor muscle tone and lethargy

LABORATORY TESTS

- CBC
- Blood, urine, and cerebrospinal fluid cultures and sensitivities
- Positive blood cultures, indicates the presence of infection/sepsis
- Chemical profile shows a fluid and electrolyte imbalance.

PATIENT-CENTERED CARE

NURSING CARE

- Determine infection risks (review maternal health record).
- Monitor for findings of opportunistic infection.
- Monitor vital signs continuously.
- Monitor I&O and daily weight.
- Monitor fluid and electrolyte status.
- Restrict any visitors with infections.
- Obtain specimens (blood, urine, stool) to assist in identifying the causative organism.
- Initiate and maintain IV therapy to administer electrolyte replacements, fluids, and prescribed medications.
- Administer medications as prescribed (broad-spectrum antibiotics prior to cultures being obtained).
- Maintain respiratory support as needed.
- Monitor IV site for evidence of infection.
- Provide newborn care to maintain temperature.
- Utilize standard precautions.
- Clean and sterilize all equipment to be used.

CLIENT EDUCATION

- Understand infection control.
  - Use clean bottles and nipples for each feeding.
  - Discard any unused formula.
  - Supervise hand hygiene.
- Demonstrate infection control measures, including proper hand washing technique.
- Ensure adequate rest for newborn, and decrease physical stimulation.
- Provide emotional support to the family.

Plagiocephaly

Plagiocephaly is an acquired condition that occurs from cranial molding in infancy. The infant's head becomes asymmetric or oblique in shape due to flattening of the occiput. Plagiocephaly is attributed to the supine sleep position, as its occurrence has increased significantly since the Safe to Sleep campaign of infants sleeping on their backs was initiated to prevent SIDS.

- The key to prevention of plagiocephaly is educating parents on the importance of allowing the infant to lie in the prone position for 30 to 60 min/day while awake. Guardians should also alternate the infant's head position each night to avoid persistent pressure on the occiput.
- Treatment for plagiocephaly includes physical therapy and the wearing of a customized helmet to reshape the skull.

DATA COLLECTION

RISK FACTORS

- Placing the infant in the supine sleep position
- Torticollis

EXPECTED FINDINGS

PHYSICAL FINDINGS
- Oblique shape of head
- Asymmetrical skull and facial features
- Flattened occiput
- Frontal and parietal bossing
- Prominent cheekbone
- Anterior displacement of an ear
- Possible decreased range of motion in neck if torticollis present

PATIENT-CENTERED CARE

NURSING CARE

- Assist with referring guardians to physical therapy for neck exercises.
- Assist guardians in the proper use of the skull-molding helmet.

CLIENT EDUCATION
- Understand the importance of daily "tummy time" when infant is awake.
- Limit the time the infant is in a car seat, bouncer, or swing.
- Understand the importance of alternating the infant's head position during sleep.
- The helmet needs to be worn 23 hr/day, usually for 3 months
- Continue to place infant in the supine position for sleep

COMPLICATIONS

- There is no evidence that positional plagiocephaly leads to permanent cognitive or neurologic damage.
- Torticollis, or tightening of the sternocleidomastoid muscle on one side of the neck, can develop. Physical therapy can successfully treat torticollis within 4 to 8 weeks.

Newborn seizures

Newborn seizures are usually a manifestation of a serious underlying disease. The most common cause for newborn seizures is hypoxic-ischemic encephalopathy (HIE), or cellular damage due to a hypoxic perinatal episode.

- Newborn seizures are divided into four subtypes: clonic, tonic, myoclonic, and subtle.
- Newborn seizures can be difficult to identify due to subtle manifestations. Seizures must be differentiated from normal newborn jitteriness and tremors. Newborns typically exhibit oral movements, oculomotor deviations and apnea during seizure activity.

DATA COLLECTION

RISK FACTORS

Metabolic: Hyperglycemia, hypoglycemia, PKU, hypocalcemia, hypomagnesemia

Toxic: Uremia, kernicterus

Prenatal infection: Toxoplasmosis, syphilis, cytomegalovirus, herpes, hepatitis

Postnatal infection: Bacterial or viral meningitis, sepsis, brain abscess

Trauma during birth: Hypoxia, intracranial hemorrhage, subarachnoid or subdural hemorrhage, intraventricular hemorrhage

Miscellaneous: Degenerative disease, narcotic withdrawal, stroke (fetal, perinatal, or neonatal), benign familial newborn seizures

EXPECTED FINDINGS

Findings vary based on type of seizure.

Clonic: Slow rhythmic jerking movements; one to three movements per second
- Focal: Involves face, or upper or lower extremities on one side of the body; can involve neck or trunk; newborn is conscious during seizure
- Multifocal: Can migrate randomly from one part of the body to another; movements can start at different times

Tonic: Extension, stiffening movements
- Generalized: Extension of all limbs; upper limbs maintain a stiffly flexed position
- Focal: Sustained posturing of one limb; asymmetric posturing of trunk or neck

Subtle: Most common in premature newborns, often overlooked
- Horizontal eye deviation, repetitive blinking, fluttering of eyelids, staring
- Sucking or other oral/buccal/tongue movements
- Arm movements resembling swimming or rowing
- Leg movements resembling pedaling
- Apnea is common

Myoclonic: Rapid jerks that involve flexor muscle groups
- Focal: Involves upper extremity flexor muscles; no changes in EEG
- Multifocal: Asynchronous twitching of several parts of the body; no changes in EEG
- Generalized: Bilateral jerks of upper and lower limbs; associated with EEG discharges

LABORATORY TESTS

- Blood glucose levels
- Blood electrolytes
- CSF analyzed for blood, protein, glucose and cultured

DIAGNOSTIC PROCEDURES

- Electroencephalogram (EEG): continuous video EEG is gold standard for diagnosis
- CT scan
- Ultrasound
- Echoencephalography

PATIENT-CENTERED CARE

NURSING CARE

- Early recognition of seizure activity.
- Monitor vital signs.
- Continue routine newborn evaluations.
- Administer antiseizure medications as prescribed.
- Administer medications as prescribed for the underlying cause.
- Respiratory support if hypoxia present.
- Encourage infant-parent bonding.

CLIENT EDUCATION
- Be aware of newborn's status and treatment plan.
- Understand home medications and safe administration.

Chromosomal abnormalities

- Genetic disorders are passed from one generation to the next due to a disorder in a gene or chromosome. Genetic disorders can occur at the moment of fusion of sperm and egg or earlier, during meiotic division of the egg or sperm. Up to 50% of miscarriages are due to chromosomal disorders.
- Mendelian laws are the principles of genetic inheritance of disease.
  - Homozygous: Two healthy genes for a like trait
  - Heterozygous: One healthy gene and one unhealthy gene for a like trait
- Different types and characteristics of genetic disorders and inheritance include autosomal dominant, autosomal recessive, X-linked dominant, X-linked recessive, mitochondrial, and multifactorial.
- Provide education and support to parents who seek genetic counseling. Nurses also play an important role in supporting parents to make an informed decision about pregnancy and future reproductive options.

DATA COLLECTION

RISK FACTORS

- Parent who has existing genetic disorder or inborn error of metabolism
- Previous child born with a genetic disorder or inborn error of metabolism
- Previous stillbirth
- A close relative with a genetic disorder or inborn error of metabolism
- Parents who are closely related

- Parent who is a known carrier of a genetic disorder
- Woman older than 35 or man older than 55 at time of conception
- Exposure to infectious or environmental toxins (cytomegalovirus, radiation, chemicals)

MODES OF INHERITANCE

Autosomal dominant

Huntington's disease, Marfan syndrome
- Males and females equally affected.
- Children of affected parent have 50% chance of being affected.
- Expression of these genes can be very minor to severe and debilitating.

Autosomal recessive

Cystic fibrosis, phenylketonuria, galactosemia, Tay-Sachs disease, sickle cell
- Males and females equally affected.
- Both males and females can be carriers.
- Carrier parents have 25% chance of having an affected child with each pregnancy.
- Carrier parents have 50% chance of having a carrier child with each pregnancy.

Sex-linked: X-linked dominant

Hypophosphatemic vitamin D-resistant rickets, incontinentia pigmenti
- All males and females who have the gene are affected.
- All daughters of an affected male have the disorder and a 50% chance of passing the defective gene to their children.
- Affected males do not transmit the defective gene to their sons.

Sex-linked: X-linked recessive

Hemophilia types A and B, Duchenne muscular dystrophy, fragile X syndrome
- Most affected persons are male; affected females are very rare.
- Parents of affected children do not have the disorder.

Mitochondrial

Leigh syndrome, Kearns-Sayre syndrome
- Male carriers cannot pass the disorder to any children.
- Female carriers will pass disorder to 100% of their children.
- Inherited solely from cytoplasm of egg.

Multifactorial (complex)

Neural tube defects, cleft lip and palate, pyloric stenosis, many congenital heart defects, diabetes mellitus type 1, pyloric stenosis
- Have a higher than usual occurrence in some families, but no specific mode of inheritance identified
- Can occur from multiple gene combinations and environmental influence

Autosomal aneuploidies

- The uneven division (nondisjunction) of a cell leading to an uneven number of chromosomes
- Frequently leads to one extra or one too few chromosomes in a cell

Trisomy 21 (Down syndrome)
- Most frequently occurring chromosomal disorder
- Broad, flat nose
- Epicanthal fold
- Protruding tongue
- Short neck with extra pad of fat
- Hypotonicity
- Low set ears
- Fifth finger curved inward
- Single palmar crease
- Mild to moderate cognitive deficits
- Cardiac anomalies common
- Altered immune system

Trisomy 18 (Edwards syndrome)
- Severe cognitive deficits
- SGA
- Low-set ears, small jaw
- Misshapen fingers and toes
- Rocker-bottom feet
- Most die in infancy

Trisomy 13 (Patau syndrome)
- Severe cognitive deficits
- Midline body disorders: cleft lip/palate, cardiac defects, abnormal genitalia
- Microcephaly
- Eyes small or missing

Klinefelter syndrome: male who has an extra X chromosome
- Characteristics not noticeable until puberty
- Testes remain small leading to sterility
- Gynecomastia
- Elongated lower limbs

Turner syndrome: Female who has only one functional X chromosome
- Short stature
- Small, nonfunctioning ovaries leading to sterility
- No secondary sex characteristics develop at puberty except pubic hair
- Neck webbed and short
- Mild learning disabilities to severe cognitive deficits

DIAGNOSTIC TESTS AND PROCEDURES

- DNA analysis of parents prior to conception
- Newborn screening

TESTS DURING PREGNANCY
- Blood AFP level (elevated in the presence of a NTD; decreased in the presence of chromosomal abnormality)
- Chorionic villus sampling
- Amniocentesis
- Ultrasonography

PATIENT-CENTERED CARE

NURSING CARE

- Obtain a complete family history.
- Provide emotional support and guidance.
- Assist with referring guardians to support groups.
- Perform physical examination of newborn for any abnormalities.
- Monitor affected infants closely, including cardiac and respiratory status, and feeding difficulties.

COMPLICATIONS

Short- and long-term complications vary based on type of chromosomal abnormality and the severity of its effects.

CLIENT EDUCATION
- Be aware of expected outcomes for infant.
- Observe for manifestations and report to the provider if necessary.

Application Exercises

1. A nurse is reviewing the medical record of a newborn who has necrotizing enterocolitis (NEC). The nurse should identify that which of the following findings is a risk factor for NEC?

   A. Macrosomia

   B. Transient tachypnea of the newborn (TTN)

   C. Maternal gestational hypertension

   D. Gestational age 36 weeks

2. A nurse is collecting data from a newborn who has congenital hypothyroidism. Which of the following findings should the nurse expect? (Select all that apply.)

   A. Hypertonicity

   B. Cool extremities

   C. Short neck

   D. Tachycardia

   E. Hyperreflexia

3. A nurse is reinforcing teaching with the parent of a newborn who has plagiocephaly. Which of the following statements by the parent indicates an understanding of the instructions?

   A. "I should put my baby to sleep on the belly during her afternoon nap."

   B. "I should ensure my baby's head is in the same position whenever sleeping."

   C. "I should have my baby wear the prescribed helmet 23 hours a day."

   D. "I should allow my baby to sleep in an infant swing."

4. A nurse is contributing to the plan of care for a newborn who has hyperbilirubinemia and is scheduled to receive phototherapy. Which of the following interventions should the nurse include?

   A. Reposition the newborn every 4 hr.

   B. Lotion the newborn's skin twice per day.

   C. Check the newborn's temperature every 8 hr.

   D. Remove the newborn's eye mask during feedings.

5. A nurse is reinforcing preconception teaching with a client who has phenylketonuria (PKU). Which of the following information should the nurse include?

   A. Follow a low-phenylalanine diet once pregnancy is confirmed.

   B. Testing of phenylalanine levels will be required one to two times per week throughout pregnancy.

   C. Increase intake of dietary proteins prior to conception.

   D. Cesarean birth will be required due to the likelihood of having a fetus with macrosomia.

Active Learning Scenario

A nurse is contributing to the plan of care for a newborn who has a myelomeningocele. What interventions should the nurse plan to include? Use the ATI Active Learning Template: System Disorder to complete this item.

NURSING CARE: Include preoperative and postoperative nursing actions for a newborn who has a myelomeningocele.

Application Exercises Key

1. A. Macrosomia does not place a newborn at risk for NEC.
   B. TTN does not place a newborn at risk for NEC.
   C. Maternal gestational hypertension does not place a newborn at risk for NEC.
   D. CORRECT: A gestational age of 36 weeks, or a preterm birth, places a newborn at risk for NEC.

   Ⓝ *NCLEX® Connection: Physiological Adaptation, Basic Pathophysiology*

2. A. Hypertonicity is not an expected finding in a newborn who has congenital hypothyroidism.
   B. CORRECT: Cool extremities are an expected finding in a newborn who has congenital hypothyroidism.
   C. CORRECT: A short neck is an expected finding in a newborn who has congenital hypothyroidism.
   D. Tachycardia is not an expected finding in a newborn who has congenital hypothyroidism.
   E. Hyperreflexia is not an expected finding in a newborn who has congenital hypothyroidism.

   Ⓝ *NCLEX® Connection: Physiological Adaptation, Basic Pathophysiology*

3. A. A newborn who has plagiocephaly should not be placed in the prone position to sleep.
   B. A newborn's head should not be placed in the same position when sleeping.
   C. CORRECT: A newborn who has plagiocephaly should wear the prescribed helmet 23 hr/day.
   D. A newborn who has plagiocephaly should not be allowed to sleep in an infant swing.

   Ⓝ *NCLEX® Connection: Physiological Adaptation, Alterations in Body Systems*

4. A. A newborn undergoing phototherapy should be repositioned every 2 hr.
   B. A newborn undergoing phototherapy should not have lotion applied to the skin because it can cause burns.
   C. A newborn undergoing phototherapy should have their temperature monitored every 4 hr.
   D. CORRECT: A newborn undergoing phototherapy should have the eye mask removed for each feeding to allow for bonding and evaluation of the newborn's eyes.

   Ⓝ *NCLEX® Connection: Physiological Adaptation, Alterations in Body Systems*

5. A. A client who has PKU should follow a low-phenylalanine diet for at least 3 months prior to conception and throughout the pregnancy.
   B. CORRECT: A client who has PKU will have phenylalanine levels monitored one to two times per week throughout pregnancy.
   C. A client who has PKU should decrease dietary intake of protein prior to conception.
   D. A client who has PKU is at no higher risk of fetal macrosomia and will not require a cesarean birth.

   Ⓝ *NCLEX® Connection: Reduction of Risk Potential, Potential for Alterations in Body Systems*

Active Learning Scenario Key

Using the ATI Active Learning Template: System Disorder

NURSING CARE

Preoperative
- Protect the sac.
- Place the infant in a radiant warmer, without clothing.
- Apply sterile, moist non-adhering dressing saturated with 0.9% sodium chloride. Re-wet as needed.
- Monitor cysts for findings of fluid leak or infection.
- Administer prescribed antibiotics.
- Avoid measuring temperature rectally.
- Prepare the parents for the newborn's surgery.

Postoperative
- Monitor vital signs.
- Monitor I&O.
- Monitor the surgical site for redness, edema, and drainage.
- Provide pain management.
- Monitor for leakage of CSF.
- Maintain prone position until other positions are prescribed.

Ⓝ *NCLEX® Connection: Safety and Infection Control, Accident/Error/ Injury Prevention*

CHAPTER 40 *Pediatric Emergencies*

In caring for children, nurses often deal with emergent care situations that require rapid data collection and intervention and offer opportunities for parent and community education.

Respiratory emergencies

Respiratory insufficiency: Increased work of breathing with mostly adequate gas exchange or hypoxia with acidosis

Respiratory failure: Inability to maintain adequate oxygenation of the blood

Apnea
- Cessation of respirations for more than 20 seconds
- Can be associated with hypoxemia or bradycardia
- Can be central or obstructive

Respiratory arrest: Complete cessation of respirations

Airway obstruction: Can be due to aspiration of a foreign body

DATA COLLECTION

RISK FACTORS

- Infants and toddlers
- Primary inefficient gas exchange due to cerebral trauma, brain tumor, toxicity, asphyxia, or CNS infection
- Obstructive lung disease caused by aspiration, infection, tumor, anaphylaxis, laryngospasm, or asthma
- Restrictive lung disease resulting from cystic fibrosis, pneumonia, or respiratory distress syndrome

EXPECTED FINDINGS

- History of illnesses (chronic or acute)
- History of events leading to respiratory emergency
- Allergies

EARLY INDICATIONS OF RESPIRATORY DISTRESS
- Restlessness
- Tachypnea
- Tachycardia
- Diaphoresis
- Nasal flaring
- Retractions
- Grunting
- Dyspnea
- Wheezing

ADVANCED HYPOXIA
- Bradypnea
- Bradycardia
- Peripheral or central cyanosis
- Stupor
- Coma

INDICATIONS OF CHOKING
- Universal choking sign (clutching neck with hands)
- Inability to speak
- Weak, ineffective cough
- High-pitched sounds or no sound
- Dyspnea
- Cyanosis

LABORATORY TESTS

Arterial blood gases (ABGs)

DIAGNOSTIC PROCEDURES

Chest x-rays

PATIENT-CENTERED CARE

NURSING CARE

- Follow the American Heart Association (AHA) guidelines for CPR for respiratory and cardiac arrest.
- Follow the facility's protocol for activating the rapid response team. Q EBP
- Use current basic life support and advanced cardiac life support guidelines for neonates and for pediatric clients.
- Position to maintain patent airway. Monitor respiratory status. Monitor vital signs.
- Administer oxygen as prescribed.
- Suction as needed.
- Assist with preparation for intubation if needed.
- Use a calm approach with the child and family.
- Administer medications, IV fluids, and emergency medications as prescribed.
- Keep the family informed of the child's status.

Obstructed airway
- Follow the AHA guidelines for a choking child.
- For infants, use a combination of back blows and chest thrusts.
- For children and adolescents, use abdominal thrusts.
- Remove any visual obstruction or large debris from the mouth, but do not perform blind finger sweep.
- Place the recovered child (one who resumes breathing) into the recovery position (side-lying position with legs bent at knees for stability).

CLIENT EDUCATION
- Observe for manifestations of respiratory distress.
- Learn CPR.
- Reinforce teaching with the family about strategies to prevent respiratory emergencies (recognizing choking hazards for toddlers).

Drowning

Asphyxiation while child is submerged in fluid can occur in any standing body of water that is at least 1 inch deep (bathtub, toilet, bucket, pool, pond, lake).

- Submersion injury (near-drowning) incidents are those in which children have survived for 24 hr after being submerged in fluid.
- Families should be taught preventive measures.

DATA COLLECTION

RISK FACTORS

- Children ages 0 to 4 years
- Swimming (can be overconfident or lack ability)
- Inadequate supervision or unattended in bathtub, pools
- Not wearing life jackets when in water
- Diving
- Child maltreatment

EXPECTED FINDINGS

- History of event including location and time of submersion
- Type and temperature of the fluid
- Respiratory evaluation (SEE RESPIRATORY EMERGENCIES)
- Body temperature (hypothermia)
- Bruising, spinal cord injury, or other physical injuries

LABORATORY TESTS

ABGs

DIAGNOSTIC PROCEDURES

Chest x-rays

PATIENT-CENTERED CARE

NURSING CARE

Based on degree of cerebral insult
- Administer oxygen.
- Monitor vital signs.
- Administer medications, IV fluids, and emergency medications as prescribed.
- Monitor for complications that can occur 24 hr after incident (cerebral edema, respiratory distress).
- Use a calm approach with the child and family.
- Keep the family informed of the child's status.

CLIENT EDUCATION

- Lock toilet seats when their child is at home.
- Do not leave the child unattended in the bathtub.
- Even a small amount of water can lead to accidental drowning.
- Do not leave the child unattended in a swimming pool, even if the child can swim.
- Make sure private pools are fenced with locked gates to prevent children from wandering into the pool area.
- Provide life jackets when boating.

Apparent life-threatening event

Sudden event where the infant exhibits apnea, change in color, change in muscle tone, and choking

DATA COLLECTION

RISK FACTORS

- Gastroesophageal reflux
- Respiratory infections
- Seizure
- Urinary tract infection (UTI)
- Sepsis
- Metabolic disorders
- Neurologic disorders
- Airway anatomy anomaly

EXPECTED FINDINGS

- Description of the event by the observer
- CPR efforts provided
- Maternal history
- Family history of seizures

EVENT: Apnea can be present during event.
- Change in color: pallor, redness, cyanosis
- Change in muscle tone: hypotonia
- Choking, gagging, coughing

LABORATORY TESTS

Blood cultures: bacterial or viral infection

Urine culture: UTI

CBC

Blood glucose

Electrolytes

DIAGNOSTIC PROCEDURES

Electrocardiogram: long QT syndrome or dysrhythmias

Electroencephalogram: epilepsy

pH study: reflux

Magnetic resonance imaging: hemorrhage or cerebral abnormalities/injuries

Sleep study: sleep apnea

PATIENT-CENTERED CARE

NURSING CARE

- Prepare the infant and family for testing.
- Monitor the infant for recurrent events.
- Encourage the family to learn CPR.

CLIENT EDUCATION: Use an apnea monitor, if prescribed.

Sudden infant death syndrome

- Sudden infant death syndrome (SIDS) is the sudden, unpredictable death of an infant without an identified cause, even after investigation and autopsy.
- Preventive measures should be reinforced to families.

DATA COLLECTION

RISK FACTORS
- Maternal smoking during pregnancy
- Secondhand smoke
- Co-sleeping with parent or adult
- Nonstandard bed (sofa, soft bedding, water beds, pillows)
- Prone or side-lying sleeping
- Low birth weight
- Prematurity
- Twin or multiple birth
- Low Apgar scores
- Viral illness
- Family history of SIDS
- Poverty
- Heart rate abnormalities

EXPECTED FINDINGS
- History of events prior to discovery of infant
- History of illnesses
- Pregnancy and birth history
- Presence of risk factors

PATIENT-CENTERED CARE

NURSING CARE

- Provide support.
- Allow the infant's family an opportunity to express feelings.
- Refer to support groups, counseling, or community groups.

CLIENT EDUCATION: Reinforce teaching with the family how to reduce the risks of SIDS.
- Place the infant on the back for sleep. Qs
- Avoid exposure to tobacco smoke.
- Prevent overheating.
- Use a firm, snug-fitting mattress in the infant's crib.
- Remove pillows, quilts, and stuffed animals from the crib during sleep.
- Ensure that the infant's head is kept uncovered during sleep.
- Offer pacifier when infant is sleeping (naps and at night).
- Encourage breastfeeding.
- Avoid co-sleeping.
- Maintain immunizations up to date.

Poisoning

- Ingestion of or exposure to toxic substances.
- Preventive measures should be reinforced to families.

DATA COLLECTION

RISK FACTORS
- Children younger than 6 years of age
- Improperly stored medications, household chemicals, and hazardous substances
- Exposure to plants, cosmetics, and heavy metals, which are potential sources of toxic substances
- Lead ingestion from lead-based paint, soil contamination

EXPECTED FINDINGS

INFORMATION REGARDING POISONOUS AGENT
- Name and location
- Amount ingested
- Time of ingestion

Specific poisons

Physical response depends on specific poison. Q EBP

Acetaminophen
- **2 to 4 hr after ingestion:** Nausea, vomiting, sweating, and pallor
- **24 to 36 hr after ingestion:** Improvement in condition
- **36 hr to 7 days or longer (hepatic stage):** Pain in upper right quadrant, confusion, stupor, jaundice, and coagulation disturbances
- **Final stage:** Death or gradual recovery

Acetylsalicylic acid (aspirin)
- **Acute poisoning:** Nausea, vomiting, disorientation, diaphoresis, tachypnea, tinnitus, oliguria, lightheadedness, and seizures
- **Chronic poisoning:** Subtle version of acute manifestations, bleeding tendencies, dehydration, and seizures more severe than acute poisoning

Supplemental iron
- **Initial period (30 min to 6 hr after ingestion):** Vomiting, hematemesis, diarrhea, gastric pain, and bloody stools
- **Latency period (2 to 12 hr after ingestion):** Improvement of condition
- **Systemic toxicity period (4 to 24 hr after ingestion):** metabolic acidosis, hyperglycemia, bleeding, fever, shock, and possible death
- **Hepatic injury period (48 to 96 hr after ingestion):** seizures or coma

Hydrocarbons: Gasoline, kerosene, lighter fluid, paint thinner, turpentine
- Gagging, choking, coughing, nausea, and vomiting
- Lethargy, weakness, tachypnea, cyanosis, grunting, and retractions

Corrosives: Household cleaners, batteries, denture cleaners, bleach
- Pain and burning in mouth, throat, and stomach
- Edematous lips, tongue, and pharynx with white mucous membranes
- Violent vomiting with hemoptysis
- Drooling
- Anxiety
- Shock

Lead
- **Low-dose exposure:** Distractibility, impulsiveness, hyperactivity, hearing impairment, and mild intellectual difficulty
- **High-dose exposure:** Cognitive delays varying in severity, blindness, paralysis, coma, seizures, and death
- **Other manifestations:** Kidney impairment, impaired calcium function, and anemia

LABORATORY TESTS

- Blood lead
- CBC with differential
- ABGs
- Blood iron
- Blood acetaminophen
- Liver function tests
- Blood alcohol and toxicology screening

PATIENT-CENTERED CARE

NURSING CARE

Depends on the poison ingested
- Monitor for ongoing changes.
- Terminate exposure.
- Provide cardiorespiratory support as needed.
- Notify local or regional poison control center.
- Assist with the administration of IV fluids.
- Assist with cardiac monitoring.
- Monitor vital signs and oxygen saturation.
- Monitor I&O.
- Administer antidote if indicated.
- Assist with gastric decontamination if indicated.
  - Activated charcoal
  - Gastric lavage
  - Increasing bowel motility
  - Syrup of ipecac is contraindicated for routine poison control treatment
- Keep the family informed of the child's condition.

Interventions for specific substances

Acetaminophen: N-acetylcysteine given orally

Acetylsalicylic acid
- Activated charcoal
- Sodium bicarbonate
- Oxygen and ventilation
- Vitamin K
- Hemodialysis for severe cases

Anticonvulsant: External cooling measures for hyperpyrexia

Supplemental iron
- Emesis or lavage
- Chelation therapy using deferoxamine mesylate

Hydrocarbons (gasoline, kerosene, lighter fluid, paint thinner, turpentine)
- Do not induce vomiting
- Treatment of chemical pneumonia

Corrosives (household cleaners, batteries, denture cleaners, bleach)
- Airway maintenance
- NPO
- No attempt to neutralize acid (corrosive)
- Do not induce vomiting
- Analgesics for pain

Lead: Chelation therapy using calcium EDTA (calcium disodium versenate)

CLIENT EDUCATION

POISON PREVENTION
- Keep toxic agents out of reach of children. Qs
- Lock cabinets containing potentially harmful substances.
- Do not take medication in front of children.
- Discard unused medications.
- When giving a child medication, do not say it is candy.
- Use non-mercury thermometers.
- Eliminate lead-based paint in the environment.
- Encourage hand hygiene prior to eating.
- Do not store food in lead-based containers.

COMPLICATIONS

Cognitive impairments

Varies with degree of anoxic insult or lead levels in blood

NURSING ACTIONS
- Reinforce prevention measures with families.
- Recommend routine screening for lead levels at 1, 2, and 3 years of age.
- Assist with case management for children who have elevated lead levels.
- Assist with making appropriate referrals (community nurse, teacher, early intervention).

Application Exercises

1. A nurse is caring for a child who is experiencing respiratory distress. Which of the following findings are early manifestations of respiratory distress? (Select all that apply.)

   A. Bradypnea

   B. Peripheral cyanosis

   C. Tachycardia

   D. Diaphoresis

   E. Restlessness

2. A nurse in an urgent-care clinic is caring for a child whose guardian reports that the child has swallowed paint thinner. The child is lethargic, gagging, and cyanotic. Which of the following actions should the nurse anticipate assisting with?

   A. Induce vomiting with syrup of ipecac.

   B. Insert a nasogastric tube, and administer activated charcoal.

   C. Prepare for intubation with a cuffed endotracheal tube.

   D. Administer chelation therapy using deferoxamine mesylate.

3. A nurse in an urgent-care clinic is admitting an infant who experienced a life-threatening event. Which of the following prescriptions by the provider should the nurse anticipate? (Select all that apply.)

   A. Electroencephalogram

   B. Electrocardiogram

   C. Urine culture

   D. Arterial blood gases

   E. Blood culture

4. A nurse is reinforcing teaching with a caregiver about acetaminophen poisoning. Which of the following information should the nurse include?

   A. Nausea begins 24 hr after ingestion.

   B. Pallor can appear as early as 2 hr after ingestion.

   C. Jaundice will appear in 12 hr if the child is toxic.

   D. Children can have 4 g/day of acetaminophen.

5. A nurse in a community center is assisting with an in-service to a group of guardians on management of airway obstructions in toddlers. Which of the following responses by one of the caregivers indicates an understanding of the information? (Select all that apply.)

   A. "I will push on my child's abdomen."

   B. "I will hyperextend my child's head to open the airway."

   C. "I will listen over my child's mouth for sounds of breathing."

   D. "I will use my finger to check my child's mouth for objects."

   E. "I will place my child in my car and take them to the closest emergency facility."

Active Learning Scenario

A nurse is reinforcing teaching with a group of caregivers about prevention of sudden infant death syndrome (SIDS). What instructions should the nurse include? Use the ATI Active Learning Template: System Disorder to complete this item.

NURSING CARE: Identify at least seven methods to reduce the risk of SIDS.

Application Exercises Key

1. A. Bradypnea is an advanced manifestation of respiratory distress.
   B. Cyanosis is an advanced manifestation of hypoxia.
   C. **CORRECT:** Tachycardia is an early manifestation of respiratory distress.
   D. **CORRECT:** Diaphoresis is an early manifestation of respiratory distress.
   E. **CORRECT:** Restlessness is an early manifestation of respiratory distress.

   Ⓝ *NCLEX® Connection: Physiological Alterations, Basic Pathophysiology*

2. A. Inducing vomiting with syrup of ipecac is contraindicated as a poison control measure.
   B. Activated charcoal is indicated for acetylsalicylic acid poisoning.
   C. **CORRECT:** Treatment for poisoning with hydrocarbons includes intubation to protect the airway before proceeding with gastric decontamination.
   D. Chelation therapy is indicated for lead poisoning.

   Ⓝ *NCLEX® Connection: Physiological Adaptation, Alterations in Body Systems*

3. A. **CORRECT:** EEG is performed to monitor for epilepsy.
   B. **CORRECT:** ECG is performed to monitor for long QT syndrome or dysrhythmias.
   C. **CORRECT:** A urine specimen is obtained for a culture to monitor for a UTI.
   D. ABGs are not routinely performed for an infant who experienced an apparent life-threatening event.
   E. **CORRECT:** A blood culture is obtained to monitor for bacterial or viral infections.

   Ⓝ *NCLEX® Connection: Physiological Adaptation, Alterations in Body Systems*

4. A. Nausea is a manifestation that begins 2 to 4 hr after ingestion.
   B. **CORRECT:** Sweating is a manifestation that starts 2 to 4 hr after ingestion.
   C. Jaundice will appear in 36 hr to 7 days.
   D. The maximum dose of acetaminophen in children 2 to 5 years of age is 720 mg/day. In children 6 to 12 years of age, it is 2.6 g/day.

   Ⓝ *NCLEX® Connection: Physiological Adaptation, Alterations in Body Systems*

5. A. **CORRECT:** Instruct the caregivers to use abdominal thrusts to open an obstructed airway in a toddler.
   B. Instruct the caregiver to position the child with the chin elevated, rather than hyperextended, to open the airway.
   C. **CORRECT:** Instruct the caregiver to look for chest motion and listen for normal breath sounds over the child's mouth and nose when evaluating for an airway obstruction.
   D. Finger sweeps to check for an impaired airway are not performed because this action can cause an object to be pushed further down into the toddler's throat, causing injury.
   E. Instruct the caregivers to attempt to clear the child's airway according to AHA guidelines and to call 911. Attempting to independently transport the child to an emergency facility delays treatment.

   Ⓝ *NCLEX® Connection: Health Promotion and Maintenance, Community Resources*

Active Learning Scenario Key

Using the ATI Active Learning Template: System Disorder

NURSING CARE: Methods to reduce the risk of SIDS
- Place the infant on the back for sleep.
- Avoid exposure to tobacco smoke.
- Prevent overheating.
- Use a firm, tight-fitting mattress in the infant's crib.
- Remove pillows, quilts, and sheepskins from the crib during sleep.
- Ensure that the infant's head is kept uncovered during sleep.
- Offer pacifier at naps and night.
- Encourage breastfeeding.
- Avoid co-sleeping.
- Maintain immunizations up to date.

Ⓝ *NCLEX® Connection: Health Promotion and Maintenance, Community Resources*

UNIT 3 OTHER SPECIFIC NEEDS

CHAPTER 41 *Psychosocial Issues of Infants, Children, and Adolescents*

Nurses care for pediatric clients who have psychosocial issues, as well as physical illness. Psychosocial issues (depressive disorder) can occur as a result of a physical illness, be independent from physical illness, or be the cause for somatic manifestations (pain due to maltreatment). A pediatric client who has a depressive disorder has a potential risk for suicide. It is important that the nurse be familiar with various psychosocial issues to ensure the child receives appropriate screenings, referrals, and treatment.

Depressive disorder

- Difficult to detect and often overlooked in school-aged children because children have limitations in expressing their feelings.
- Findings must be present for 1 year to diagnose major depressive disorder in children and adolescents.

DATA COLLECTION

RISK FACTORS
- Family history
- Traumatic event

EXPECTED FINDINGS
- Sad facial expressions
- Tendency to remain alone
- Withdrawn from family, friends, and activities
- Fatigue
- Tearful/crying
- Ill feeling
- Feelings of worthlessness
- Weight loss or gain
- Alterations in sleep
- Lack of interest in school, drop in performance in school
- Statements regarding low self-esteem
- Hopelessness
- Suicidal ideation
- Constipation

PATIENT-CENTERED CARE

NURSING CARE
- Plan care that is individualized.
- Obtain health history and growth and development information.
- Monitor for substance use.
- Monitor for actual or potential risk to self (including a suicide plan, lethality of the plan, and the means to carry out the plan).
- Assist with coping strategies.
- Encourage peer group discussions, mentoring, and counseling.
- Interview the child.

MEDICATIONS

Tricyclic antidepressants or selective serotonin reuptake inhibitors (SSRIs)

Trazodone, sertraline, paroxetine, bupropion, venlafaxine

NURSING ACTIONS
- Monitor for adverse effects.
- Monitor for suicidal ideation.

CLIENT EDUCATION
- Observe for adverse effects.
- Therapeutic effectiveness can take up to 2 weeks.
- Do not abruptly discontinue the medication.

COMPLICATIONS

Suicide

EXPECTED FINDINGS
- Monitor carefully for verbal and nonverbal clues. It is essential to ask the client if he is thinking of suicide. This will not give the client the idea
- Suicidal comments usually are made to someone that the client perceives as supportive.
- Comments or signals can be overt (direct) or covert (indirect).
  - Overt comment: "There is just no reason for me to go on living."
  - Covert comment: "Everything is looking pretty grim for me."
- Determine the client's suicide plan.
  - Does the client have a plan?
  - How lethal is the plan?
  - Can the client describe the plan exactly?
  - Does the client have access to the intended method?
  - Has the client's mood changed? A sudden change in mood from sad and depressed to happy and peaceful can indicate a client's intention to commit suicide.

PHYSICAL FINDINGS: Lacerations, scratches, and scars that could indicate previous attempts at self-harm

Posttraumatic stress disorder

Develops following a traumatic or catastrophic event

DATA COLLECTION

RISK FACTORS

- Potential genetic predisposition
- Traumatic incident
- Repeated trauma
- Psychiatric disorder
- Natural disaster
- Sexual abuse
- Witness to homicide, suicide or other violent act

EXPECTED FINDINGS

INITIAL RESPONSE
- Lasts a few minutes to 2 hr
- Increased stress hormones (fight or flight)
- Psychosis

SECOND PHASE
- Lasts approximately 2 weeks
- Period of calm (feeling of numbness, denial)
- Defense mechanisms decrease

THIRD PHASE (COPING)
- Extends 2 to 3 months
- Client gets worse instead of better.
- Depression, phobias, anxiety, conversion reactions, repetitive movements, flashbacks, or obsessions

PATIENT-CENTERED CARE

NURSING CARE

- Refer to psychotherapy services.
- Monitor for behavior changes/problems.
- Assist the client and family with coping strategies.
- Allow the client and family to express their feelings.
- Prevent or reduce long-term effects.

MEDICATIONS

Selective norepinephrine reuptake inhibitors can be used on an individual basis.

Attention-deficit/ hyperactivity disorder

- Inattentiveness, hyperactivity, and impulsiveness usually revealed prior to age 7.
- Common in childhood and can persist into adulthood.
- A child must meet diagnostic criteria for diagnosis of attention-deficit hyperactivity disorder (ADHD).
  - Manifestations are present between the ages of 4 and 18 years.
  - Manifestations are present in more than one setting.
  - Evidence of social or academic impairment.
  - Six or more findings from a category are present (inattention or hyperactivity-impulsivity).

DATA COLLECTION

RISK FACTORS

- Can be a familial tendency
- Exposure to toxins or medicines
- Chronic otitis media, meningitis, or head trauma

EXPECTED FINDINGS

INATTENTION
- Failing to pay close attention to detail or making careless mistakes
- Blocking incoming stimuli
- Difficulty sustaining attention
- Does not seem to listen
- Failing to follow through on instructions
- Difficulty organizing activities
- Avoiding or disliking activities that require mental effort for a period of time (reading)
- Losing things
- Easily distracted
- Forgetfulness

HYPERACTIVITY
- Fidgeting
- Failing to remain seated
- Inappropriate running
- Difficulty engaging in quiet play
- Seeming to be busy all the time
- Talking excessively

IMPULSIVITY
- Blurting out responses before questions are asked
- Difficulty waiting turns
- Interrupting often
- Striking out, biting, shouting

PATIENT-CENTERED CARE

NURSING CARE

- Obtain medical, developmental, or behavioral history.
- Use behavioral checklists with adaptive scales.
- Use a calm, firm, respectful approach with the child.
- Use modeling to demonstrate acceptable behavior.
- Obtain the child's attention before giving directions. Provide short and clear explanations.
- Set clear limits on unacceptable behaviors and be consistent.
- Plan physical activities through which the child can use energy and obtain success.
- Focus on the child's and family's strengths, not just the problems.
- Support the caregivers' efforts to remain hopeful.
- Provide a safe environment for the child and others.
- Provide the child with specific positive feedback when expectations are met.
- Identify issues that result in power struggles.
- Assist the child in developing effective coping mechanisms.
- Encourage the child to participate in a form of group, individual, or family therapy.
- Assist the family with behavioral strategies.
  - Positive reinforcement
  - Rewards for good behavior
  - Age-appropriate consequences
- Assist the family with modification of the environment to help the child become successful.
  - Structured environment
  - Charts to assist with organization
  - Decreasing stimuli in the environment
  - Consistent study area
  - Modeling positive behaviors
  - Using steps when assigning chores
  - Using pastel colors
- Assist with appropriate classroom placement in the school.
  - Collaborate with the school nurse.
  - Allow more time for testing.
  - Place in classroom that has order and consistent rules.
  - Offer verbal instruction combined with visual cues.
  - Plan academic subjects in the morning.
  - Include regular breaks.
  - Provide for small classroom settings or work groups.

MEDICATIONS

Methylphenidate, dextroamphetamine

Psychostimulant, which increases dopamine and norepinephrine levels

NURSING ACTIONS

- Gradually increase dose to reach therapeutic results.
- Give last dose of the day prior to 1800 to prevent insomnia.
- Monitor for adverse effects, including insomnia, anorexia, nervousness, hyper/hypotension, tachycardia, and anemia.
- Avoid caffeine.
- Store properly. The medication has potential for misuse by others.
- Tricyclic antidepressants are used as adjunct therapy to treat insomnia.

Atomoxetine

Selective norepinephrine reuptake inhibitor

NURSING ACTIONS

- Gradual increase in dose to reach therapeutic results.
- Monitor for adverse effects (suicidal ideation).

Autism spectrum disorder

Complex neurodevelopmental disorders with spectrum of behaviors affecting the ability to communicate, learn, and interact with others in a social setting. This disorder begins in early childhood and lasts throughout an individual's life. It includes what was once referred to as pervasive developmental disorder and Asperger syndrome.

DATA COLLECTION

RISK FACTORS

- Possible genetic component
- Exact cause unknown

EXPECTED FINDINGS

- Delays in at least one of the following
  - Social interaction
  - Social communication
  - Imaginative play prior to age 3 years
- Distress when routines are changed
- Unusual attachments to objects
- Inability to start or continue conversation
- Using gestures instead of words
- Delayed or absent language development
- Grunting or humming
- Inability to adjust gaze to look at something else
- Not referring to self correctly
- Withdrawn, labile mood
- Lack of empathy
- Decreased pain sensation
- Spending time alone rather than playing with others
- Avoiding eye contact
- Withdrawal from physical contact
- Heightened or lowered senses
- Not imitating actions of others
- Minimal pretend play
- Exhibiting repetitive movements
- Typical IQ less than 70

PATIENT-CENTERED CARE

NURSING CARE

- Assist with screening evaluation tools, such as the Checklist for Autism in Toddlers (CHAT) or Pervasive Developmental Disorders Screening Test.
- Refer to early intervention, physical therapy, occupational therapy, and speech and language therapy.
- Assist with behavior modification program.
  - Promote positive reinforcement.
  - Increase social awareness.
  - Reinforce verbal communication.
  - Decrease unacceptable behaviors.
  - Set realistic goals.
  - Structure opportunities for small successes.
  - Set clear rules.
- Decrease environmental stimulation.
- Assist with nutritional needs.
- Introduce the child to new situations slowly.
- Monitor for behavior changes.
- Encourage age appropriate play.
- Communicate at an age-appropriate level (brief and concrete).
- Provide support to the family.
- Encourage the child and family to attend support groups.

MEDICATIONS

Used on an individual basis to control aggression, anxiety, hyperactivity, irritability, mood swings, compulsions, and attention problems.
- SSRIs can decrease aggression.
- Antipsychotics and melatonin can help with insomnia.

Intellectual disability

- Also known as cognitive impairment
- Previously called mental retardation

DATA COLLECTION

RISK FACTORS

- Familial, social, environmental, organic or other unknown causes
- Infections (congenital rubella, syphilis)
- Fetal alcohol syndrome
- Chronic lead ingestion
- Trauma to the brain
- Gestational disorders
- Pre-existing disease (Down syndrome, psychiatric disorders, microcephaly, hydrocephaly, metabolic disorders, cerebral palsy)

EXPECTED FINDINGS

- Can range from mild to severe
- Delayed developmental milestones
- Inability to reason or problem solve

EARLY MANIFESTATIONS
- Abnormal eye contact
- Feeding difficulties
- Language difficulties
- Fine and gross motor delays
- Decrease alertness
- Unresponsive to contact
- Reduced response to name
- Decreased response to social cues
- Echolalia
- Clients "lose" milestones between 15 to 30 months (Autism regression)

PATIENT-CENTERED CARE

NURSING CARE

- DSM-5 used to diagnose.
- Determine the child's deficiency.
- Care and instruction should be individualized to the client's needs.
- Make appropriate referrals (early intervention program, social work, speech therapy, physical therapy, and occupational therapy).
- Add visual cues with verbal instruction.
- Give one-step instructions.
- Assist the family in teaching the child self-cares.
- Assist the family in promoting development.
- Encourage play.
- Assist the family with selecting activities and toys.
- Assist with communication skills.
- Encourage social activities.

Failure to thrive

Inadequate growth resulting from the inability to obtain or use calories required for growth. It is usually described in an infant or child who falls below the fifth percentile for weight (and possibly for height) or who has persistent weight loss. Failure to thrive (FTT) can be classified according to the cause:
- Inadequate caloric intake (incorrect formula prep, breastfeeding difficulties, or excessive juice consumption)
- Inadequate absorption (cystic fibrosis, celiac or Crohn's disease)
- Increased metabolism (hyperthyroidism)
- Defective utilization (Down syndrome)

DATA COLLECTION

RISK FACTORS

- Preterm birth with low birth weight or intrauterine growth restriction
- Parental neglect, lack of parental knowledge, or disturbed maternal–child attachment
- Poverty
- Health or childrearing beliefs
- Family stress
- Feeding resistance

ORGANIC CAUSES: Cerebral palsy, chronic kidney failure, congenital heart disease, hyperthyroidism, cystic fibrosis, celiac disease, hepatic disease, Down syndrome, prematurity, and gastroesophageal reflux

EXPECTED FINDINGS

- Less than the fifth percentile on the growth chart for weight
- Malnourished appearance
- Poor muscle tone, lack of subcutaneous fat
- No fear of strangers
- Minimal smiling
- Decreased activity level
- Withdrawal behavior
- Developmental delays
- Feeding disorder
- Wide-eyed gaze, absent eye contact
- Stiff or flaccid body

PATIENT-CENTERED CARE

NURSING CARE

- Child may need to be removed from guardians' care in order to evaluate carefully and receive therapy.
- Obtain a nutritional history.
- Observe parent-child interactions.
- Obtain accurate baseline height and weight. Observe for low weight, malnourished appearance, and manifestations of dehydration.
- Weigh the child daily without clothing or a diaper.
- Maintain I&O and calorie counts as prescribed.
- Establish a routine for eating that encourages usual times, duration, and setting.
- Reinforce proper positioning, latching on, and timing for children who are breastfed.
- Provide 24 kcal/oz formula as prescribed.
- Provide high-calorie milk supplements for children.
- Administer multivitamin supplements including zinc and iron.
- Limit juice to 4 oz/day.
- Provide developmental stimulation.
- Nurture the child (rocking and talking to the child).

- Encourage caregivers to do the following.
  - Maintain eye contact and face-to-face posture during feedings.
  - Talk to the infant while feeding.
  - Burp the infant frequently.
  - Keep the environment quiet and avoid distractions.
  - Be persistent, remaining calm during 10 to 15 min of food refusal.
  - Introduce new foods slowly.
  - Never force the infant to eat.

CLIENT EDUCATION

- Recognize and respond to the infant's cues of hunger.
- Mix formula properly according to provided step-by-step written instructions

COMPLICATIONS

Extreme malnourishment

NURSING ACTIONS: Prepare the client and guardians for tube feedings or IV therapy.

Maltreatment of infants and children

Maltreatment of infants and children is attributed to a variety of predisposing factors, which include parental, child, and environmental characteristics. Child maltreatment can occur across all economic and educational backgrounds and racial/ethnic/religious groups.

Maltreatment of children is made of several specific types of behaviors.
- **Physical:** causing pain or harm to a child (shaken baby syndrome, fractures, factitious disorder imposed on another)
- **Sexual:** occurring when sexual contact takes place without consent, whether or not the victim is able to give consent (includes any sexual behavior toward a minor and dating violence among adolescents)
- **Emotional:** humiliating, threatening, or intimidating a child (includes behavior that minimizes an individual's feelings of self-worth)
- **Neglect:** includes failure to provide the following.
  - **Physical care:** feeding, clothing, shelter, medical or dental care, safety, education
  - **Emotional care** and/or stimulation to foster normal development: nurturing, affection, attention

DATA COLLECTION

RISK FACTORS

CAREGIVER CHARACTERISTICS
- Younger parents
- Having a partner unrelated to the child
- Social isolation
- Low-income situation
- Lack of education
- Low self-esteem
- Lack of parenting knowledge
- Substance use disorder
- History of having been abused
- Lack of support systems

CHARACTERISTICS OF THE CHILD
- Child 1 year old or younger is at greater risk due to the need for constant attention and increased demands of caregiving.
- Infants and children who are unwanted, hyperactive, or who have physical or mental disabilities are at risk due to their increased demands and need for constant attention.
- Premature infants are at risk due to the possible failure of parent-child bonding at birth.

ENVIRONMENTAL CHARACTERISTICS
- Chronic stress
- Divorce, alcohol or substance use disorder, poverty
- Unemployment, inadequate housing, crowded living conditions
- Substitute caregivers

EXPECTED FINDINGS

WARNING INDICATORS OF MALTREATMENT
- Physical evidence of maltreatment
- Vague explanation of injury
- Other injuries discovered that are not related to the original client concern
- Delay in seeking care
- Statement of possible maltreatment from a caregiver or client
- Inconsistencies between the caregiver's report and the child's injuries
- Inconsistency between nature of injury and developmental level of the child
- Repeated injuries requiring emergency treatment
- Inappropriate responses from the parents or child

Physical neglect
- Failure to thrive, malnutrition
- Lack of hygiene
- Frequent injuries
- Delay in seeking health care
- Dull affect
- School absences
- Self-stimulating behaviors

Physical maltreatment
- Bruises, welts in various stages of healing
- Bruising in a non-mobile client
- Multiple fractures at different stages of healing
- Burns
- Fractures
- Lacerations
- Fear of parents
- Lack of emotional response/reaction
- Superficial relationships
- Withdrawal
- Aggression

Emotional neglect
- Failure to thrive
- Eating disorder
- Enuresis
- Sleep disturbances
- Self-stimulating behaviors
- Withdrawal
- Lack of social smile (infant)
- Extreme behaviors
- Delayed development
- Attempts suicide
- Caregiver behaviors: rejecting, isolating, terrorizing, ignoring, verbally assaulting, or overpressuring the child

Sexual maltreatment defined as the employment, use, persuasion, or inducement of a child to engage in any sexually explicit conduct. Examples include pedophilia, prostitution, incest, molestation, and pornography.
- Bruises, lacerations
- Bleeding of genitalia, anus, or mouth
- Sexually transmitted infection
- Difficulty walking or standing
- UTI
- Regressive behavior
- Withdrawal
- Personality changes
- Bloody, torn, or stained underwear
- Unusual body odor

Shaken baby syndrome or abusive head trauma:
Shaking can cause intracranial hemorrhage. Caregiver's frustrations with persistent crying can lead to this.
- Can have no external manifestations of injury
- Vomiting, poor feeding, and listlessness
- Respiratory distress
- Bulging fontanels
- Retinal hemorrhages
- Seizures
- Posturing
- Alterations in level of consciousness
- Apnea
- Bradycardia
- Blindness
- Unresponsiveness
- Bruising in an infant before 6 months of age, should be deemed suspicious by the nurse

LABORATORY TESTS

CBC, urinalysis, and other tests that determine if the child has sexually transmitted infections or bleeding

DIAGNOSTIC PROCEDURES

Depend upon the injuries and findings during the examination
- Radiograph
- Computed tomography or magnetic resonance imaging scan

PATIENT-CENTERED CARE

NURSING CARE

- Identify abuse as soon as possible. Conduct detailed history and physical examination.
- The nursing priority is to have the child removed from the abusive situation.
- Mandatory reporting is required of all health care providers, including suspected cases of child abuse. There are civil and criminal penalties for not reporting.
- Monitor for unusual bruising on the abdomen, back, and buttocks. Document thoroughly with size, shape, and color. Use diagrams to represent location.
- Determine the mechanism of injury, which might not be congruent with the physical appearance of the injury. Many bruises at different stages of healing can indicate ongoing beatings.
- Observe for bruises or welts in the shape of a belt buckle or other objects.
- Observe for burns that appear glove- or stocking-like on hands or feet, which can indicate forced immersion into boiling water. Small, round burns can be caused by lit cigarettes. Document detailed descriptions of all findings.
- Note fractures that have unusual features (forearm spiral fractures) which could be caused by twisting the extremity forcefully. The presence of multiple fractures is suspicious.
- Check the child for head injuries. Determine the child's level of consciousness, making sure to note equal and reactive pupils. Monitor for nausea/vomiting.
- Clearly and objectively document information obtained in the interview and during the physical examination.
- Photograph and detail all visible injuries, if possible, including measuring devices to show size of injuries.
- Conduct the interview with the child and guardians individually.
- Be direct, honest, and professional.
- Use language the child understands.
- Be understanding and attentive.
- Client circumstances are case-sensitive, and referrals are made to always keep the client safe. When applicable, explain the process if a referral is made to child or adult protective services.
- Monitor surroundings for safety and reduce danger for the victim.
- Use open-ended questions that require a descriptive response. These questions are less threatening and elicit more relevant information.

- Provide support for the child and parents.
- Demonstrate behaviors for child-rearing with the parents and child.
- Provide consistent care to the child.
- Avoid asking the child probing questions.
- Promote self-esteem.
- Assist with alleviating feelings of shame and guilt.
- Assist the child with grieving the loss of parents, if indicated.
- Discharge can begin once legal determination of placement has been decided.

INTERPROFESSIONAL CARE

Initiate appropriate referrals for social services.

Bullying behavior

Physical, verbal, or emotional maltreatment that is intentional and repetitive by a person to another person with the intent to establish power and dominance with intimidation. This could be with or without face-to-face contact.

SETTINGS: school, playground, bus, texting, or online

DATA COLLECTION

RISK FACTORS

PERPETRATORS OF BULLYING BEHAVIOR
- Male sex
- Depression
- Decreased academic performance
- Decreased social involvement with peers
- Exposure to spouse or partner violence
- Conduct problems
- Criminal acts
- Dropping out of school

RECIPIENTS OF BULLYING BEHAVIOR
- Low self-esteem
- Loneliness
- Somatic reports
- Anxiety
- Depression

PATIENT-CENTERED CARE

CLIENT EDUCATION

- Observe for manifestations and be inquisitive.
- Obtain support from the family.
- Refer to counseling and bully prevention programs.
- Follow procedures for investigating and reporting.
- Refer for psychiatric evaluation because bullying can be an early indication of psychiatric disorders.

Application Exercises

1. A nurse is reinforcing teaching with a group of guardians about characteristics of infants who have failure to thrive. Which of the following characteristics should the nurse include?

   A. Intense fear of strangers

   B. Increased risk for childhood obesity

   C. Inability to form close relationships with siblings

   D. Developmental delays

2. A nurse is reinforcing teaching with the teacher of a child who has attention-deficit/hyperactivity disorder (ADHD). Which of the following classroom strategies should the nurse include? (Select all that apply.)

   A. Eliminate testing.

   B. Allow for regular breaks.

   C. Combine verbal instruction with visual cues.

   D. Establish consistent classroom rules.

   E. Increase stimuli in the environment.

3. A nurse is reinforcing teaching with a guardian about posttraumatic stress disorder (PTSD). Which of the following information should the nurse include? (Select all that apply.)

   A. Children who have PTSD can benefit from psychotherapy.

   B. A manifestation of PTSD is phobias.

   C. Personality disorders are a complication of PTSD.

   D. PTSD develops following a traumatic event.

   E. There are six stages of PTSD.

4. A nurse is reinforcing teaching with the guardian of a child about risk factors for attention-deficit/hyperactivity disorder (ADHD). Which of the following risk factors should the nurse include?

   A. Formula-feeding as an infant

   B. History of head trauma

   C. History of postterm birth

   D. Child of a single guardian

5. A nurse is caring for a child who has a depressive disorder. Which of the following findings should the nurse expect? (Select all that apply.)

   A. Prefers being with peers

   B. Weight loss or gain

   C. Reports low self-esteem

   D. Sleeps more than usual

   E. Hyperactivity

Active Learning Scenario

A nurse is reinforcing teaching with a group of caregivers about shaken baby syndrome. What manifestations should the nurse include in this presentation? Use the ATI Active Learning Template: Basic Concept to complete this item.

UNDERLYING PRINCIPLES: Include seven manifestations.

Application Exercises Key

1. A. These infants do not exhibit the expected fear of strangers.
   B. These infants are not at an increased risk for childhood obesity.
   C. These infants are able to form close relationships with siblings.
   D. **CORRECT:** These infants can exhibit developmental delays due to decreased nutritional intake needed for brain development.

   Ⓝ *NCLEX® Connection: Reduction of Risk Potential, Potential for Alterations in Body Systems*

2. A. Allowing for added time when testing can assist the client who has ADHD to be successful.
   B. **CORRECT:** Allowing for regular breaks will assist the client who has ADHD to focus on the required tasks.
   C. **CORRECT:** Combining verbal instruction with visual cues will assist the client who has ADHD with learning information.
   D. **CORRECT:** Providing consistent classroom rules will assist the client who has ADHD to become successful.
   E. Stimuli in the environment distract the client who has ADHD, so it should be decreased.

   Ⓝ *NCLEX® Connection: Psychosocial Integrity, Behavioral Management*

3. A. **CORRECT:** Children who have PTSD should be referred to psychotherapy to assist with resolution of the traumatic event.
   B. **CORRECT:** The child who is experiencing PTSD often has new phobias that can be related to the traumatic event.
   C. Personality disorders are not a complication of PTSD.
   D. **CORRECT:** PTSD develops following a traumatic event (assault, serious injury, or a life-threatening episode).
   E. PTSD has three stages: the initial response, and second and third phase.

   Ⓝ *NCLEX® Connection: Psychosocial Integrity, Behavioral Management*

4. A. Being formula-fed as an infant is not a risk factor for the development of ADHD.
   B. **CORRECT:** History of head trauma is a risk factor for the development of ADHD.
   C. History of a post-term birth is not a risk factor for the development of ADHD.
   D. Being the child of a single guardian does not increase the risk of development of ADHD.

   Ⓝ *NCLEX® Connection: Health Promotion and Maintenance, Health Promotion/Disease Prevention*

5. A. A preference for being alone is a finding associated with depression.
   B. **CORRECT:** Weight loss or gain are findings associated with depression.
   C. **CORRECT:** Low self-esteem is a finding associated with depression.
   D. **CORRECT:** Sleeping more than usual is a finding associated with depression.
   E. Fatigue is a finding associated with depression.

   Ⓝ *NCLEX® Connection: Physiological Adaptation, Basic Pathophysiology*

Active Learning Scenario Key

Using the ATI Active Learning Template: Basic Concept

UNDERLYING PRINCIPLES
- Vomiting, poor feeding, and listlessness
- Respiratory distress
- Bulging fontanels
- Retinal hemorrhages
- Seizures
- Posturing
- Alterations in level of consciousness
- Apnea
- Bradycardia

Ⓝ *NCLEX® Connection: Health Promotion and Maintenance, Community Resources*

References

Centers for Disease Control and Prevention. (2019). Vaccine schedules for child-adolescent. Retrieved from https://www.cdc.gov/vaccines/schedules/hcp/imz/child-adolescent.html

Centers for Disease Control and Prevention. (2019). Possible side-effects from vaccines. Retrieved from https://www.cdc.gov/vaccines/vac-gen/side-effects.htm

Hockenberry, M. J., Wilson, D., & Rodgers, C. (2019). *Wong's nursing care of infants and children* (11th ed.). St. Louis, MO: Mosby.

Pagana, K. D. & Pagana, T. J. (2018). Mosby's manual of diagnostic and laboratory tests (6th ed.). St. Louis: Elsevier.

Silbert-Flagg, J., & Pillitteri, A. (2018). *Maternal & child health nursing: Care of the childbearing and childrearing family* (8th ed.). Philadelphia: Wolters Kluwer.

Taketomo, C. K., Hodding, J. H., & Kraus, D. M. (2018). *Lexicomp pediatric & neonatal dosage handbook with international trade names index: A global resource for clinicians treating pediatric and neonatal patients (pediatric dosage handbook)* (25th ed.). Hudson, Ohio: Wolters Kluwer Clinical Drug Information, Inc.

Vallerand, A. H., Sanoski, C. A. & Deglin, J. H. (2019). *Davis's drug guide for nurses* (16th ed.). Philadelphia.

STUDENT NAME _____

CONCEPT_____   REVIEW MODULE CHAPTER_____

Related Content

(E.G., DELEGATION,
LEVELS OF PREVENTION,
ADVANCE DIRECTIVES)

Underlying Principles

Nursing Interventions

WHO? WHEN? WHY? HOW?

STUDENT NAME _____

PROCEDURE NAME _____   REVIEW MODULE CHAPTER _____

Description of Procedure

Indications

CONSIDERATIONS

Nursing Interventions (pre, intra, post)

Interpretation of Findings

Client Education

Potential Complications

Nursing Interventions

Growth and Development

STUDENT NAME _____

DEVELOPMENTAL STAGE _____ REVIEW MODULE CHAPTER_____

EXPECTED GROWTH AND DEVELOPMENT

Physical Development	Cognitive Development	Psychosocial Development	Age-Appropriate Activities

Health Promotion

Immunizations	Health Screening	Nutrition	Injury Prevention

STUDENT NAME _____

MEDICATION _____ REVIEW MODULE CHAPTER_____

CATEGORY CLASS_____

PURPOSE OF MEDICATION

Expected Pharmacological Action

Therapeutic Use

Complications

Medication Administration

Contraindications/Precautions

Interactions

Nursing Interventions

Client Education

Evaluation of Medication Effectiveness

STUDENT NAME _____

SKILL NAME_____ REVIEW MODULE CHAPTER_____

Description of Skill

Indications

CONSIDERATIONS

Nursing Interventions (pre, intra, post)

Outcomes/Evaluation

Client Education

Potential Complications

Nursing Interventions

STUDENT NAME _____

DISORDER/DISEASE PROCESS _____ REVIEW MODULE CHAPTER_____

Alterations in Health (Diagnosis)	Pathophysiology Related to Client Problem	Health Promotion and Disease Prevention

ASSESSMENT

Risk Factors

Expected Findings

Laboratory Tests

Diagnostic Procedures

SAFETY CONSIDERATIONS

PATIENT-CENTERED CARE

Nursing Care

Medications

Client Education

Therapeutic Procedures

Interprofessional Care

Complications

STUDENT NAME _____

PROCEDURE NAME _____ REVIEW MODULE CHAPTER_____

Description of Procedure

Indications

CONSIDERATIONS

Nursing Interventions (pre, intra, post)

Outcomes/Evaluation

Client Education

Potential Complications

Nursing Interventions

STUDENT NAME _____

CONCEPT ANALYSIS_____

Defining Characteristics

Antecedents

(WHAT MUST OCCUR/BE IN PLACE FOR
CONCEPT TO EXIST/FUNCTION PROPERLY)

Negative Consequences

(RESULTS FROM IMPAIRED ANTECEDENT —
COMPLETE WITH FACULTY ASSISTANCE)

Related Concepts

(REVIEW LIST OF CONCEPTS AND IDENTIFY, WHICH
CAN BE AFFECTED BY THE STATUS OF THIS CONCEPT
— COMPLETE WITH FACULTY ASSISTANCE)

Exemplars